Spacecraft Collision Probability

Spacecraft Collision Probability

F. Kenneth Chan

The Aerospace Press • El Segundo, California

American Institute of Aeronautics and Astronautics, Inc. • Reston, Virginia

The Aerospace Press
2350 E. El Segundo Boulevard
El Segundo, California 90245-4691

American Institute of Aeronautics and Astronautics, Inc.
1801 Alexander Bell Drive
Reston, Virginia 20191-4344

Library of Congress Cataloging-in-Publication Data

Chan, F. Kenneth.
Spacecraft collision probability / F. Kenneth Chan.
p. cm.
Includes bibliographical references and index.
ISBN-13: 978-1-884989-18-6 (alk. paper)
ISBN-10: 1-884989-18-7 (alk. paper)
1. Space debris. 2. Space vehicle accidents--Mathematical models. 3. Space vehicles--Protection. 4. Probabilities. 5. Mathematical statistics. I. Title.

TL1499.C48 2007
363.12'2--dc22

2007024163

Cover design by Karl Jacobs

Dedicated to

Mr. Ambrose J. Dairiam
My teacher at St. Paul's Institution
Seremban, Malaysia

Dr. Melvin C. Molstad
My mentor at the University of Pennsylvania

Dr. Wallace D. Hayes
My advisor at Princeton University

Dr. Thomas J. Eisler
My colleague of more than four decades

Contents

Preface

The amount of debris in space has recently been growing at an alarming rate, giving rise to increased concern about the collision of operational spacecraft with orbiting debris in the Earth's environment. This book, the outgrowth of my research during the past two decades, treats the probability of such a collision of a spacecraft with another orbiting object. It analyzes the probability of collisions when measurements (with inherent errors) are obtained of the orbits of two approaching objects. Its primary objective is to derive analytical solutions that are fairly simple in nature but still capture the essence of the problem. The approach ensures that the logic is mathematically correct and the assumptions are physically meaningful. It also discusses the accuracies of the models and the limitations of these analytical solutions.

In the last few years, many papers have dealt with the methodology of computing the collision probability in the "encounter region." They have implicitly assumed that the encounter is a flyby and is "short-termed," wherein the trajectories of the objects can be represented by straight lines. They have not given sufficient attention to fundamental concepts such as the extent of the encounter region and the transit time through it. Eventually, this model fails to deal with the "long-termed" case of two objects that spend a protracted period in the vicinity of each other.

For short-term encounters, most researchers take an approach based on several assumptions. First is the idea that the nominal trajectories of the approaching objects are straight lines in the encounter region. This assumption leads to a nominal rectilinear relative motion of one object with respect to the other. Associated with each trajectory is a covariance describing the uncertainty of the nominal position. Moreover, it is assumed that these covariances are constant during the encounter.

An assumption is also made that the trajectories are determined from uncorrelated or independent measurements. Thus, the covariance of the relative position is given by the sum of the two individual covariances. A three-dimensional Gaussian probability density function (pdf*) is assumed for the relative position. Because the combined covariance is constant during the encounter, the spatial Cartesian variables (x, y, z) can be taken to be random variables.

The next assumption is that both objects are spherical so that a collision occurs when their centers lie within a sphere of radius equal to their combined radii. The region generated by the rectilinear relative motion of this combined sphere is a circular cylinder with cross section of the same radius. The probability

*This book follows the common convention of printing acronyms in uppercase format, with the exception of pdf (probability density function), which is shown in lowercase type throughout to avoid confusion with PDF (probability distribution function).

of collision of the two objects is then given by a three-dimensional integral of the pdf in the circular cylindrical volume that (for reasons somehow mysteriously included in the process) is assumed to be infinitely long. Integration along the direction of the cylindrical axis reduces the three-dimensional collision integral to a two-dimensional one.

The NASA computation of the probability of collision of the International Space Station (ISS) is based on Foster's 1992 formulation of a two-dimensional integral evaluated numerically. Subsequently, several researchers (Chan in 1995, 1997, and 2001; Patera in 2000 and 2006; and Alfano in 2002) have reduced the two-dimensional integral to a one-dimensional one. Unlike Patera's and Alfano's formulations in which the collision probability is evaluated numerically, my formulation converts the two-dimensional Gaussian integral to the one-dimensional Rician integral and yields analytical expressions for the collision probability. For a wide range of realistic collision parameters (nominal distance of closest approach, collision cross-sectional radius, and standard deviations of relative positions), these four formulations yield numerical results that agree to at least two or three significant figures.

Auxiliary to the main theme of this book are two topics: the Rician integral and the method of equivalent cross-section area (MECSA). The Rician pdf arises frequently in the detection of signals in the presence of noise. It also arises in target detection by pulsed radar, noncoherent detection of band-passed binary signals, accuracy of unguided ballistic bombs, and artillery effectiveness of fragmentation bombs. Now, we find that it arises in spacecraft collision probability for the special isotropic case. The Rician integral is a one-dimensional integral and is exactly equal to the integral of a two-dimensional isotropic Gaussian pdf over a circle displaced from the center. MECSA is a method of determining an equivalent circular area for the integral of a two-dimensional isotropic Gaussian pdf over an ellipse displaced from the center. It can also be extended to the case for which the area of integration is not elliptical but of an arbitrary shape (such as a triangle or quadrilateral) that is not too elongated.

Thus, it is possible to model the ISS not simply as a sphere but according to its actual shape, component by component. Chapter 6 of this book is devoted to this particular topic and to the subject of detailed computation of a more realistic collision probability. This comprehensive chapter should be of great value to personnel working with the ISS. Moreover, because the huge solar panels are always sun-pointing, it is necessary to develop a sufficiently accurate algorithm for computing the sun vector that can be used in-line without resorting to table lookup and interpolation. This requirement has resulted in the creation of an algorithm accurate to four thousandths of a degree using for inputs the time of vernal equinox and the day plus decimal part of interest. This algorithm is sufficient to meet the accuracy requirements of most applications and certainly the sun-pointing of ISS solar panels.

Long-term encounters are typified by certain pairs of geosynchronous satellites observed with low relative velocity (low enough to be measured in meters per second) so that the time they spend in the encounter region is appreciable. During this period, which can extend to considerably more than a day, neither the direction of the relative velocity nor the combined covariance error ellipsoid can be treated as constant. In contrast to the existing short-term encounter models for which the assumption of constant relative velocity is valid, a different approach must be used for computing the collision probability. In order to analyze the general case of long-term encounter, we must account for the covariance error ellipsoid changing in shape, size, and orientation. Thus, we can no longer consider the three spatial Cartesian coordinates (x, y, z) representing the relative position uncertainty as random variables. Instead, we must choose three different random variables (x^*, y^*, z^*) as a common basis so that we have a time-independent pdf and can meaningfully compute the collision probability. This probability is determined by evaluating a three-dimensional integral over the appropriate region V^* in the space of the random variables. (Formulations based on the incremental addition of probability as a function of time and time-dependent pdf are at variance with the crux of probability theory.) The computation of collision probability for long-term encounters finds application in constellations flying in formation.

A chapter is included on the collision probability of a spacecraft moving within a spherical layer of orbiting secondary objects such as debris from earlier on-orbit explosions. These secondary objects are grouped into different classes. The objects in each class have circular orbits and lie within small tolerances about a specific altitude and inclination. All the secondary objects in a class have ascending nodes uniformly distributed around the equator, and they have phase angles uniformly distributed within an orbital plane. This model closely resembles the steady-state debris cloud after explosion. We can use an equivalent isotropic Gaussian pdf in the encounter plane because the direction of encounter is random. Thus, the problem is again reduced to the one (involving the Rician integral) that already has been considered. This approach is different from that used by the European Space Agency (ESA), which is based on the kinetic theory of gases and the Poisson distribution. As this book goes to press, I have also completed the formulation for computing the probability of collision of a spacecraft with a partially dispersed cloud of debris.

The book concludes with a chapter that briefly describes the Excel macros I have developed to obtain all the numerical tables and graphical plots appearing herein. The software is available on the Web site of the American Institute of Aeronautics and Astronautics (AIAA) and may be downloaded for the reader's private use. (See the "Supporting Materials" page at the end of this book for downloading instructions.) The equations and the variable names used in the code follow very closely the corresponding ones used in each chapter. This practice eliminates the need to have mathematical specifications and documentation of the software. The tabulated results serve as benchmarks that the reader may wish to retain to check the algorithms.

—Fu-Kiong Kenneth Chan

Acknowledgments

First of all, I am indebted to The Aerospace Press of The Aerospace Corporation for funding during the preparation of the book. In particular, I express my gratitude to Donna Born, Gabriel Spera, and Nancy Profera for their constant encouragement, and Jon Bach for his masterful editing.

From the corporation's Graphics & Design Department, I thank Karl Jacobs for his imaginative cover design, as well as John Hoyem and John Griffith for their superb technical illustrations.

I thank Drs. Sal Alfano, Glenn Peterson, Todd Cerven, Roger Thompson, and Scott Zimmer for painstakingly reading the whole manuscript, and Tim Meisenhelder, Rob Kalinowsky, and Darryl Branting for reading selected portions.

My first spacecraft collision analysis dealt with the impact of dust particles on the International Cometary Explorer Spacecraft, work that I performed for Tom Stengle of the NASA Goddard Space Flight Center in 1984. I owe very much of my continuing research in spacecraft collision to the far-sighted sponsorship of Joe Pizzicaroli while I was on the Iridium Program at Motorola in Chandler, Arizona, from 1995 to 1996. In addition, I thank Al Treder of Barrios Technology for directing me to the NASA Web site from which I gathered much of the information on the International Space Station.

I appreciate the moral support given me by Ted Muelhaupt, associate director of The Aerospace Corporation's System Analysis and Simulation Subdivision, during the last many years. I also acknowledge the financial support from Dr. William Ailor, director of the Center for Orbital and Reentry Debris Studies during the years 1999 and 2000.

I am grateful to Felicia Bagby of The Aerospace Corporation's Lauritsen Library for all the help she provided when I urgently needed material for the preparation of this book as well as the assistance I needed for all my other projects. I also wish to thank Jorgen Olsen, Shirley Tanaka, Joan Tseng, Sandra Dennis, Benita Campbell, Shirley McElroy, Tanisha Church, and the rest of the library staff for promptly gathering information that I much needed.

Finally, I wish to acknowledge the immense sacrifices made by my family—Lai-Koon, Brian, Smart, and Trixie—so that I could devote time to my work. I value very much the kindness and understanding shown me by Alethea, Fleur, Rosalie, Kelly, Sue, and Valerie over many decades of friendship. I treasure the many helpful conversations with Drs. David Blanchard, Richard Brown, Val Chobotov, Larry Delaney, and Rob Moffatt during my career.

Sources

Approximately half of this book is based on papers I presented at various conferences in the past decade, but the contents of these papers have been augmented and reorganized to form a more coherent whole. The remaining half comes from research done at other times in the past two decades, particularly in the past two years while I was preparing the manuscript.

Specifically, acknowledgment of the following copyrighted materials is in order:

The seed paper of the Rician integral approach to computing spacecraft collision probability (Chapter 4 of this book, "The Isotropic Problem") was originally presented at the 7th International Space Conference of Pacific-Basin Societies, held 15–18 July 1997 in Nagasaki, Japan, and was originally published in the AAS publication, "Space Cooperation into the 21st Century" (edited by Peter M. Bainum et al.), American Astronautical Society (AAS) Advances in the Astronautical Sciences, Vol. 96, 1997, pp. 1033–1048, Paper AAS 97-491, "Collision Probability Analyses for Earth Orbiting Satellites," by Ken Chan. (Copyright © 1997 by AAS Publications Office, P.O. Box 28130, San Diego, CA 92198, U.S.A.; Web site: http://www.univelt.com. All rights reserved. This material is reprinted with permission of the AAS.)

Chapter 5 of this book, "Analytical Expressions for Short-Term Encounters," was originally presented at the AAS/AIAA Space Flight Mechanics Meeting held 9–13 February 2003 in Ponce, Puerto Rico, and was originally published in the AAS publication "Astrodynamics 2003" (edited by Daniel J. Scheeres et al.), AAS Advances in the Astronautical Sciences, Vol. 114, 2003, pp. 1197–1216, Paper AAS 03-184, "Improved Analytical Expressions for Computing Spacecraft Collision Probabilities," by Ken Chan. (Copyright © 2003 by AAS Publications Office, P.O. Box 28130, San Diego, CA 92198, U.S.A.; Web site: http://www.univelt.com. All rights reserved. This material is reprinted with permission of the AAS.)

Chapter 7, "Spacecraft Maneuvers to Mitigate Potential Collision," was originally presented at the AIAA/AAS Astrodynamics Specialist Conference held 5–8 August 2002 in Monterey, California, and was originally published in the American Institute of Aeronautics and Astronautics (AIAA) publication, "A Collection of Technical Papers: AIAA Astrodynamics Specialist Conference 2002" (edited by James V. McAdams et al.), Paper AIAA 2002-4629, "Spacecraft Maneuvers to Mitigate Potential Collision," by Ken Chan. (Copyright © 2002 by AIAA Publications Office, 1801 Alexander Bell Drive, Suite 500, Reston, VA 20191-4344, U.S.A.; Web site: http://www.aiaa.org. The author holds the copyright to this paper. All rights reserved.)

Chapter 8, "Analytical Spacecraft Collision Probability for Long-Term Encounters," was originally presented at the AAS/AIAA Space Flight Mechanics Meeting held 3–7 August 2003 in Big Sky, Montana, and was originally published in the AAS publication "Astrodynamics 2003" (edited by Jean de Lafontaine et al.), AAS Advances in the Astronautical Sciences, Vol. 116, 2004, pp. 769–784, Paper AAS 03-549, "Spacecraft Collision Probability for Long-Term Encounters," by Ken Chan. (Copyright © 2004 by AAS Publications Office, P.O. Box 28130,

San Diego, CA 92198, U.S.A.; Web site: http://www.univelt.com. All rights reserved. This material is reprinted with permission of the AAS.)

Chapter 9, "Short-Term vs. Long-Term Spacecraft Encounters," was originally presented at the AIAA/AAS Space Flight Mechanics Meeting held 16–19 August 2004 in Providence, Rhode Island, and was originally published in the AIAA publication "A Collection of Technical Papers: AIAA Astrodynamics Specialist Conference 2004" (edited by Craig A. Kluever et al.), Paper AIAA 2004-5460, "Short-Term vs. Long-Term Spacecraft Encounters," by Ken Chan. (Copyright © 2004 by AIAA Publications Office, 1801 Alexander Bell Drive, Suite 500, Reston, VA 20191-4344, U.S.A.; Web site: http://www.aiaa.org. All rights reserved. This material is reprinted with permission of the American Institute of Aeronautics and Astronautics, Inc.)

Chapter 10, "Formation Flying," was originally presented at the NASA/Goddard Space Flight Center (GSFC) 2003 Flight Mechanics Symposium held 28–30 October 2003 in Greenbelt, Maryland, and was originally published in the (CD-ROM) NASA CP-2003-212246 publication "2003 Flight Mechanics Symposium" (edited by John P. Lynch et al.), Paper No. 11, "Formation Flying: Collision Assessment, Pre-emptive Maneuvers and Safe IIaven Parking," by Kcn Chan. (Flight Dynamics Analysis Branch, Goddard Space Flight Center, Greenbelt, MD 20771; Web site: http://www.fdab.gsfc.nasa.gov. The author holds the copyright to this paper. All rights reserved.)

Chapter 12, "Close Encounters with Multiple Satellites," was originally presented at the AAS/AIAA Space Flight Mechanics Meeting held 27–30 January 2002 in San Antonio, Texas, and was originally published in the AAS publication "Astrodynamics 2002" (edited by Kyle T. Alfriend et al.), AAS Advances in the Astronautical Sciences, Vol. 112, 2002, pp. 281–300, Paper AAS 02-120, "Close Encounters with Multiple Satellites," by Ken Chan. (Copyright © 2002 by AAS Publications Office, P.O. Box 28130, San Diego, CA 92198, U.S.A.; Web Site: http://www.univelt.com. All rights reserved. This material is reprinted with permission of the AAS.)

Chapter 1: Overview

1.1 Introduction

The exploitation of the near-Earth space environment by commercial, military, and scientific interests during the last 50 years has led to the increasing likelihood of collisions between orbiting objects. Because their positions are not known to extremely high precision, the inevitable question of collision probability becomes one of great interest. In such an encounter, one of the orbiting objects is usually an operational spacecraft and is referred to as the primary object. The other, referred to as the secondary object, can be an active, inactive, or even a rogue spacecraft; it may be a piece of orbiting debris of natural or man-made origin.

The timely publication of this book serves the needs of the space community by exploring the subject of collision probability. This first chapter summarizes the topics that appear in the remainder of the book, including subjects such as different types of encounters; the extent of encounter regions and transit times; probabilities of collisions for a variety of orbits and circumstances, including encounters with multiple objects; and evasive maneuvers. This chapter introduces the concepts and analyses, the problems and solutions that will be developed more rigorously and comprehensively in the later chapters. Each section that follows corresponds to a different chapter.

In order to compute the probability of collision, we need to formulate the problem rigorously within the framework of probability theory. If we know the probability density functions (pdf) describing the uncertainties of the positions of the two objects, we can determine the probability that they are within a specified volume. If we assume that the random variables associated with these pdfs are independent (or less stringently uncorrelated), then we can take the product of these pdfs to obtain the joint pdf. We can then integrate over the product space of random variables that corresponds to the specified volume of interest. Even for simple pdfs, this approach is rather involved.

Another approach is to consider the relative position of one object with respect to the other and obtain the pdf describing the uncertainty of their relative positions. We can then integrate over the region of space swept out by the volume of interest as one object moves relative to the other. This is the approach taken in this book.

Until around 1990, most analyses[1.1-1.5] on spacecraft collision probability were concerned with a spacecraft going through a layer of orbiting space debris. They have been based on the Poisson distribution (i.e., they modeled the process as in the kinetic theory of gases, in which the gas molecules move along straight lines with random directions and their number density is statistically uniform). The general applicability of this model is questionable because the orbiting objects move in essentially Keplerian orbits and their number density varies from the equator to their inclination latitude (the highest latitude reached during an orbit), where the statistical density is several orders of magnitude higher.

Most present analyses[1.6-1.14] on spacecraft collision probability are concerned with close encounters between two orbiting objects. They are based on the Gaussian distribution because the primary spacecraft and secondary space objects can be tracked and their positions determined to within the errors associated with the corresponding position covariance ellipsoids. The collision probability is then computed using this information.

1.2 Spacecraft Encounters

Chapter 2 addresses the mathematical and physical formulation of an encounter between two orbiting objects. If we assume that the positional uncertainties of the two objects are uncorrelated, we may simply add the two covariances to obtain the combined covariance of the relative position. To facilitate the formulation of the collision probability computation, an encounter coordinate system is defined at the instant of "nominal" closest approach. In this system, the origin is at the secondary object, the y-axis is in the direction of the relative velocity, the x-axis is in the direction of the primary, and the z-axis completes the right-handed triad. The (x, z)-plane is defined as the encounter plane. This definition of the encounter system is applicable to the case of most spacecraft in low Earth orbits (LEOs) with large relative velocities engaged in short-term encounters whereby they experience a flyby lasting for only a few seconds. It is also true that in such cases the relative motion is essentially rectilinear in the encounter region.

Of special significance is the unstable behavior of such an encounter coordinate system when the relative velocity is small (sometimes a few meters per second). Because the relative velocity can change in direction, the coordinate axes so defined change direction drastically and the elements of the combined covariance fluctuate violently. This radical behavior precludes the encounter system from being used for long-term encounters because they are characterized by small relative velocities and nonrectilinear relative motion in the encounter region. This is the case with some pairs of spacecraft, located in geosynchronous orbits (GEOs), that can spend close to a day in the vicinity of each other.

Thus, two different methods must be used to study these two significantly different problems. Hitherto, analyses on collision probabilities have assumed that the encounters are of the short-term nature without explicitly stating as much. This book formulates the theory and the algorithms for computing the collision probabilities for these two cases and also presents results illustrating the salient differences between them.

1.3 The Encounter Region

Chapter 3 explains how the extent of the encounter region and the transit time are determined. For any object orbiting Earth, we know that the trajectory is curved as a result of the effects of gravitational forces. Thus, in general, the relative motion of one object with respect to another will be a curved line. However, under certain circumstances, it may be unnecessary to account for the details of the nonlinear relative motion when computing the probability of collision between them. Thus, in the vicinity of the point of closest approach for the case of short-term encounters, we assume that the two objects move along straight lines so that their relative motion is also described by a straight line. The question is: When can we make this assumption? Stated in another way, what is the extent of this region for which the orbits can be considered to be straight lines? It is important to determine the extent of the encounter region.

In computing the probability of collision, we need to integrate over the region of random variables that corresponds to a collision. For simplicity, we assume that both the objects are spherical. Let r_p and r_s respectively denote the radius of the primary and the secondary object. Then, if the secondary comes within a sphere with radius $r_A = r_p + r_s$ centered at the primary, there will be a physical overlap between them.

We have stated that we base the collision probability integral on the relative position covariance. It is a three-dimensional integral that can be time-consuming to evaluate. If we make the assumption of rectilinear relative motion, then the volume swept out by the sphere of radius r_A is a long cylinder extending along the y-direction from $-\infty$ to $+\infty$. The outcome of this process is that, instead of having to deal with a cumbersome three-dimensional pdf, we now consider the corresponding marginal two-dimensional pdf. The volume integration over an infinitely long circular cylinder is replaced by the area integration over a circular cross section. Let σ be the standard deviation along the relative velocity direction. If we perform numerical analysis, we obtain a requirement of 17σ for the approximating straight-line path to achieve a 17-digit accuracy and a requirement of 6σ for the approximating straight-line path to achieve a 2-digit accuracy. These lengths are used to estimate the extent of the encounter region for which the relative motion may be regarded as rectilinear.

We can also obtain the time to traverse the encounter region. For large angles of approach, the transit time is relatively small so that the approximation becomes valid. However, for small approach angles, the relative velocity of transit is very small and the transit time is very large. Consequently, the rectilinear relative motion approximation is invalid and it is not possible to reduce the three-dimensional collision integral to a two-dimensional one.

1.4 The Isotropic Problem

Even after transitioning to a two-dimensional integral, we find that there is no known closed-form solution when the integrand is a bivariate Gaussian pdf, that is, the two standard deviations σ_x and σ_z are not equal. However, for the isotropic Gaussian pdf for which $\sigma_x = \sigma_z \equiv \sigma$, we can transform the two-dimensional integral exactly to a one-dimensional integral involving the Rician pdf as the integrand. Chapter 4 examines this isotropic case.

The Rician pdf arises frequently in the detection of signals in the presence of noise. It also arises in target detection by pulsed radar, noncoherent detection of band-passed binary signals, accuracy of unguided ballistic bombs hitting their targets, and artillery effectiveness of fragmentation bombs. Now, we find that it arises in spacecraft collision probability for the special isotropic case.

It is possible to derive an analytical expression for the Rician integral in the form of an infinite series that is convergent for all values of the input collision parameters. This infinite series yields the zeroth-order and first-order approximations for the collision probability by retaining respectively one or two terms in the series. The Rician integral forms an important topic of this book.

For simplicity, we shall take σ to be between 1 km and 10 km for LEOs. For most spacecraft dimensions, we can safely take the radius r_A up to 100 m. (Most large spacecraft are at most 40 m and the International Space Station is approximately 100 m at the largest dimension, so that r_A is, in these cases, respectively 20 m and 50 m.) For encounters between two orbiting objects, we can take the miss distance x_e up to 100 km, which is more than we really need to consider. Hence, we can establish the following present limits for our collision parameters:

$$0 < \left(\frac{r_A}{\sigma}\right) \le 10^{-1} \qquad \text{and} \qquad 0 \le \left(\frac{x_e}{\sigma}\right) \le 100 \tag{1.1}$$

For some future systems, we may have very accurate orbit determinations and thus σ may lie between 10 m and 100 m. Accordingly, we may consider miss distance up to 100 m. Therefore, the future limits become

$$0 < \left(\frac{r_A}{\sigma}\right) \le 10 \qquad \text{and} \qquad 0 \le \left(\frac{x_e}{\sigma}\right) \le 10 \tag{1.2}$$

We find that the first three orders of approximation yield sufficient accuracy for the present range of collision parameters but that substantially higher orders are needed for the anticipated future range of parameters. Specifically, for most present-day applications (for which the combined object radius is approximately less than one-tenth the standard deviation), the zeroth-order and first-order approximations provide collision probabilities accurate to within 1% error.

1.5 Analytical Expressions for Short-Term Encounters

Whereas Chapter 4 considers an isotropic Gaussian pdf in the encounter (x, z)-plane, even though we might have started with a three-dimensional covariance that is not necessarily isotropic, Chapter 5 considers the nonisotropic case for which the two standard deviations σ_x and σ_z are not equal in the two-dimensional

Gaussian pdf used in computing the collision probability. The covariance C, in general, contains an off-diagonal term with a nonzero correlation coefficient ρ_{xz}.

To handle this case, we rotate the (x, z)-coordinate axes to new (x', z')-coordinate axes so that the new covariance C' has only diagonal terms $\sigma_{x'}^2$ and $\sigma_{z'}^2$. We then transform the (x', z')-coordinate axes to new (x'', z'')-coordinate axes so that the new covariance C'' has equal diagonal terms $\sigma_{x''}^2$ and $\sigma_{z''}^2$. In this process, the circular cross section becomes an elliptical cross-sectional area of integration.

Next, if we approximate this elliptical cross section by an equivalent circular one having the same area and the same centroid, then we convert the probability problem into the isotropic one already solved. Thus, we are able to use all the previous results of the isotropic problem already available for the collision probability. The approximation in representing the elliptical cross section by a circular cross section ultimately determines the accuracy of using the Rician pdf in our modeling. The requirement is basically that the combined object radius r_A is approximately less than one-tenth the standard deviation $\sigma \equiv \sqrt{(\sigma_{x'}\sigma_{z'})}$ and the encounter plane elliptic aspect ratio $1 \leq (\sigma_{x'}/\sigma_{z'}) \leq 10$.

To obtain a measure of accuracy, we compare this formulation (Chan) with three other well-known formulations for use in computing spacecraft collision probability. These are the Foster (used by NASA), Patera, and Alfano formulations. We compare the numerical results over a very wide range of input collision parameters: miss distance x_e, cross-sectional radius r_A, and standard deviations $\sigma_{x'}$ and $\sigma_{z'}$. It is found that, over the present limits of the collision parameter ratios, the four formulations yield collision probabilities agreeing to at least 1% for the case of circular collision cross section. The NASA model is strictly applicable to the case of circular cross section, whereas the other three may be extended in principle to noncircular areas.

From the standpoint of the number of function evaluations, the Chan method is 1000 times faster than the Patera and the Alfano methods and 10,000 times faster than the NASA method. If collision probability is used in screening thousands of pairs of orbiting objects that are candidates for potential collision, this difference in computation speed is an important factor to be considered.

In addition, we also compare the collision probabilities for triangular and rectangular cross sections using the Chan, Patera, and Alfano formulations. Again, we find that the numerical results agree to two or three significant digits.

1.6 International Space Station Collision Probability

A little consideration reveals that it is possible to compute the collision probabilities for complex spacecraft structures having geometrical components such as plates, discs, spheres, ellipsoids, cylinders, cones, and parallelepipeds if self-shadowing is ignored. The approach is to obtain the collision cross section of each component and convert it to an equivalent circle having the same area and the same centroid. We shall refer to this as the method of equivalent cross section area (MECSA).

Presently, NASA models the International Space Station (ISS) as a sphere with radius of approximately 60 m. With the capability provided by MECSA, we may now model the ISS in greater detail. Instead of modeling every minute detail, we shall just model the solar panels and shields as flat rectangular plates, the main cross boom as a rectangular cylinder, and the other modules as circular cylinders. As before, we shall take the origin of the encounter system to be at the secondary object (an inactive or rogue spacecraft, or debris). Each component of the ISS is regarded as a primary object. The orientation and centroid of each of these components are known in the ISS body system. They are easily transformed to the encounter system by known orthogonal transformation matrices. It now makes sense why we conveniently chose the origin of the encounter system to be at the secondary.

In Chapter 6, using MECSA, we compute the collision probability between the ISS and an oncoming object for three case studies: head-on collision, broadside collision, and overhead collision. If the huge solar panels are tilted at 30 deg with respect to the relative velocity, we find that the collision probability for the broadside collision is one or two orders of magnitude smaller than that obtained for a spherical model.

1.7 Maneuvers to Mitigate Potential Collision Threats

Closely related to the problem of computing the collision probability between two orbiting objects is that of deciding, planning, and implementing maneuvers so that the two objects will have a reduced chance of colliding. Chapter 7 looks at these processes. The primary object is assumed to be an active controllable spacecraft. The secondary may not be controllable, as in the case of a rogue satellite or space debris. Suppose we are faced with a situation of high imminent collision probability or one that is greater than a specified acceptable threshold value. We wish to perform an orbit maneuver that is optimal in the sense that it requires the minimum velocity change to mitigate the potential collision threat and reduce the collision probability accordingly.

Because we have the zeroth-order expression for collision probability in terms of closest distance of approach, it is possible to invert this equation to yield the latter in terms of the former. Thus, if we specify a sufficiently low collision probability, we can compute the requisite separation at closest approach. From this, we can obtain intrack thrusting so as to decrease the collision probability to that specified acceptable threshold value. The analysis is simple and the maneuver is also simple to perform. Alternatively, we can also derive the equations for general thrusting with crosstrack and radial components. The analysis is complicated and the maneuver is difficult to perform.

The point to bear in mind is that, except for cases of immediate exigency, we should not base a maneuver only on myopic considerations of near-term reduction of collision probability, but we must also take into consideration subsequent scenarios. In whatever situation, we recommend performing a simple intrack thrusting.

1.8 Analytical Expressions for Long-Term Encounters

Certain pairs of geosynchronous satellites have been observed to have low relative velocity (so low it is measured in units of meters per second) so that the time they spend in the encounter region is appreciable. During this period, which can extend to well in excess of a day, neither the relative velocity can be considered constant in direction nor can the combined covariance error ellipsoid be treated as constant. In contrast to the existing short-term encounter models for which the assumption of constant relative velocity is valid, the long-term encounter model requires that a different approach be used for computing collision probability. Chapter 8 explores this approach.

In order to analyze the general case of long-term encounter, we must account for the covariance error ellipsoid changing in shape, size, and orientation. Thus, we can no longer consider the three Cartesian coordinates (x, y, z) representing the relative position uncertainty as random variables. Instead, we must choose three different random variables (x^*, y^*, z^*) as a common basis so that we can meaningfully compute the collision probability. This probability is determined by evaluating a three-dimensional integral over the appropriate region V^* corresponding to the values of the random variables. This is the crux of probability theory.

We can derive equations for the transformation of a sphere of radius r_A in the (x, y, z)-space to the (x^*, y^*, z^*)-space. We also need the relative motion of the primary in the physical space consistent with the laws of dynamics. As a first approximation, the relative motion is given by the well-known Clohessy-Wiltshire equations.

Next, we need to derive the equation of an envelope generated by a sphere of radius r_A moving in the three-dimensional space (x, y, z). The volume enclosed by this envelope is denoted by V. This volume is then mapped into the corresponding volume V^* in the (x^*, y^*, z^*)-space and is used for integration to obtain the collision probability. In general, the region of integration V^* is very complicated, being a tube with a curved axis and varying cross section. It may not be simply connected such as a torus, an elliptical doughnut, or even a pretzel. The collision probability in most cases must be determined by numerical integration.

1.9 Short-Term vs. Long-Term Spacecraft Encounters

Most encounters between spacecraft are short-term in duration, but it would be misleading to treat all of them as such. There are encounters that are of the long-term nature. By using equations for the two types of encounters, Chapter 9 examines cases to elucidate the differences between their results.

Three illustrative cases of long-term encounters are studied in detail in this chapter to compare the results of the correct long-term formulation with those obtained by inappropriately using the erroneous short-term formulation. For specific cases, one collision probability can be greater than the other or vice versa, depending on the range of collision parameters under consideration. Until the requisite computations are performed, it is difficult to make any a priori conclusions from an intuitive point of view.

In the first case study, we consider a family of in-plane concentric ellipses. Each ellipse describes the relative motion of a secondary spacecraft around the primary spacecraft. We find that the erroneous short-term encounter collision probability is larger than the correct value obtained for the long-term encounter when $(A/\sigma) < 0.5$ and smaller when $(A/\sigma) > 0.5$. The variable A is the semimajor axis of the ellipse, and σ is the standard deviation of an isotropic Gaussian pdf.

In the second case study, we consider a family of fixed-size in-plane ellipses along a straight line. Each ellipse describes the relative motion of a secondary spacecraft with reference to the primary spacecraft. We find that the erroneous short-term encounter collision probability is always larger than the correct value obtained for the long-term encounter.

In the third case study, we consider a family of variable-size in-plane ellipses with a common apsidal point. Each ellipse describes the relative motion of a secondary spacecraft with reference to the primary spacecraft. We find that the erroneous short-term encounter collision probability is larger than the correct value obtained for the long-term encounter when $(A/\sigma) < 0.6$ and smaller when $(A/\sigma) > 0.6$.

These three cases illustrate the fallacy of using the short-term encounter formulation to compute the collision probability when the relative motion does not meet the criteria of rectilinear motion.

1.10 Formation Flying

Chapter 10 describes onboard procedures to assess probable collisions between spacecraft flying in formation and between the constellation members and other orbiting objects. In addition to making these assessments, we would like to minimize collision risk by performing evasive maneuvers, and to design contingency plans for safe haven parking and subsequent system recovery. These efforts should draw on the analytical expressions derived previously for computing collision probability.

First and foremost in formation flying, we need to assess the collision between members of the constellation during flight. During normal times of operation, the satellite positions can be obtained by using the Global Positioning System (GPS) and intersatellite range measurements. During times of system failure resulting from malfunction of any spacecraft sensor, it is desirable to have other backup means of orbit determination for that particular space vehicle. The use of intersatellite ranging by the other functioning constellation members should provide this information.

For evasive maneuvers, we advocate using intrack thrusting for mitigating potential collision threats because it is much simpler to implement and execute operationally for spacecraft maneuvers. After the close encounter, it could be used again to regain the proper phasing of the spacecraft in its nominal trajectory. This is especially important if the primary spacecraft is one member of a large constellation moving in some prescribed configuration.

It is desirable to have contingency plans and to devise a safe haven configuration whereby we can set the system up for eventual recovery operations. Safe haven parking in times of emergencies should take advantage of the information provided by the estimation, guidance, and control systems from the running archives available on board.

For subsequent system recovery, we recommend that the onboard system make use of the information provided by the relative trajectory estimations of the satellites' state vectors during times of nominal operational conditions. In times of emergencies, the onboard system will take advantage of the information provided by the estimation, guidance, and control systems.

1.11 Maximum Probability of Collision

Chapter 11 considers the following problem: Suppose we are given the Gaussian pdf in the two-dimensional encounter plane. However, we are not given the standard deviations σ_x and σ_z and the cross-correlation coefficient ρ_{xz} or, equivalently, the two standard deviations $\sigma_{x'}$ and $\sigma_{z'}$ in the principal directions. All we know are the distance of closest approach x_e on the x-axis and the combined circular collision cross-sectional area of radius r_A with center $(x_e, 0)$. We would like to determine the maximum probability that can be obtained by assigning different values to $\sigma_{x'}$ and $\sigma_{z'}$ in the $(\sigma_{x'}, \sigma_{z'})$-plane. There are two approaches: the maximum likelihood method and the maximum probability method.

The first of these is an approximation. The principle of maximum likelihood can be used to obtain a quick estimate of the maximum probability when the pdf does not vary much over the combined circular collision cross-sectional area.

The second approach is an exact analysis of the problem as stated and depends only on the accuracy of the analytical expression for the collision probability previously derived. Thus, if we use the zeroth approximation of the collision probability, we expect approximately 1% accuracy for the present limits of the collision parameter ratios.

The numerical results obtained from the two approaches agree to two significant figures or approximately 1% over much of the range of applications interest. Thus, the simpler method of maximum likelihood can be treated as being of comparable accuracy for the present limits of the collision parameter ratios.

1.12 Close Encounters with Multiple Satellites

We are next concerned, in Chapter 12, with a detailed calculation of the probability of collision between the primary spacecraft and numerous secondary orbiting objects during a period of time. These secondary objects are grouped into different classes. The objects in each class have circular orbits and lie within small tolerances about a specific altitude and inclination; the value of the latter parameter can be different from that of the primary spacecraft. All the secondary objects in this class have ascending nodes uniformly distributed around the equator and have phase angles uniformly distributed within an orbital plane. Each class also has an associated number density of orbiting objects.

We can approximate the bivariate Gaussian pdf by an isotropic pdf because the angular direction with respect to the ellipse's principal axes is not known. Thus, the problem is again reduced to that involving the Rician integral. From this, we obtain the equation giving the number of collisions per orbit for each class of secondary objects in terms of its equatorial density, inclination, orbital period, relative velocity, and other collision parameters.

Next, we consider the geometry of the encounters in terms of the inclinations of the primary and secondary objects and the latitude of the encounter. We also categorize the collisions into approaching and trailing. For collisions of the primary spacecraft with all the secondary objects of a given class, computations reveal that the predominant contribution to the collision integral comes from encounters near the inclination latitude. (The inclination latitude is defined to be the highest or the lowest latitude reached during an orbit.) The contribution of the last 2 deg to the value of the approaching collision integral I_A is substantially larger in proportion to the rest of the contribution. The same statement holds for the trailing collision integral I_T. For most of these cases, this contribution is approximately 25% or more. This larger contribution means that there is a greater probability of collision near the inclination latitude.

1.13 Instantaneous Probability of Collision

Up till this point, we have considered the probability of collision between two orbiting objects during a time interval, whether it is the case of short-term or long-term encounter. The probability integral was performed over a volume of the random variable space correspondingly swept out by the motion of a sphere of combined radius $r_A = (r_p + r_s)$ in the physical three-dimensional space. In the case of short-term encounters, the volume of integration was an infinitely long circular cylinder. In the case of long-term encounters, the volume was more complicated, being that contained in the enveloping surface traced out by a time-varying ellipsoid. We used a torus and an elliptical doughnut as simple illustrative examples.

Chapter 13 addresses the idea that, in certain other applications, we may be required to determine the probability of collision at a specific instant of time. In this case, the volume of integration is a sphere of radius R that may be the combined radius r_A or some other parameter such as an effective "event radius" r_E. This event may be the sudden misbehavior of a rogue spacecraft or the explosion of a nearby orbiting object producing many fragments. Inside a sphere of radius r_E, an object can be considered as being impacted by the rogue spacecraft or exploding fragments within a very short time interval.

A little consideration will reveal that the analysis given here is not restricted just to the probability of collision between two orbiting objects. It is equally applicable to other three-dimensional phenomena, such as the explosion of a fragmentation bomb near Earth's surface.

To compute the probability of collision, we can generalize the previous approach by using the transformation of a Gaussian pdf to a Rician pdf and introducing the concept of equivalent volume. It is found that the accuracy is within 1% throughout a wide range of collision parameters. On the basis of the number of function evaluations, which is an indication of computing time, this method is found to be approximately 65,000 times faster than the high-precision brute-force method of numerically evaluating the three-dimensional Gaussian integral.

1.14 Spherical Error Probability Computation

Suppose we are given a pdf and a spherical volume of a certain radius. We can determine the collision probability by evaluating a three-dimensional integral either analytically or numerically as we have just done. This is known as the direct problem. However, we may be given the inverse problem: We need to determine the radius of the spherical region when the collision probability is specified. This problem is known as spherical error probability (SEP). Chapter 14 focuses on computing it.

Six parameters are input to the problem: three standard deviations of the Gaussian pdf, and the three components of the displacement vector of the center of the sphere of consideration. The most obvious approach to determining SEP is to perform many time-consuming numerical evaluations of three-dimensional integrals and then interpolate to obtain the desired result.

The approach here is radically different from that just described, in that we use concepts from statistics to invert an expression involving a particular type of integral. It is based on first formulating the problem in terms of the cumulative noncentral chi-square distribution; then appropriately choosing the degree n' of a central chi-square distribution to approximate the noncentral one; and last, in a second transformation, transforming the central distribution to a Gaussian distribution. The degree n' is chosen so that the first three moments are satisfied. The transformation from central chi-square to Gaussian distribution is accomplished using an expression derived by Wilson and Hilferty. The radius of the sphere is obtained through the use of the inverse error function.

Numerical results are presented for more than 200 benchmark cases. Comparison with several cases of known exact analytical solutions indicates that this method is generally accurate to approximately 1% for probabilities greater than 0.5 and approximately 10% for probabilities between 0.1 and 0.5. This level of accuracy meets the requirements of most applications.

It is recommended that this analytical approximation be used when it is necessary to evaluate very high-dimensional integrals of this nature arising in statistical analysis and signal detection.

1.15 References

[1.1] M. Hechler and J. C. Van der Ha, "Probability of Collisions in the Geostationary Ring," *J. Spacecraft* **18** (4), 361–366 (1981).

[1.2] K. Takahashi, "Collision between Satellites in Stationary Orbits," IEEE Trans. Aerospace and Electronic Systems AES-17 (4), 591–596 (1981).

[1.3] V. A. Chobotov, "Classification of Orbits with Regard to Collision Hazard in Space," *J. Spacecraft* **20** (5), 484–490 (1983).

[1.4] D. J. Kessler, "Orbital Debris Issues," *Advances in Space Research* **5** (2), 3–10 (1985).

[1.5] D. S. McKnight and P. D. Anz-Meador, "Historical Growth of Quantities Affecting On-Orbit Collision Hazard," *J. Spacecraft and Rockets* **30** (1), (1993).

[1.6] J. L. Foster and H. S. Estes, "A Parametric Analysis of Orbital Debris Collision Probability and Maneuver Rate for Space Vehicles," NASA/JSC-25898 (August 1992).

[1.7] Z. N. Khutorovsky, V. F. Boikov, and S. Y. Kamensky, "Direct Method for the Analysis of Collision Probability of Artificial Space Objects in LEO: Techniques, Results and Applications," *Proceedings of the First European Conference on Space Debris, European Space Agency*, Vol. SD-01 (1993), pp. 491–508.

[1.8] F. K. Chan, "Collision Probability Analyses for Earth-Orbiting Satellites," *Proceedings of the 7th International Space Conference of Pacific Basin Societies*, (Nagasaki, Japan, July 1997). (Work performed for the Iridium Program at Motorola, Inc., in 1995.)

[1.9] G. Bollenbacher and J. D. Guptill, "Launch Collision Probability," NASA/TP-1999-208852 (Glenn Research Center, September 1999).

[1.10] N. Berend, "Estimation of the Probability of Collision between Two Catalogued Orbiting Objects," *Advances in Space Research* **23** (1), 342–247 (1999).

[1.11] K. T. Alfriend, M. R. Akella, J. Frisbee, J. L. Foster, D. J. Lee, and M. Wilkins, "Probability of Collision Error Analysis," *J. Space Debris* **1**, 21–35 (1999).

[1.12] R. P. Patera, "A General Method for Calculating Satellite Collision Probability," AAS/AIAA Space Flight Mechanics Meeting (Clearwater, FL, January 2000).

[1.13] R. A. LeClair, "Probability of Collision in the Geosynchronous Orbit," *Space Control Conference* (MIT Lincoln Laboratory, Lexington, MA, April 2000).

[1.14] S. Alfano, "Aerospace Support to Space Situation Awareness," *MIT Lincoln Laboratory Satellite Operations and Safety Workshop* (Haystack Observatory, Chelmsford, MA, October 2002).

Chapter 2: Spacecraft Encounters

It was mentioned in Chapter 1 that the Gaussian distribution is used for analyzing spacecraft collision probability because the primary spacecraft and secondary space objects can be tracked and their positions determined to within the errors associated with the corresponding position covariance ellipsoids. Figure 2.1 illustrates the general case of the two 1-σ covariance ellipsoids for which the velocities are not exactly aligned with their major principal axes.

For emphasis, this illustration exaggerates the actual lack of perfect velocity alignment with the covariance ellipsoids. In most cases for almost-circular orbits, the velocities of spacecraft or orbiting objects are essentially in the directions of the major principal axes, and the corresponding ellipsoids have aspect ratios of approximately 10:2:1 along the intrack, crosstrack, and radial directions. For some cases, these aspect ratios may be even 20:2:1. It is possible that for still other cases, these aspect ratios are in the 5:2:1 range.

2.1 Covariance Ellipsoids

The relative position covariance of the two objects may be obtained as follows: Let C_p' denote the covariance matrix for the primary spacecraft defined in its radial,

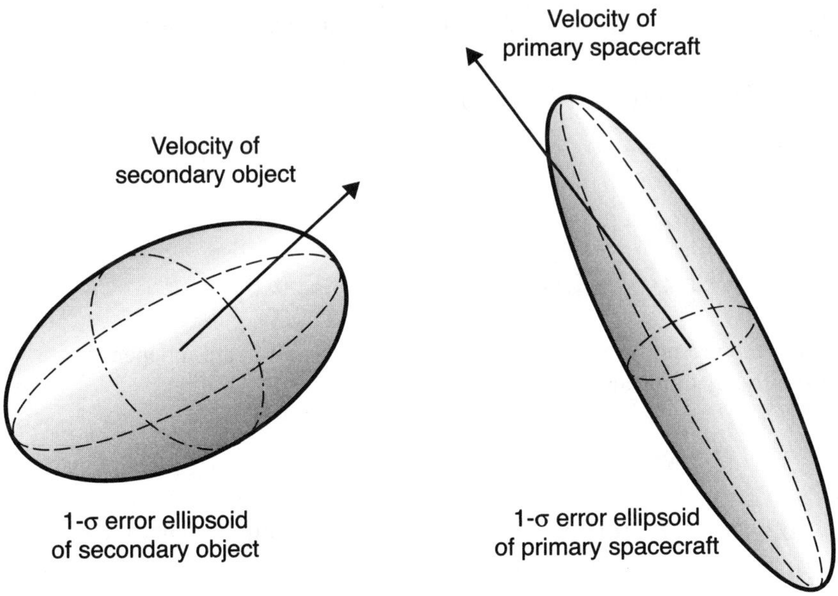

Figure 2.1. Covariance ellipsoids of primary spacecraft and secondary space object.

intrack, and crosstrack (RIC) system; let T_p denote the matrix that governs the transformation from this system to some other system that may be inertial, Earth-fixed rotating, or even the RIC system of one of the two objects. Similarly, let C_s'' and T_s denote the corresponding covariance and transformation matrices for the secondary orbiting object. Then, the covariances C_p and C_s in the common system are given by

$$C_p = T_p C_p' T_p^T \tag{2.1}$$

$$C_s = T_s C_s'' T_s^T \tag{2.2}$$

where the superscript T denotes the transpose. Thus, we now have a common basis to exhibit the two covariance ellipsoids.

Next, let $E[q]$ denote the expectation of a random variable q and the mean $\bar{q} \equiv E[q]$. Let x_i denote any of the three coordinates of the primary spacecraft. Similarly, let y_i denote the corresponding coordinate of the secondary object. Let $\alpha_i \equiv (x_i - \bar{x}_i)$ denote any of the three positional random variables about the mean associated with the primary spacecraft. Similarly, let $\beta_j \equiv (y_j - \bar{y}_j)$ denote any of the three positional random variables about the mean associated with the secondary object. Let $\mathbf{r}_p$ and $\mathbf{r}_s$ be the respective positions of the primary and the secondary. The relative position of the primary with respect to the secondary is $(\mathbf{r}_p - \mathbf{r}_s)$ and the mean relative position is $E[\mathbf{r}_p - \mathbf{r}_s]$. Then, the deviation from the mean is $\{(\mathbf{r}_p - \mathbf{r}_s) - (\bar{\mathbf{r}}_p - \bar{\mathbf{r}}_s)\}$. The relative position covariance C is defined by

$$\begin{aligned} C &\equiv E\left[\{(x_i - y_i) - (\bar{x}_i - \bar{y}_i)\}\{(x_j - y_j) - (\bar{x}_j - \bar{y}_j)\}\right] \\ &= E\left[\{(x_i - \bar{x}_i) - (y_i - \bar{y}_i)\}\{(x_j - \bar{x}_j) - (y_j - \bar{y}_j)\}\right] \\ &= E\left[(\alpha_i - \beta_i)(\alpha_j - \beta_j)\right] \\ &= E\left[\alpha_i\alpha_j\right] + E\left[\beta_i\beta_j\right] - E\left[\alpha_i\beta_j\right] - E\left[\alpha_j\beta_i\right] \end{aligned} \tag{2.3}$$

For the present, suppose for simplicity that α_i and β_j are independent or, less stringently, that they are uncorrelated. Then,

$$E\left[\alpha_i\beta_j\right] = E\left[\alpha_i\right]E\left[\beta_j\right] \tag{2.4}$$

By definition, $E[\alpha_i] = 0$ and $E[\beta_j] = 0$. Therefore, Eq. (2.3) becomes

$$C = E\left[\alpha_i\alpha_j\right] + E\left[\beta_i\beta_j\right] - 0 - 0 \tag{2.5}$$

It follows that, under the assumption in Eq. (2.4) that the uncertainties are uncorrelated, the relative position covariance (also referred to as the combined covariance) C is given by the sum of the individual covariances, all expressed in the same coordinate system:

$$C = C_p + C_s \tag{2.6}$$

In Section 2.6, we will discuss the case for which the assumption of Eq. (2.4) is not invoked.

2.2 Combined Covariance Ellipsoids

Consider the primary spacecraft and secondary object with velocities $\mathbf{v}_p$ and $\mathbf{v}_s$ in a small region of three-dimensional space called the encounter region. (We shall rigorously define this encounter region in Chapter 3. When the two objects are in this region, they are said to be in conjunction.) We take the vector cross product $\mathbf{n} \equiv \mathbf{v}_p \times \mathbf{v}_s$ and project the two velocities onto a plane perpendicular to $\mathbf{n}$ as depicted in Fig. 2.2. Note that, in general, $\mathbf{n}$ is not necessarily vertical and the projection plane orthogonal to $\mathbf{n}$ is not necessarily horizontal.

Let (X', Y', Z') be a coordinate system associated with the primary spacecraft and let $\hat{\mathbf{Y}}'$ be defined parallel to $\hat{\mathbf{v}}_p$. (The "hat" symbol will henceforth denote a unit vector.) Similarly, let (X'', Y'', Z'') be a coordinate system associated with the secondary object and let $\hat{\mathbf{Y}}''$ be defined parallel to $\hat{\mathbf{v}}_s$. Moreover, let $\hat{\mathbf{Z}}'$ and $\hat{\mathbf{Z}}''$ be defined parallel to $\mathbf{n}$. Finally, let $\hat{\mathbf{X}}'$ and $\hat{\mathbf{X}}''$ be defined in the usual sense to form a right-handed triad in their respective coordinate systems.

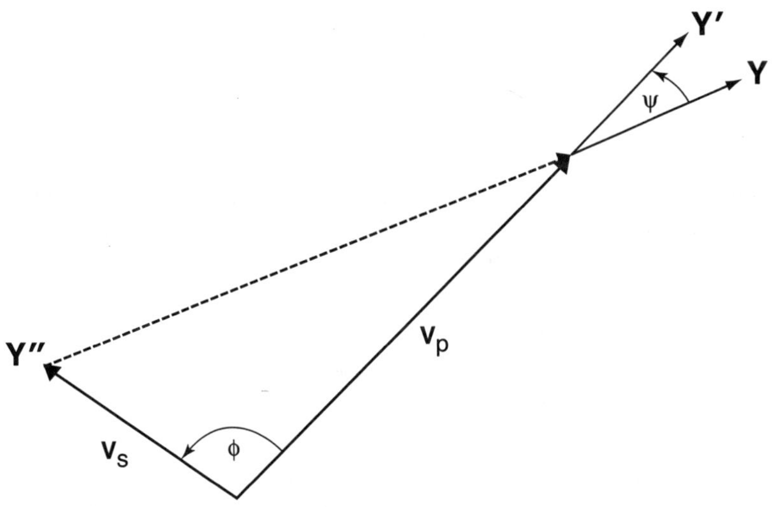

Figure 2.2. Projection plane perpendicular to $\mathbf{n} \equiv \mathbf{v}_p \times \mathbf{v}_s$.

The relative velocity $\mathbf{v}_{ps}$ of the primary with respect to the secondary is given by $\mathbf{v}_{ps} = \mathbf{v}_p - \mathbf{v}_s$. This vector is also projected onto the projection plane. Let $\hat{\mathbf{Y}}$ be defined in the direction of $\mathbf{v}_{ps}$. Moreover, let $\hat{\mathbf{Z}}$ be defined parallel to $\mathbf{n}$ and let $\hat{\mathbf{X}}$ be defined to form a right-handed triad with $\hat{\mathbf{Y}}$ and $\hat{\mathbf{Z}}$.

Let ϕ be the angle measured from $\hat{\mathbf{Y}}'$ to $\hat{\mathbf{Y}}''$ as illustrated in Fig. 2.2. It is positive counterclockwise and negative clockwise around the $\mathbf{n}$-axis. Because the vector cross product $\mathbf{v}_p \times \mathbf{v}_s$ is defined from $\mathbf{v}_p$ to $\mathbf{v}_s$ by the right-hand rule, therefore ϕ is by definition always positive. It is computed from

$$\cos\phi = \widehat{\mathbf{v}_p} \cdot \widehat{\mathbf{v}_s} \tag{2.7}$$

If the right-hand side (RHS) of Eq. (2.7) is positive, then $0 \le \phi < \pi/2$; if it is negative, then $\pi/2 < \phi \le \pi$. Hence, the range is $0 \le \phi \le \pi$.

Similarly, let ψ be the angle measured from $\hat{\mathbf{Y}}$ to $\hat{\mathbf{Y}}'$. A little consideration of Fig. 2.2 reveals that ψ is always positive regardless of ϕ being acute or obtuse. It is computed from

$$\cos\psi = \widehat{\mathbf{v}_{ps}} \cdot \widehat{\mathbf{v}_p} \tag{2.8}$$

If the RHS of Eq. (2.8) is positive, then $0 \le \psi < \pi/2$; if it is negative, then $\pi/2 < \psi \le \pi$. Hence, the range is $0 \le \psi \le \pi$.

Let $\mathbf{r}'$ be any point referenced to (X', Y') on the projection plane and let $\mathbf{r}''$ be the same point referenced to (X'', Y'') on the projection plane. Then, we have the following transformation from the (X', Y') system to the (X'', Y'') system.

$$\mathbf{r}'' = T^*_{ps}\,\mathbf{r}'$$
$$T^*_{ps} = \begin{bmatrix} \cos\phi & \sin\phi \\ -\sin\phi & \cos\phi \end{bmatrix} \tag{2.9}$$

Similarly, let $\mathbf{r}$ be any point referenced to (X, Y) on the projection plane and let $\mathbf{r}'$ be the same point referenced to (X', Y') on the projection plane. Then, we have the following transformation from the (X, Y) system to the (X', Y') system.

$$\mathbf{r}' = T^*\,\mathbf{r}$$
$$T^* = \begin{bmatrix} \cos\psi & \sin\psi \\ -\sin\psi & \cos\psi \end{bmatrix} \tag{2.10}$$

We shall next assume that the major axis of the covariance ellipsoid C_p' for the primary is aligned with the velocity vector $\mathbf{v}_p$ (which is in the direction of $\hat{\mathbf{Y}}'$ by definition). This is a very reasonable assumption, because much of the spacecraft positional uncertainty is along this direction. We know that the three principal axes of the covariance ellipsoid are mutually orthogonal. For simplicity, we shall also assume that the other two principal axes are aligned with $\hat{\mathbf{X}}'$ and $\hat{\mathbf{Z}}'$. In the same way, for the secondary object, we shall make similar assumptions about the covariance ellipsoid C_s'' in the (X'', Y'', Z'') system.

This alignment of the covariance ellipsoid with the coordinate axes for both the objects is referred to as the "general simplified model." It is called general because the velocity magnitudes and the covariances of the primary and the secondary objects are not assumed to be equal, as depicted in Fig. 2.2.

In considering almost-circular orbits much of the time, we note that the intermediate axis is essentially (but not exactly) aligned in the crosstrack direction and the minor axis is essentially (but not exactly) aligned in the radial direction. These simplifying assumptions about the alignment of axes greatly reduce an exorbitant amount of algebraic manipulation and still retain the essential features of the combined covariance that we wish to illustrate.

Hence, in the (X', Y', Z') system, the covariance C_p' of the primary object is given by

$$C_p' = \begin{bmatrix} a_p^2 & 0 & 0 \\ 0 & b_p^2 & 0 \\ 0 & 0 & c_p^2 \end{bmatrix} \tag{2.11}$$

where a_p^2, b_p^2, and c_p^2 are respectively the crosstrack, intrack, and radial variances with $b_p^2 > a_p^2 > c_p^2$. Similarly, in the (X'', Y'', Z'') system, the covariance C_s'' of the secondary object is given by

$$C_s'' = \begin{bmatrix} a_s^2 & 0 & 0 \\ 0 & b_s^2 & 0 \\ 0 & 0 & c_s^2 \end{bmatrix} \tag{2.12}$$

where a_s^2, b_s^2, and c_s^2 are respectively the crosstrack, intrack, and radial variances with $b_s^2 > a_s^2 > c_s^2$. Let C_s' denote the covariance of the secondary in the (X', Y', Z') system. Therefore, we have

$$C_s' = T_{ps}^T \, C_s'' \, T_{ps} \tag{2.13}$$

where

$$T_{ps} = \begin{bmatrix} \cos\phi & \sin\phi & 0 \\ -\sin\phi & \cos\phi & 0 \\ 0 & 0 & 1 \end{bmatrix} \tag{2.14}$$

Note that Eq. (2.13) is consistent with Eq. (2.2). This is because T^*_{ps} appearing in Eq. (2.9) is the transformation matrix from the (X', Y') system to the (X'', Y'') system. Consequently, T_{ps} in Eq. (2.13) is the transformation matrix from the (X', Y', Z') system to the (X'', Y'', Z'') system, whereas T_s^T used in Eq. (2.2) is the inverse of this transformation. Note that, because the transformation is orthogonal, the inverse is also equal to the transpose.

Substituting Eq. (2.14) into Eq. (2.13), we see it follows that

$$C_s' = \begin{bmatrix} \left(a_s^2 \cos^2\phi + b_s^2 \sin^2\phi\right) & \left(\frac{1}{2}(a_s^2 - b_s^2)\sin 2\phi\right) & 0 \\ \left(\frac{1}{2}(a_s^2 - b_s^2)\sin 2\phi\right) & \left(a_s^2 \sin^2\phi + b_s^2 \cos^2\phi\right) & 0 \\ 0 & 0 & c_s^2 \end{bmatrix} \tag{2.15}$$

By Eq. (2.6), therefore the combined covariance C' in the (X', Y', Z') system is

$$C' = C_p' + C_s' \tag{2.16}$$

By substituting Eqs. (2.11) and (2.15) into Eq. (2.16), we obtain

$$C' = \begin{bmatrix} C'_{11} & C'_{12} & 0 \\ C'_{21} & C'_{22} & 0 \\ 0 & 0 & C'_{33} \end{bmatrix} \tag{2.17}$$

where

$$\begin{aligned} C'_{11} &= a_p^2 + a_s^2 \cos^2\phi + b_s^2 \sin^2\phi \\ C'_{12} &= C'_{21} = \frac{1}{2}(a_s^2 - b_s^2)\sin 2\phi \\ C'_{22} &= b_p^2 + a_s^2 \sin^2\phi + b_s^2 \cos^2\phi \\ C'_{33} &= c_p^2 + c_s^2 \end{aligned} \tag{2.18}$$

This is the combined covariance in the (X', Y', Z') system. If we wish to obtain the combined covariance C in the (X, Y, Z) system, then we have

$$C = T^T \, C' \, T \tag{2.19}$$

where

$$T = \begin{bmatrix} \cos\psi & \sin\psi & 0 \\ -\sin\psi & \cos\psi & 0 \\ 0 & 0 & 1 \end{bmatrix} \tag{2.20}$$

By substituting Eq. (2.20) into Eq. (2.19), we see it follows that

$$C = \begin{bmatrix} C_{11} & C_{12} & 0 \\ C_{21} & C_{22} & 0 \\ 0 & 0 & C_{33} \end{bmatrix} \tag{2.21}$$

where

$$\begin{aligned} C_{11} &= C'_{11}\cos^2\psi + C'_{22}\sin^2\psi - C'_{12}\sin 2\psi \\ C_{12} &= C_{21} = \frac{1}{2}(C'_{11} - C'_{22})\sin 2\psi + C'_{12}\cos 2\psi \\ C_{22} &= C'_{11}\sin^2\psi + C'_{22}\cos^2\psi + C'_{12}\sin 2\psi \\ C_{33} &= C'_{33} \end{aligned} \tag{2.22}$$

Note that the combined covariance C given by Eq. (2.22) is subject only to the assumptions that the major principal axes of the primary and the secondary are aligned with the velocities $\mathbf{v}_p$ and $\mathbf{v}_s$ and that the other principal axes of C_p' and C_s'' are aligned with the X', Z', X'', and Z'' axes. There are no restrictions imposed on the velocities $\mathbf{v}_p$ and $\mathbf{v}_s$.

Next, we shall investigate the special case of $\mathbf{v}_p$ and $\mathbf{v}_s$ having essentially the same magnitude. This condition is not very restrictive because we are considering objects in near-circular orbits encountering each other at essentially the same altitude. We shall also assume that their covariances are essentially alike. Specifically, let us consider the "special simplified model" for which the velocity magnitudes and covariances of the primary and the secondary are assumed to be equal.

$$\begin{aligned} v &= v_p = v_s \\ a &= a_p = a_s \\ b &= b_p = b_s \\ c &= c_p = c_s \end{aligned} \tag{2.23}$$

where a^2, b^2, and c^2 are respectively the crosstrack, intrack, and radial variances with $b^2 > a^2 > c^2$. We observe that we now have an isosceles triangle. Figure 2.3 illustrates this case.

Consequently, the angle ψ is now independent of the magnitude of the velocities $\mathbf{v}_p$ and $\mathbf{v}_s$. Thus,

$$\begin{aligned} \psi &= \pi/2 - \phi/2 \\ \sin\psi &= \cos(\phi/2) \\ \cos\psi &= \sin(\phi/2) \\ \sin 2\psi &= \sin\phi \\ \cos 2\psi &= -\cos\phi \end{aligned} \tag{2.24}$$

If we substitute Eqs. (2.23) and (2.24) into Eq. (2.18), we obtain

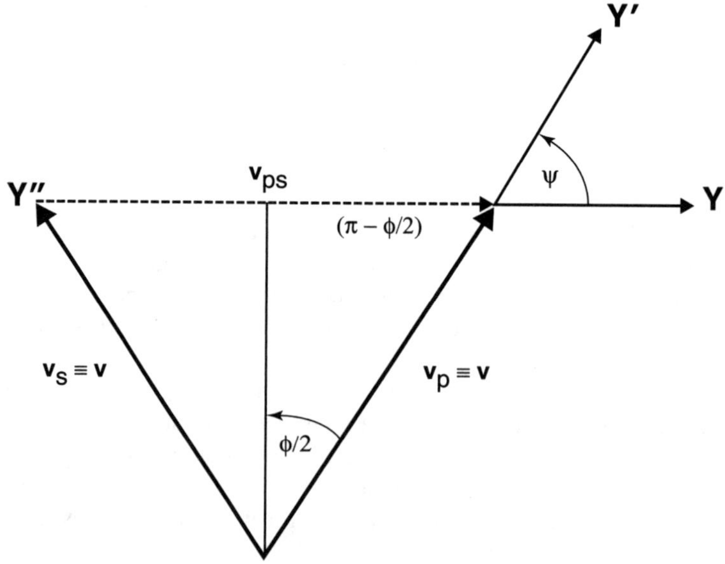

Figure 2.3. Special simplified model with equal velocity magnitudes and covariances.

$$\begin{aligned} C'_{11} &= a^2(1+\cos^2\phi)+b^2\sin^2\phi \\ C'_{12} &= C'_{21} = \frac{1}{2}(a^2-b^2)\sin 2\phi \\ C'_{22} &= a^2\sin^2\phi + b^2(1+\cos^2\phi) \\ C'_{33} &= 2c^2 \end{aligned} \tag{2.25}$$

If we now substitute Eq. (2.25) into (2.22), we have

$$\begin{aligned} C_{11} &= 2\cos^2\phi\left[a^2\sin^2(\phi/2)+b^2\cos^2(\phi/2)\right]+(a^2+b^2)\sin^2\phi-\frac{1}{2}(a^2-b^2)\sin\phi\sin 2\phi \\ C_{22} &= 2\cos^2\phi\left[b^2\sin^2(\phi/2)+a^2\cos^2(\phi/2)\right]+(b^2+a^2)\sin^2\phi-\frac{1}{2}(b^2-a^2)\sin\phi\sin 2\phi \\ C_{33} &= 2c^2 \\ C_{12} &= C_{21} \equiv 0 \end{aligned} \tag{2.26}$$

We observe from Eq. (2.26) that the combined covariance C in the (X, Y, Z) system is precisely diagonal for all values of the intersection angle ϕ:

$$C = \begin{bmatrix} C_{11} & 0 & 0 \\ 0 & C_{22} & 0 \\ 0 & 0 & C_{33} \end{bmatrix} \tag{2.27}$$

This property is a direct consequence of the assumptions of the special simplified model. It is not surprising in view of the assumption in Eq. (2.23) that the primary and secondary covariances are the same. Hence, the two angular bisectors of the velocity projections on the (X, Y)-plane become lines of symmetry of the combined covariance. We recall that the Y-axis is defined to be in the direction of the relative velocity $\mathbf{v}_{ps}$ of the primary with respect to the secondary. Hence, if $\pi/2 < \phi \le \pi$, then the major axis of the combined covariance ellipsoid is along the Y-axis and the intermediate axis is along the X-axis. However, if $0 < \phi < \pi/2$, then the major axis of the combined covariance ellipsoid is along the X-axis and the intermediate axis is along the Y-axis. That is, the situation gets switched. This is illustrated in Fig. 2.4.

We next show rigorously that the first two diagonal elements in the matrix of Eq. (2.27) are always larger than the third. By judicious rearrangement of terms, we obtain

$$\begin{aligned} C_{11} &= 2\cos^2\phi\left[a^2+(b^2-a^2)\cos^2(\phi/2)\right]+2a^2\sin^2\phi+(b^2-a^2)\sin^2\phi(1+\cos\phi) \\ &= 2a^2+(b^2-a^2)\left[2\cos^2\phi\cos^2(\phi/2)+\sin^2\phi(1+\cos\phi)\right] \end{aligned} \tag{2.28}$$

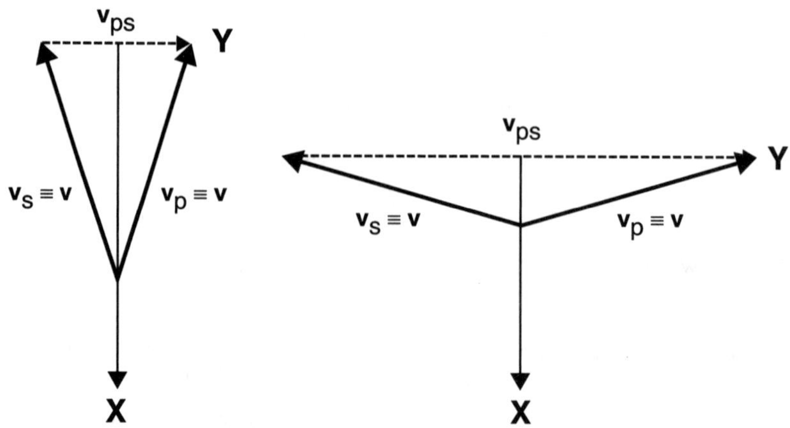

Figure 2.4. Switching of major and intermediate covariance axes for Y.

Because the second term in Eq. (2.28) is always positive for all values of ϕ, therefore

$$C_{11} > 2a^2 > 2c^2 = C_{33} \tag{2.29}$$

Similarly, we obtain

$$\begin{aligned} C_{22} &= 2\cos^2\phi\left[a^2 + (b^2 - a^2)\sin^2(\phi/2)\right] + 2a^2\sin^2\phi + (b^2 - a^2)\sin^2\phi(1-\cos\phi) \\ &= 2a^2 + (b^2 - a^2)\left[2\cos^2\phi\sin^2(\phi/2) + \sin^2\phi(1-\cos\phi)\right] \end{aligned} \tag{2.30}$$

Again, the second term in Eq. (2.30) is always positive for all values of ϕ; therefore

$$C_{22} > 2a^2 > 2c^2 = C_{33} \tag{2.31}$$

The results in Eqs. (2.29) and (2.31) are not surprising, because the covariance associated with the minor axis of the combined covariance ellipsoid is derived from the sum of the two radial variances. However, this observation does not constitute a derivation. One must be cautious about making such arguments as a substitute for a rigorous proof. For instance, one can say that the second diagonal term C_{22} in the matrix of Eq. (2.27) is derived mainly from the two intrack variances. Hence, it is expected that $C_{22} > C_{11}$, which is derived mainly from the two crosstrack variances. This is a fallacious conclusion, as we have just noted, regarding the *Y*-axis switching from the major axis of the combined covariance ellipsoid when $\pi/2 < \phi \le \pi$ to the intermediate axis when $0 < \phi < \pi/2$. We shall see this again in the examples that follow.

To illustrate some of the subtle properties associated with the combined covariance, we next study some special cases in detail.

2.2.1 Case 1: $\phi = \pi$

In this case, the two orbiting objects are headed directly toward each other. It is easy to show that Eq. (2.26) yields

$$[C]_{\phi=\pi} = \begin{bmatrix} 2a^2 & 0 & 0 \\ 0 & 2b^2 & 0 \\ 0 & 0 & 2c^2 \end{bmatrix} \tag{2.32}$$

This is not surprising because the two individual prolate covariance ellipsoids are aligned to produce a bigger prolate combined covariance ellipsoid, as illustrated in Fig. 2.5. However, the corresponding major, intermediate, and minor axes are each increased only by a factor of $\sqrt{2}$.

2.2.2 Case 2: $\phi = \pi/2$

In this case, the two orbiting objects are approaching each other broadside. It is easy to show that Eq. (2.26) yields

$$[C]_{\phi=\pi/2} = \begin{bmatrix} (a^2+b^2) & 0 & 0 \\ 0 & (a^2+b^2) & 0 \\ 0 & 0 & 2c^2 \end{bmatrix} \tag{2.33}$$

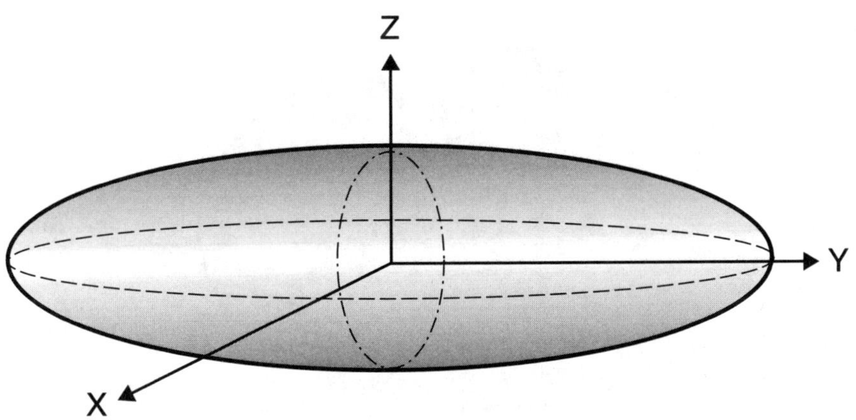

Figure 2.5. Prolate combined covariance ellipsoid.

The two individual prolate covariance ellipsoids are aligned at right angles to produce an oblate combined covariance ellipsoid with rotational symmetry about the *Z*-axis, as illustrated in Fig. 2.6. This may be a bit surprising if examined without going through the process of the analysis given here.

It may be shown using Eq. (2.26) that these two geometrical shapes represent the extreme cases that the combined covariance ellipsoid can take. Some papers on spacecraft encounters have stated that the elongation of the combined covariance ellipsoid is much less than the elongations of the individual ellipsoids whenever the symmetry axes do not align. This is true only if the two orbiting objects are approaching broadside with large angles near 90 deg between the two velocity vectors. For smaller angles, this statement is not true, because the combined covariance ellipsoid is between the two individual covariance ellipsoids in geometrical shape.

It is easy to give numerical examples using Eq. (2.22) to illustrate this point. In fact, without resorting to this equation, we can give the following simple counter-example: Consider an ellipsoid with major axis of 2 units and the other two axes 1 unit of length. Consider another ellipsoid with major axis $(1 + \varepsilon)$ units and the other two axes 1 unit of length, tilted at an angle ε radians with respect to the major axis of the first ellipsoid, ε being a small positive number. Then, the aspect ratio of the combined ellipsoid is $[\sqrt{5/2} + O(\varepsilon)]$, and this is between the aspect ratio of 2 for the first ellipsoid and the aspect ratio of $(1 + \varepsilon)$ for the second ellipsoid.

2.2.3 Case 3: Limiting Case of $\phi \to 0$

When ϕ is small, the two orbiting objects are headed almost in the same direction. It is easy to show that Eq. (2.26) yields

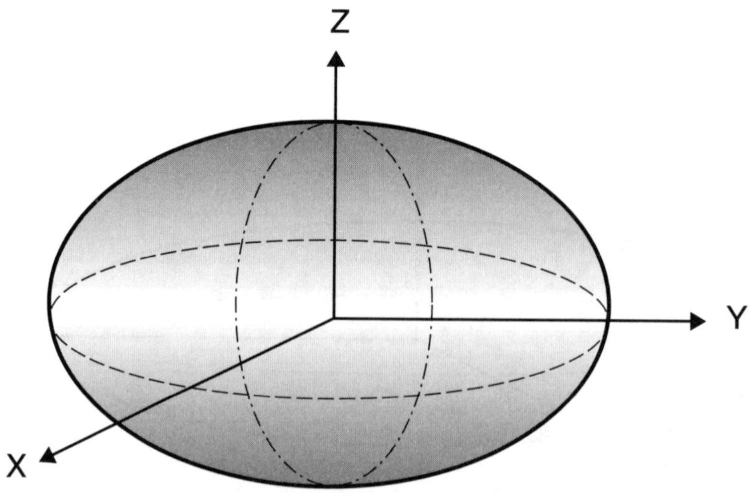

Figure 2.6. Oblate combined covariance ellipsoid with rotational symmetry around the Z-axis.

$$\lim_{\phi\to 0}\left[C\right]=\begin{bmatrix} 2b^2 & 0 & 0 \\ 0 & 2a^2 & 0 \\ 0 & 0 & 2c^2 \end{bmatrix} \tag{2.34}$$

This is rather surprising, because even though the two individual prolate covariance ellipsoids are aligned to produce a bigger prolate combined covariance ellipsoid, the *X*-axis and the *Y*-axis have switched roles compared to case 1. This is because the *Y*-axis is defined to be in the direction of the relative velocity $\mathbf{v}_{ps}$. Thus, the *Y*-axis is now associated with the intermediate axis and the *X*-axis with the major axis of the combined covariance ellipsoid.

We stress that Eq. (2.26) applies to the special simplified model for arbitrary angles $0 < \phi \le \pi$. The special case of $\phi = 0$ is strictly omitted from consideration, because there can be no direction for the relative zero velocity to uniquely define the *Y*-axis. However, this pathological case cannot happen in a realistic situation, because the two velocity magnitudes, being physical quantities, cannot be exactly mathematically equal. Any difference between these two, no matter how small, will yield a relative velocity either parallel or antiparallel to the direction of $\mathbf{v}_p$ and $\mathbf{v}_s$. That is, for the case of $\phi = 0$, the direction of the relative velocity vector $\mathbf{v}_{ps}$ is very unstable, for it can just switch directions depending on whether the ratio of the two velocities $\lambda \equiv \mathbf{v}_s/\mathbf{v}_p$ is greater or less than unity. For small values of ϕ, the direction of $\mathbf{v}_{ps}$ is transverse to the direction of $\mathbf{v}_p$ and $\mathbf{v}_S$. Thus, in the regime of small relative velocities, we expect that any formulation based on the *Y*-axis being defined in the direction $\mathbf{v}_{ps}$ will experience not only mathematical but also physical difficulties.

In anticipation of the next section, an encounter coordinate system will be defined based on choosing the *Y*-axis along the direction of $\mathbf{v}_{ps}$. It follows from this discussion that such an encounter coordinate system cannot be meaningfully defined in the regime of small relative velocities. This point is borne out more specifically and succinctly in the differences between short-term encounters and long-term encounters. Encounters of the first type are typified by flybys, as with low Earth orbits (LEOs), and they last only for a relatively short period, perhaps a few seconds. Encounters of the second type are characterized by the two orbiting objects spending an appreciable period in the same vicinity, close to each other, as with some geosynchronous orbits (GEOs), and these encounters can last for a whole day.

Table 2.1 and Fig. 2.7 show values of the three diagonal terms of the combined covariance of the special simplified model computed using Eqs. (2.26) and (2.27) for various angles ϕ and using the values of $a = 2$, $b = 10$, and $c = 1$ units of length for the crosstrack, intrack, and radial semiaxes. It is noted that the *X*-axis and the *Y*-axis switch roles (the major axis and the intermediate axis) as the angle ϕ goes through 90 deg as anticipated in the discussion here. Moreover, the ellipse obtained by slicing the combined covariance ellipsoid by the (*X*, *Z*)-plane has an

Table 2.1. Combined Covariance and Encounter Plane Ellipse Aspect Ratio

ϕ (deg)	C_{11}	C_{22}	C_{33}	Encounter Plane Ellipse Aspect Ratio
0.00	200.00	8.00	2.00	10.00
20.00	194.21	13.79	2.00	9.85
40.00	177.54	30.46	2.00	9.42
60.00	152.00	56.00	2.00	8.72
80.00	120.67	87.33	2.00	7.77
90.00	104.00	104.00	2.00	7.21
100.00	87.33	120.67	2.00	6.61
120.00	56.00	152.00	2.00	5.29
140.00	30.46	177.54	2.00	3.90
160.00	13.79	194.21	2.00	2.63
180.00	8.00	200.00	2.00	2.00

aspect ratio ρ given in the last column and illustrated in Fig. 2.8. We note that $\rho = 10$ when $\phi \to 0$ deg. When the two objects approach each other broadside, $\phi = 90$ deg and $\rho = 7.21$. When they approach directly head-on, $\phi = 180$ deg and $\rho = 2$. We note that when 90 deg $\leq \phi \leq$ 180 deg, ρ is much smaller than 10. As we shall see in Chapters 3 and 4, this ellipse in the (X, Z)-plane is more important than the other two ellipses obtained by slicing the combined ellipsoid by the (X, Y)-plane or the (Y, Z)-plane, because it is used in computing the probability of collision between the two objects for the case of short-term encounters.

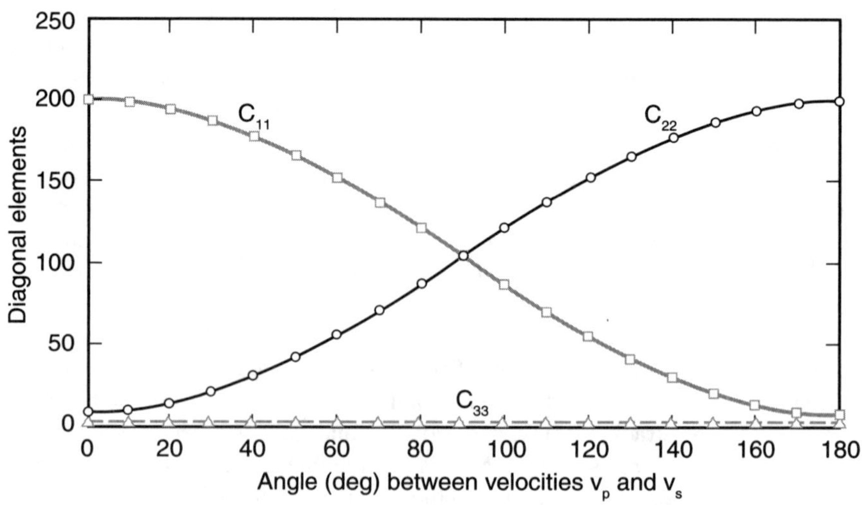

Figure 2.7. Combined covariance diagonal elements.

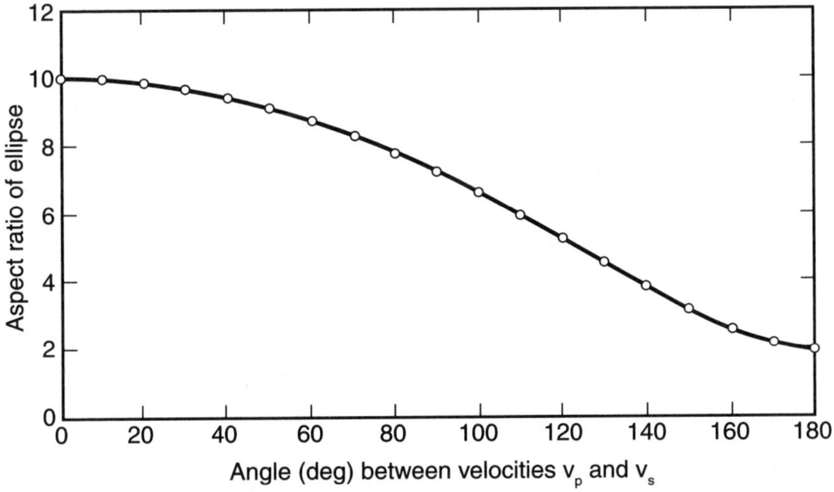

Figure 2.8. Encounter plane ellipse aspect ratio.

2.3 Encounter Coordinate System

At a conjunction involving a flyby (which holds for most encounters except possibly for some infrequent ones involving geosynchronous satellites), an encounter coordinate system (x, y, z) is defined for convenience: The origin is taken to be at either one of the two orbiting objects. In conformance to most current usage, we shall choose the secondary. Let the y-axis be along the relative vector $\mathbf{v}_{ps}$. Then, the (x, z)-plane is normal to this vector. At the instant of "nominal" closest approach, let the x-axis be defined such that the primary spacecraft is nominally at the point $(x_e, 0, 0)$. This is illustrated in Fig. 2.9. Thus, x_e is the "nominal" distance of closest approach. Other designations are "nominal" minimum separation and "nominal" miss distance. The (x, z)-plane is called the encounter plane. It must be emphasized that the encounter coordinate system and the encounter plane are defined only at the instant of nominal closest approach. Henceforth, whenever we omit the word "nominal" for convenience, we shall implicitly keep this connotation in mind.

The y-axis is the same as the Y-axis. In general, the x-axis and the z-axis do not coincide with the X-axis and the Z-axis even though the (x, z)-plane coincides with the (X, Z)-plane previously defined in Section 2.2. Thus, the (X, Z)-plane is also the encounter plane but only at the time of closest approach. Both these planes intersect the 1-σ combined covariance ellipsoid and produce the same 1-σ ellipse.

Let us study some cases to illustrate the relation between the x-axis and the X-axis and their relation to this ellipse. For simplicity of visualization, we shall implicitly consider almost-circular orbits. Hence, the (X, Y)-plane containing the projections of the two velocities is essentially horizontal and the Z-axis is essentially in the

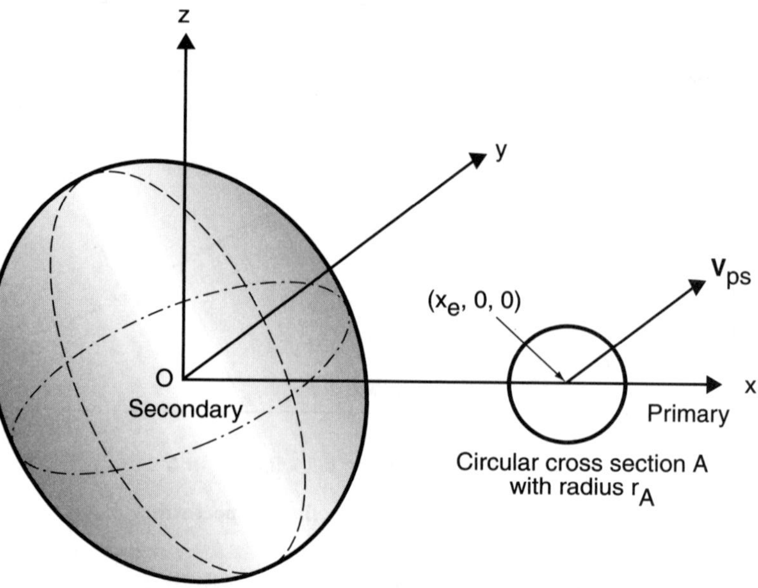

Figure 2.9. Combined error ellipsoid and collision cross section in encounter coordinate system.

outward radial direction. For more general orbits, the generalization is not difficult but the visualization is.

2.3.1 Case 1: Overhead Encounter

Suppose at the instant of closest approach, the primary object is directly above the secondary. That is, the x-axis is in the direction of the positive Z-axis and the z-axis is in the direction of the negative X-axis. By Eqs. (2.29) and (2.31), the minor axis of the combined covariance ellipsoid in the general (hence also special) simplified model is always along the Z-axis. Therefore, the x-axis is along the minor axis of the 1-σ ellipse. Let θ denote the "elevation" angle between the vector $\mathbf{r}_{\min}$ of minimum separation x_e and the major axis of the 1-σ ellipse. This major axis is also the X-axis. For the case of direct overhead encounter, we have $\theta = 90$ deg. (At the instant of closest approach, if the primary is directly below the secondary so that we have a direct "underfoot" encounter, then the x-axis is in the direction of the negative Z-axis and the z-axis is in the direction of the positive X-axis. Note that, by definition, we have $\theta = -90$ deg because it is referenced to the major axis of the 1-σ ellipse.)

2.3.2 Case 2: Oblique Encounter

Suppose the two velocities $\mathbf{v}_p$ and $\mathbf{v}_s$ are the same as before but there is a slight delay in one of the two conjoining objects. Then, obviously, the miss distance is different. Instead of experiencing a direct overhead or underfoot encounter, the vector $\mathbf{r}_{min}$ makes a different angle with the X-axis where $0 < \theta < \pi/2$.

Let us specifically consider the following simple example. Suppose the primary P and the secondary S approach each other with equal speeds v at an angle $\phi = 90$ deg in the projection (X, Y)-plane. In the case of an overhead encounter, P is directly above S at the instant of closest approach, say $t = 0$. Let this point on the (X, Y)-projection plane be denoted by Q. Next, suppose P is delayed by a time T.

Then, a little consideration involving symmetry reveals that the minimum separation occurs when P and S make an isosceles triangle with Q on the projection (X, Y)-plane at time $T/2$, as illustrated in Fig. 2.10. During this time interval, P and S would each have traveled a distance $vT/2$ so that both are now at the same distance $vT/2$ from Q and $vT/\sqrt{2}$ from each other.

Because we are implicitly considering almost-circular orbits, the two horizontal planes (one containing $\mathbf{v}_p$ and the other containing $\mathbf{v}_s$) are separated by the same vertical height H. Therefore, the minimum separation x_e and the elevation angle θ between $\mathbf{r}_{min}$ and the X-axis are given by

$$x_e = \sqrt{H^2 + \left(vT/\sqrt{2}\right)^2} \tag{2.35}$$

$$\theta = \tan^{-1}\left(\frac{\sqrt{2}H}{vT}\right) \quad \text{where} \quad -\pi/2 \le \theta \le \pi/2 \tag{2.36}$$

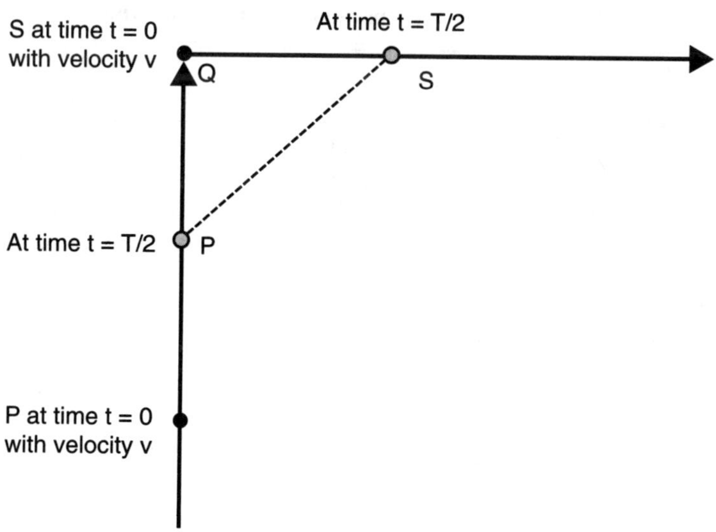

Figure 2.10. Projection plane for an oblique encounter.

Table 2.2 and Fig. 2.11 show values of the minimum separation x_e and the elevation angle θ computed using Eqs. (2.35) and (2.36) for various time delays t of the primary. The primary and the secondary are chosen to have circular orbits of 705 and 695 km altitude respectively. Thus, their corresponding velocities are 7.502 and 7.506 km/sec. Initial conditions are such that they enter the encounter region broadside and conjoin at 10 km minimum separation with the primary directly overhead.

Suppose the primary is delayed 1 sec; then $x_e = 11.32$ km and $\theta = 62.06$ deg. If the primary is delayed 10 sec, then $x_e = 54.0$ km and $\theta = 10.68$ deg. It is observed from Fig. 2.11 that it would take a long delay to reduce θ to a value close to zero. By then, x_e would have become very large. That is, we would no longer have a close encounter. This discussion is based on introducing a delay time of one of the two conjoining objects to study the effect on the minimum separation and the elevation angle. However, we could construct an artificial example to illustrate the case of $\theta = 0$ deg by specifying that they must be in exactly the same horizontal plane at conjunction but at some distance apart. Moreover, their velocities must also lie in the same horizontal plane at that instant. That is, there can be no vertical height between the horizontal plane containing $\mathbf{v}_p$ and that containing $\mathbf{v}_s$.

2.4 Minimum Separation at Conjunction

To obtain the minimum separation, one approach is to perform high-precision orbit propagations of the two objects, then compare the distance between them at closely spaced instants of time to determine the instant of closest approach, and then obtain the corresponding minimum distance. This is the basic approach taken in most systems already implemented for collision studies.

Table 2.2. Minimum Separation and Elevation Angle

Time (sec)	x_e (km)	θ (deg)
0	10.00	90.00
1	11.32	62.06
2	14.58	43.31
3	18.79	32.15
4	23.45	25.24
5	28.34	20.66
6	33.35	17.45
7	38.45	15.08
8	43.59	13.26
9	48.77	11.83
10	53.97	10.68

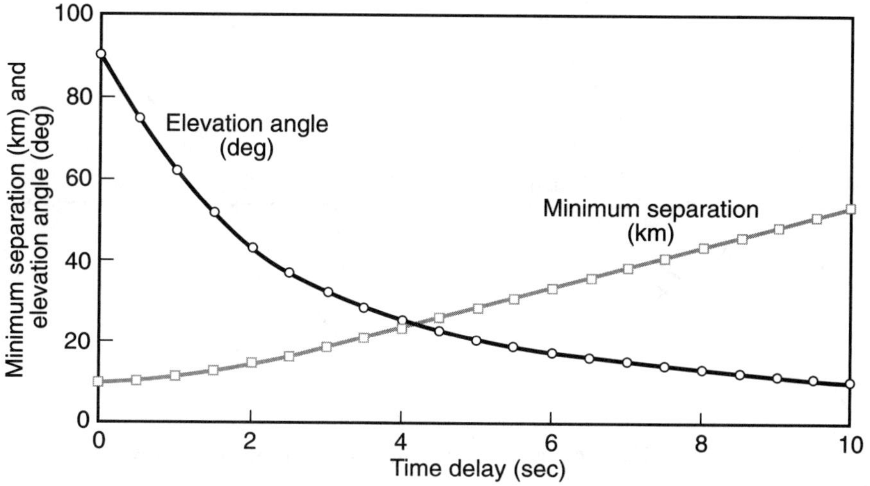

Figure 2.11. Minimum separation and elevation angle.

Unfortunately, these computations are rather time-consuming, especially when there are many pairs of orbiting objects for consideration. Attempts to optimize the procedure have involved first using larger integration step-sizes to arrive near the conjunction and then refining the computations with smaller step-sizes in the encounter region. The approach presented here, which circumvents such laborious computations, is based on techniques of projective geometry and three-dimensional analytical geometry. In Chapter 3, we discuss the conditions for approximating the orbits by rectilinear motion in the encounter region. With this assumption of linear motion, we may construct a general approach for determining the minimum separation when the state vectors (position and velocity) are given for the two orbiting objects at time t_0 in the encounter region.

As before, let $\mathbf{v}_p$ and $\mathbf{v}_s$ respectively denote the velocities of the primary object P and the secondary object S. Let $\mathbf{n}$ denote the vector defined by the cross product of these two vectors, which are assumed to be nonparallel. (The case of mathematically parallel velocity vectors is virtually nonexistent and may be circumvented by delaying the instant specifying the initial conditions of the approach to the encounter region.) Thus, we may construct two planes perpendicular to $\mathbf{n}$: one containing the vector $\mathbf{v}_p$ and the other containing the vector $\mathbf{v}_s$. Let H denote the distance (height) between these two planes.

Next, let us project $\mathbf{v}_s$ onto the plane containing $\mathbf{v}_p$. As the secondary moves along $\mathbf{v}_s$, its projected S_{image} moves along the projected $\mathbf{v}_s$ in the plane containing $\mathbf{v}_p$. Let Q denote the intersection point between $\mathbf{v}_p$ and the projected $\mathbf{v}_s$, and let ϕ denote the angle between them. This scenario is illustrated in Fig. 2.12. This illustration depicts P and S_{image} at any instant of time t where I and J respectively denote their distances from the point Q for two different cases depending on the

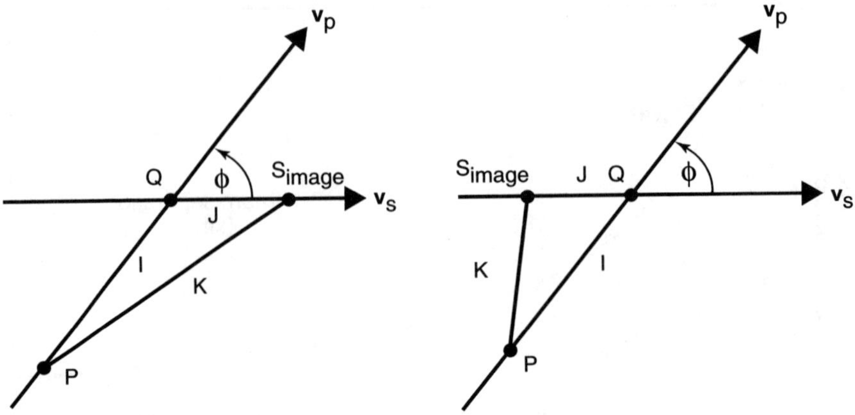

Figure 2.12. Two basic configurations in the projective plane.

initial conditions of the encounter. Therefore, the distance K between P and S_{image} is given by

$$K^2 = I^2 + J^2 \pm 2IJ\cos\phi \tag{2.37}$$

In Eq. (2.37) and all subsequent geometric equations involving triangles, the top and bottom signs apply respectively to the first and second cases shown. For minimum K, we have

$$\frac{dK}{dI} = 0 \tag{2.38}$$

If the magnitudes of $\mathbf{v}_p$ and $\mathbf{v}_s$ are related by the scalar λ, that is,

$$v_s = \lambda v_p \tag{2.39}$$

so that

$$\frac{dJ}{dI} = \mp\lambda \tag{2.40}$$

then, by substituting Eqs. (2.37) and (2.40) into Eq. (2.38), we obtain the following condition for minimum separation in the projective plane:

$$\frac{I^*}{J^*} = \pm\left(\frac{\lambda - \cos\phi}{1 - \lambda\cos\phi}\right) \equiv \pm\eta(\lambda,\phi) \tag{2.41}$$

where I^* and J^* respectively denote the value of I and J at minimum separation. Because I^* and J^* are positive by definition, therefore η is positive in the first case and negative in the second. Moreover, for specified values of λ and ϕ but different approach times of P and S in the encounter region, Eq. (2.41) states that the ratio I^*/J^* depends only on λ and ϕ but not on the approach time. Hence, at the minimum separation, the points P, Q, and S_{image} form a set of similar triangles. Thus, we may state the following:

THEOREM 2.1. *If a pair of orbiting objects P and S have velocities* $\mathbf{v}_p$ *and* $\mathbf{v}_s$ *specified (i.e.,* λ *and* ϕ *are fixed) but have various approach times to the encounter region for which the rectilinear motion approximation is valid, then the configuration* PQS_{image} *in the projection plane forms a set of similar triangles when P and S are at minimum separation.*

This is a very important result that greatly simplifies all subsequent analysis by circumventing a tremendous amount of unnecessary algebraic manipulations. If we next substitute for J^* using Eq. (2.41) into Eq. (2.37), we obtain for both cases

$$K^{*2} = \kappa^2 I^{*2} \tag{2.42}$$

where K^* denotes the value of K at minimum separation and

$$\kappa^2 \equiv 1 + \left(\frac{1-\lambda\cos\phi}{\lambda-\cos\phi}\right)^2 + 2\left(\frac{1-\lambda\cos\phi}{\lambda-\cos\phi}\right)\cos\phi \tag{2.43}$$

Let t_Q denote the time of transit of S_{image} through the point Q. At this instant, P is at some point on the straight line $\mathbf{v}_p$ at a distance L from Q. For simplicity of discussion, we shall assume that it is at a distance L heading toward Q. (The same equations also apply for the case in which P reaches Q ahead of S_{image}.) From Fig. 2.12, a little consideration reveals that we have

$$L = I^* \pm \left(\frac{J^*}{v_s}\right) v_p = I^* \pm \frac{J^*}{\lambda} \tag{2.44}$$

We shall next consider the encounter between the primary P and the secondary S in the three-dimensional region. Let M denote the minimum separation between them. Because the distance H between the planes does not change because of the assumption of linear motion, it follows that

$$M^2 = H^2 + K^{*2} \tag{2.45}$$

The following discussion gives the details for computing I^*, J^*, K^*, M, and L from initial conditions when the primary and secondary objects ingress the encounter region. These are obtained from high-precision orbit propagators. Consider Fig. 2.13, which illustrates the initial conditions in the encounter region for which the approximation of linear motion is valid.

At time t_0, let the primary P and the secondary image S_{image} be at distances L_p and L_s from the point Q. Let t_m denote the time corresponding to minimum separation. Therefore, by equating the times for the two objects to reach the minimum separation, we obtain

$$\frac{L_p - I^*}{v_p} = \frac{L_s \pm J^*}{v_s} \tag{2.46}$$

which yields, in view of Eq. (2.39),

$$L_p - I^* = \frac{1}{\lambda}\left(L_s \pm J^*\right) \tag{2.47}$$

By substituting Eq. (2.41) into Eq. (2.47), we can see it follows that

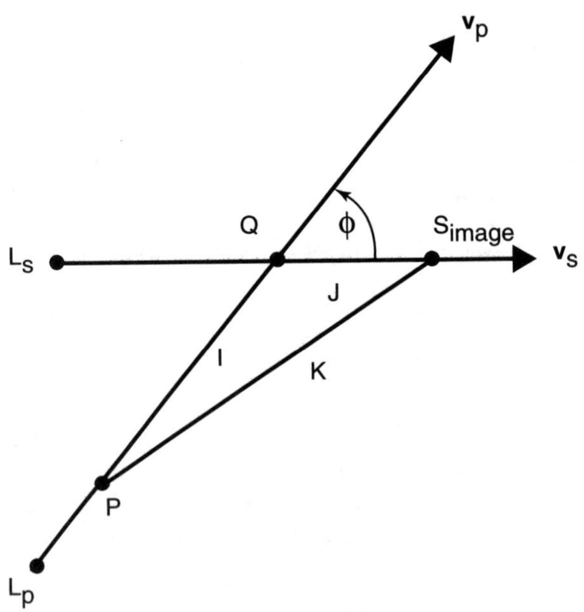

Figure 2.13. Initial conditions for encounter region.

$$L_p - I^* = \frac{1}{\lambda}\left[L_s + I^*\left(\frac{1-\lambda\cos\phi}{\lambda-\cos\phi}\right)\right] = \frac{1}{\lambda}\left(L_s + \frac{I^*}{\eta}\right) \tag{2.48}$$

which is solved for I^* in terms of known quantities:

$$I^* = \frac{(\lambda L_p - L_s)(\lambda - \cos\phi)}{(1 - 2\lambda\cos\phi + \lambda^2)} \tag{2.49}$$

The time t_m when minimum separation occurs is given by

$$t_m = t_0 + \left(\frac{L_p - I^*}{v_p}\right) \tag{2.50}$$

We shall next compute the distances L_p and L_s of the primary P and the secondary image S_{image} at time t_0 from the point Q. These are obtained from the initial conditions as the two objects ingress the encounter region or are already within it. At time t_0, let the positions and velocities of P and S be denoted by $\mathbf{r}_p$, $\mathbf{r}_s$, $\mathbf{v}_p$, and $\mathbf{v}_s$, which are obtained from high-precision orbit propagators. We note that, in the three-dimensional physical space, $\mathbf{v}_p$ passes through $\mathbf{r}_p$ and $\mathbf{v}_s$ passes through $\mathbf{r}_s$. These vectors are referenced to some coordinate system (x, y, z) such as the inertial system. (This should not be confused with the encounter system (x, y, z), which also happens to be an inertial frame of reference.)

We recall that $\mathbf{n} \equiv \mathbf{v}_p \times \mathbf{v}_s$. If we denote $\mathbf{v}_p \equiv (u_p, v_p, w_p)$ and $\mathbf{v}_s \equiv (u_s, v_s, w_s)$, then

$$\mathbf{n} = (v_p w_s - w_p v_s)\hat{\mathbf{i}} + (w_p u_s - u_p w_s)\hat{\mathbf{j}} + (u_p v_s - v_p u_s)\hat{\mathbf{k}} \tag{2.51}$$

In the coordinate system (X, Y, Z), already defined in Section 2.3, we have

$$\hat{\mathbf{Y}} \equiv \widehat{\mathbf{v}_p}, \quad \hat{\mathbf{Z}} \equiv \hat{\mathbf{n}} \quad \text{and} \quad \hat{\mathbf{X}} \equiv \hat{\mathbf{Y}} \times \hat{\mathbf{Z}} \tag{2.52}$$

Let T be the matrix governing the transformation from (x, y, z) to (X, Y, Z). Therefore, we have

$$\begin{aligned} \mathbf{R}_p &= T\mathbf{r}_p \\ \mathbf{R}_s &= T\mathbf{r}_s \\ \mathbf{V}_p &= T\mathbf{v}_p \\ \mathbf{V}_s &= T\mathbf{v}_s \end{aligned} \tag{2.53}$$

where

$$T = \begin{bmatrix} \hat{\mathbf{x}}\cdot\widehat{\mathbf{X}} & \hat{\mathbf{y}}\cdot\widehat{\mathbf{X}} & \hat{\mathbf{z}}\cdot\widehat{\mathbf{X}} \\ \hat{\mathbf{x}}\cdot\widehat{\mathbf{Y}} & \hat{\mathbf{y}}\cdot\widehat{\mathbf{Y}} & \hat{\mathbf{z}}\cdot\widehat{\mathbf{Y}} \\ \hat{\mathbf{x}}\cdot\widehat{\mathbf{Z}} & \hat{\mathbf{y}}\cdot\widehat{\mathbf{Z}} & \hat{\mathbf{z}}\cdot\widehat{\mathbf{Z}} \end{bmatrix} \tag{2.54}$$

The vectors $\mathbf{r}_p \equiv (x_p, y_p, z_p)$ and $\mathbf{r}_s \equiv (x_s, y_s, z_s)$ are projected onto the (X, Y)-plane. These projections are obtained by dropping the Z components in $\mathbf{R}_p \equiv (X_p, Y_p, Z_p)$ and $\mathbf{R}_s \equiv (X_s, Y_s, Z_s)$. Let these projected points be denoted by $A \equiv (X_p, Y_p)$ and $B \equiv (X_s, Y_s)$. Similarly, the vectors $\mathbf{v}_p$ and $\mathbf{v}_s$ are projected onto the (X, Y)-plane and have directional components (U_p, V_p) and (U_s, V_s) respectively. Thus, we have two straight lines on the projection plane. The first passes through the point A and has directions (U_p, V_p). The second passes through the point B and has directions (U_s, V_s). The equations of these lines are respectively

$$\begin{aligned} Y &= \frac{V_p}{U_p}(X - X_p) + Y_p \\ Y &= \frac{V_s}{U_s}(X - X_s) + Y_s \end{aligned} \tag{2.55}$$

These lines intersect at the point $D \equiv (X_i, Y_i)$. Using these two equations, we may solve for X_i to obtain

$$X_i = \frac{\left(Y_s - Y_p\right) + \left[\left(\dfrac{V_p}{U_p}\right)X_p - \left(\dfrac{V_s}{U_s}\right)X_s\right]}{\left[\left(\dfrac{V_p}{U_p}\right) - \left(\dfrac{V_s}{U_s}\right)\right]} \tag{2.56}$$

The result is substituted into Eq. (2.55) to obtain Y_i. Next, the distances L_p and L_s from the point Q are computed from

$$\begin{aligned} L_p &= \sqrt{\left[(X_i - X_p)^2 + (Y_i - Y_p)^2\right]} \\ L_s &= \sqrt{\left[(X_i - X_s)^2 + (Y_i - Y_s)^2\right]} \end{aligned} \tag{2.57}$$

These results are then substituted into Eq. (2.49) to obtain I^*, which, in turn, is substituted into Eq. (2.42) to obtain the minimum separation K^* in the projection plane. The distance (height) H between the two planes orthogonal to $\mathbf{n}$ (containing $\mathbf{v}_p$ and $\mathbf{v}_s$ respectively) is given by

$$H = \left| \hat{\mathbf{n}} \cdot (\mathbf{r}_p - \mathbf{r}_s) \right| \tag{2.58}$$

The minimum separation M in the three-dimensional space (also minimum separation x_e in Section 2.3) is obtained from the equation

$$x_e = \sqrt{H^2 + K^{*2}} \tag{2.59}$$

It must be stressed that the results on minimum separation obtained so far in this section are general and are valid to the extent that the assumption of rectilinear motion in the encounter region is applicable. There has been no assumption about the nature of the individual covariance ellipsoids of the primary and the secondary. Neither has there been any assumption about their principal axes aligning with their radial, intrack, and crosstrack coordinate axes. Additionally, there has been no assumption about the lack of correlation between the two covariances.

However, if we now invoke the general simplified model for any value of ϕ, then the angle θ between the vector of minimum separation $\mathbf{r}_{\min}$ and the major axis of the 1-σ ellipse in the encounter plane is given by

$$\theta = \tan^{-1}\left(\frac{H}{K^*}\right) \quad \text{where} \quad -\pi/2 \le \theta \le \pi/2 \tag{2.60}$$

Equations (2.59) and (2.60) are applicable when the velocity magnitudes and covariances for the primary and secondary are different. They are the generalizations of Eqs. (2.35) and (2.36) that are applicable only to the special simplified model with equal velocity magnitudes and covariances and $\phi = 90$ deg.

2.5 Additional Discussion on the Combined Covariance

For computing the elements of the combined covariance, Eq. (2.22) is the generalization of Eq. (2.26) in that it allows for the velocities and the covariances of the primary and secondary to be different. For a realistic conjunction involving almost-circular orbits, these velocities are very close in magnitude. However, the individual covariances may be very different because of various methods of tracking. Illustrative cases were studied to show how the combined covariance is affected by these inputs. In the first example, the primary and the secondary objects are chosen to have circular orbits of 705 and 695 km altitude respectively.

Thus, their corresponding velocities are 7.502 and 7.506 km/sec. The covariances of the primary and the secondary respectively are computed by using the values of $a_p = 2$, $b_p = 10$, $c_p = 1$, $a_s = 2$, $b_s = 20$, and $c_s = 1$ units of length for the crosstrack, intrack, and radial semiaxes.

Table 2.3 and Fig. 2.14 show values of the elements of the combined covariance of the general simplified model computed using Eqs. (2.21) and (2.22).

It is seen that when compared to Fig. 2.7, the covariance element C_{33} has remained the same as expected. However, C_{11} and C_{22} have increased because of the increase in b_s from 10 to 20 units of length. Moreover, the off-diagonal element C, which is 0 by definition for the special simplified model, is now apparent in Fig. 2.14. It is 0 when $\phi = 0$ deg and 180 deg and reaches a maximum of 150 when $\phi = 90$ deg.

Figure 2.15 shows the aspect ratio ρ of the ellipse obtained by slicing the combined covariance ellipsoid by the (X, Z)-plane. We note that $\rho = 15.8$ for small values of ϕ (but not values that are close to 0). When the two objects approach each other broadside, $\phi = 90$ deg and $\rho = 11.27$. Again, when they approach directly head-on, $\phi = 180$ deg and $\rho = 2$. We note that when 90 deg $\leq \phi \leq$ 180 deg, ρ is much smaller than 16.

Unfortunately, because these figures are plotted on a comparatively large grid, they do not tell the whole story when ϕ approaches 0. Because $\mathbf{v}_s$ (= 7.506 km/sec) is larger than $\mathbf{v}_p$ (= 7.502 km/sec), it follows that when $\phi = 0$ deg the relative velocity $\mathbf{v}_{ps}$ is antiparallel to $\mathbf{v}_p$ and $\mathbf{v}_s$ and is parallel to the Y-axis by definition. Because this is also the case when $\phi = 180$ deg, therefore the Y-axis is now the major axis of

Table 2.3. Combined Covariance and Encounter Plane Ellipse Aspect Ratio

ϕ (deg)	C_{11}	C_{22}	C_{33}	C_{12}	Encounter Plane Ellipse Aspect Ratio
0.2	488.63	19.37	2.00	73.92	15.63
20.00	485.01	22.99	2.00	52.00	15.57
40.00	442.31	65.69	2.00	96.69	14.87
60.00	376.88	131.12	2.00	130.02	13.73
80.00	296.62	211.38	2.00	147.75	12.18
90.00	253.92	254.08	2.00	150.00	11.27
100.00	211.22	296.78	2.00	147.70	10.28
120.00	130.96	377.04	2.00	129.87	8.09
140.00	65.53	442.47	2.00	96.38	5.72
160.00	22.83	485.17	2.00	51.28	3.38
180.00	8.00	500.00	2.00	0.00	2.00

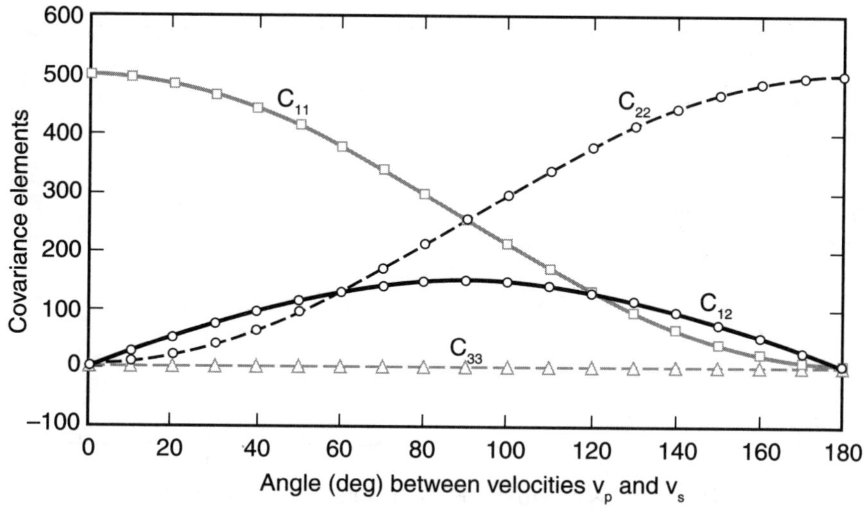

Figure 2.14. Combined covariance elements.

the combined covariance ellipsoid when $\phi = 0$ deg. Then, the ellipsoid should have the combined covariance elements $C_{11} = 8$, $C_{22} = 500$, $C_{12} = 0$, and $\rho = 2$, as shown in the last line of Table 2.3 for the case of $\phi = 180$ deg. From Section 2.3, we know that the *Y*-axis switches from the major axis when $\pi/2 < \phi \leq \pi$ to the intermediate axis when $0 < \phi < \pi/2$. From Figs. 2.14 and 2.15, we observe that the *Y*-axis is still the intermediate axis at $\phi = 10$ deg. Hence, once again, it has to switch

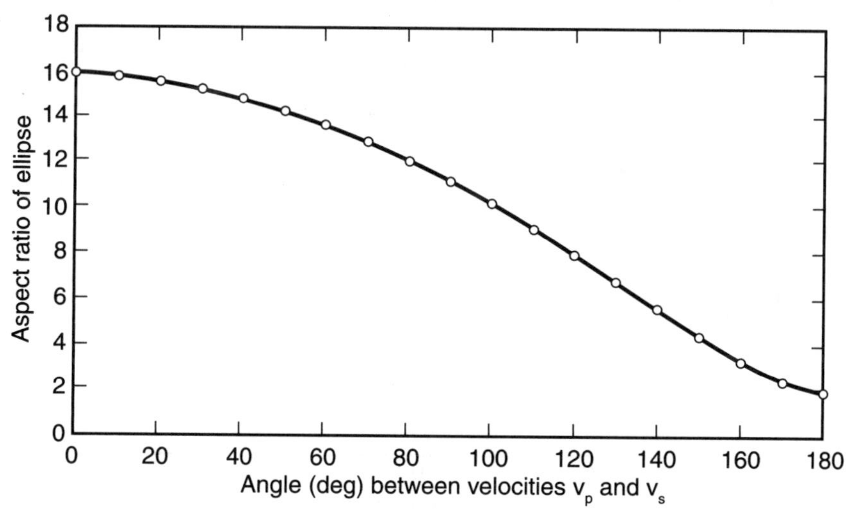

Figure 2.15. Encounter plane ellipse aspect ratio.

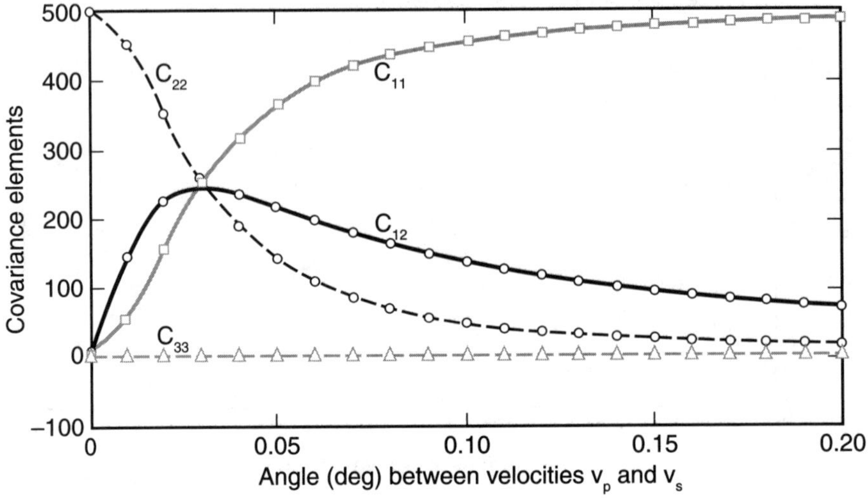

Figure 2.16. Combined covariance elements in ultrasmall region near $\phi = 0$ deg for $v_s > v_p$.

and become the major axis in a small neighborhood of $\phi = 0$ deg. This abrupt change of behavior is depicted in Figs. 2.16 and 2.17, which are plotted in an ultrasmall region near $\phi = 0$ deg.

In the second example, the primary and secondary objects are chosen to have circular orbits of 685 and 695 km altitude respectively. Thus, their corresponding velocities are 7.510 and 7.506 km/sec. That is, the velocity of the primary is chosen

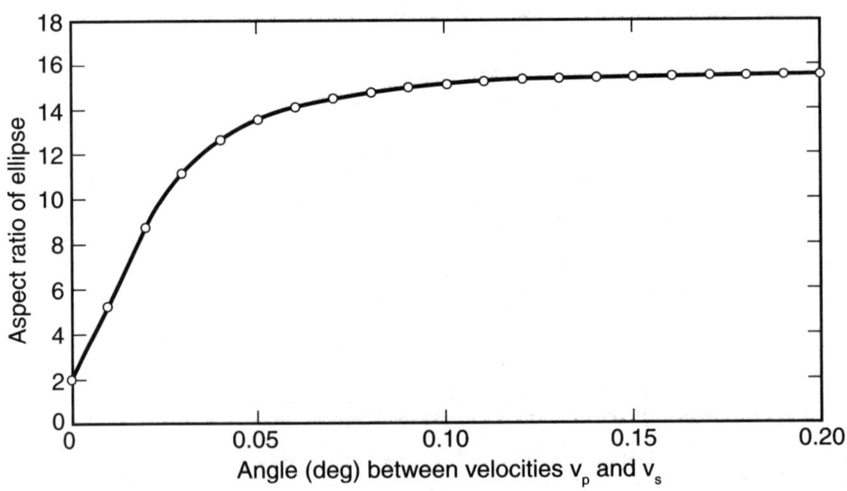

Figure 2.17. Encounter plane ellipse aspect ratio in ultrasmall region near $\phi = 0$ deg for $v_s > v_p$.

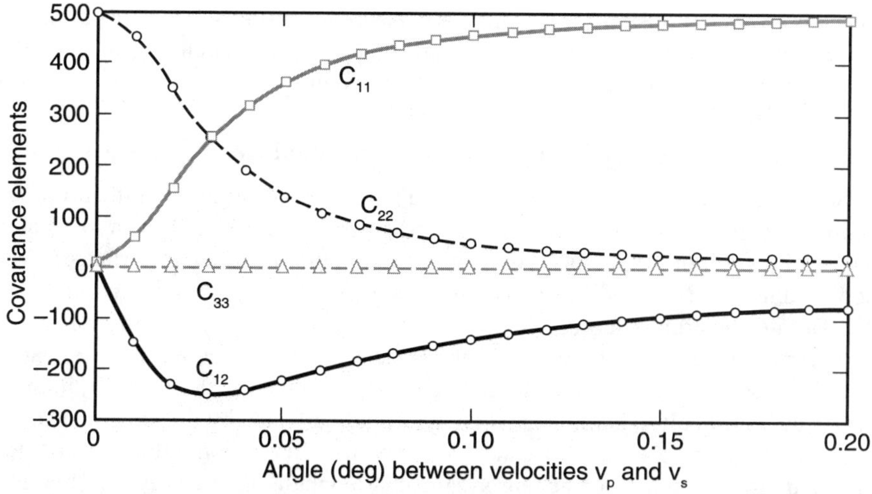

Figure 2.18. Another example of combined covariance elements in ultrasmall region near $\phi = 0$ deg; here, for $v_p > v_s$, velocity of primary object greater than that of secondary.

to be greater than that of the secondary. In this case, when $\phi = 0$ deg the relative velocity $\mathbf{v}_{ps}$ is parallel to $\mathbf{v}_p$ and $\mathbf{v}_s$. The covariances of the primary and the secondary respectively remain the same and are computed by using the values of $a_p = 2$, $b_p = 10$, $c_p = 1$, $a_s = 2$, $b_s = 20$, and $c_s = 1$ units of length for the crosstrack, intrack, and radial semiaxes.

Figures 2.18 and 2.19 show values of the elements of the combined covariance and the encounter plane ellipse aspect ratio. Again, we observe the abrupt change

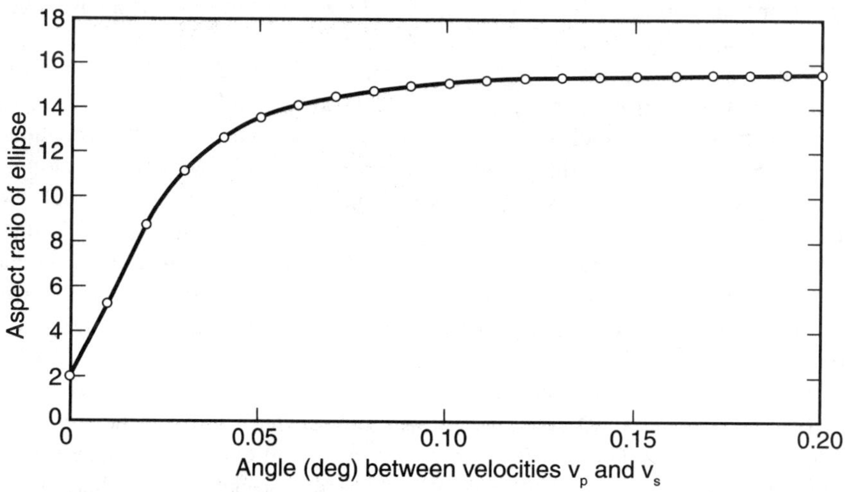

Figure 2.19. Another example of encounter plane ellipse aspect ratio in ultrasmall region near $\phi = 0$ deg; here, for $v_p > v_s$, velocity of primary object greater than that of secondary.

in behavior in an ultrasmall region near $\phi = 0$ deg. The unstable behaviors in these two illustrative cases underscore the fundamental problems in defining an encounter system when the relative velocity $\mathbf{v}_{ps}$ is very small.

2.6 Effects of Correlation on Combined Covariance

In Section 2.1, we assumed that the individual position covariances of the primary and the secondary objects were uncorrelated so that we could add them to obtain the relative position covariance (also referred to as the combined covariance). We now resume discussion of this topic and investigate the effects of correlation.

Even if the orbit determination process were performed on two different systems for these two objects, there would still be correlation between the covariances because of common force modeling parameters such as drag, which, in theory, is quite difficult to compute and is also greatly affected by the uncertain state of the atmosphere. Additionally, there is a contribution to correlation from data obtained from a common tracking system that contains inherent system biases. The contribution of drag is mostly apparent in the intrack component of the covariance and to a lesser degree, the crosstrack and the radial components.

Thus, if two orbiting objects approach each other almost head-on (or with the angle ϕ between the two velocity vectors close to 180 deg), the uncertainty of their relative intrack separation is less than the sum of their individual uncertainties. This means that the correlated combined covariance ellipsoid is less elongated than the uncorrelated combined covariance ellipsoid. On the other hand, the other two axes are less affected because of the lesser contribution of the drag on them.

In general, the correlated and the uncorrelated combined ellipsoids are not exactly aligned, because the two primary and the secondary ellipsoids are not aligned and also are not of the same shape and size. However, in most cases, this misalignment is only a few degrees.

Figure 2.20 illustrates these two combined ellipsoids for $\pi/2 < \phi \leq \pi$ with major axis of the ellipsoids along the Y-axis as discussed in Section 2.2. The relative velocity $\mathbf{v}_{ps}$ is parallel to the Y-axis by definition. Therefore, the encounter plane is the (X, Z)-plane as discussed in Section 2.3. It is unaffected by the elongation of either ellipsoid. Thus, the cross sections derived from them are almost identical in shape and size. That is, the 1-σ ellipses in their respective encounter planes are almost the same. Hence, we expect to obtain approximately the same probability density function (pdf) at the point of closest approach in the uncorrelated and correlated cases. This is basically the conclusion obtained in a numerical study made by Coppola, Woodburn, and Hujsak.[2.1]

For the case of $0 < \phi < \pi/2$, we recall from Section 2.2 that the Y-axis is the intermediate axis and the X-axis is pointing along the major axis of the combined covariance ellipsoid. The (X, Z)-plane now contains an elongated ellipse for the uncorrelated case and a less elongated ellipse for the correlated case. There seems to be a difference of some concern arising between the two cases.

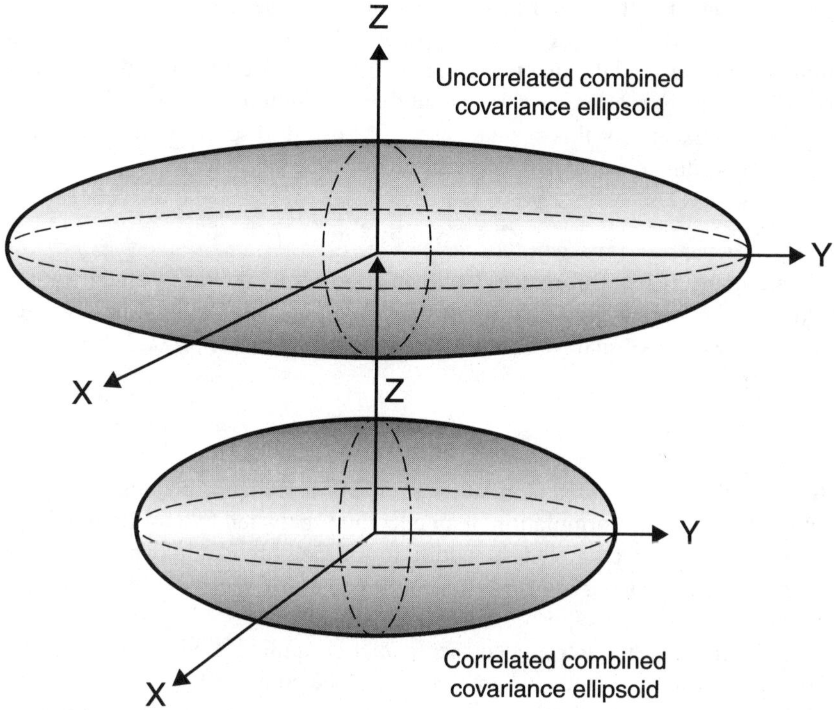

Figure 2.20. Uncorrelated and correlated combined covariance ellipsoids.

However, the analysis does not stop here. At the instant of closest approach, if the elevation angle θ is high (say, greater than 45 deg, as evident from an examination of Fig. 2.20), then there is again not much difference in the pdf at the point of closest approach in the two cases. For low elevation angles ($0 \le \theta < 45$ deg), it is expected that there can be significant difference (at the point of closest approach) in the pdf associated with the uncorrelated and the correlated covariances.

2.7 Discussion

Throughout this chapter, we emphasized that the encounter system is defined only at the instant of nominal closest approach. For short-term encounters, whether we have the rectilinear approximation or realistic curved orbits, there can be only one such instant because there is only one point of closest approach. However, for long-term encounters, it is possible that we have more than one such point. To illustrate this, let us model the orbital motion of two nearby objects as purely Keplerian and consider the relative motion by invoking the idealistic Clohessy-Wiltshire equations over one orbital period and assume that there is no drift. (See Chapter 8 for long-term encounters.) We obtain the following result: One of the objects is situated at the center of an ellipse and the other moves around it so that there are only two points of closest approach. However, in the special case for which the relative orbital plane is inclined at 60 deg, this ellipse of relative motion becomes a circle of relative motion so that there are infinitely many points of closest approach. Except for this special case, it is absurd to speak of the existence of encounter coordinate systems at every instant of time.

2.8 Conclusion

There are many salient differences between short-term and long-term encounters. The differences are so great that it is imperative to divide the treatment into two different types. As we shall see, the first type is easier and the second type is much more complicated.

2.9 Summary

In this chapter, we discussed at great length the underlying principles of the mathematical and physical formulation of an encounter between two orbiting objects.

In Section 2.1, we derived the additivity of the individual covariances of the primary and the secondary to form the combined covariance, which describes the uncertainty of the relative position of the two objects.

In Section 2.2, we introduced the special simplified model and the general simplified model to illustrate salient features of the combined covariance. In these models, the individual covariances have only diagonal terms in their respective radial-intrack-crosstrack coordinate systems. The differences between the models are in the equality of the individual velocity magnitudes and the covariances. Analytical expressions are derived for computing the combined covariances for these two models. Of special importance is the observation that mathematical and physical difficulties arise when the relative velocity between the two objects is small.

In Section 2.3, an encounter coordinate system was defined at the instant of closest approach. In this system, the origin is at the secondary object, the y-axis is in the direction of the relative velocity, the x-axis is in the direction of the primary object, and the z-axis completes the right-handed triad. Equations were derived to compute the minimum separation and elevation angle for a simple case of conjunction. This definition of the encounter system is applicable to the case of most LEOs with large relative velocities engaged in short-term encounters whereby they experience a flyby lasting only a few seconds.

In Section 2.4, equations were derived to compute these two quantities, minimum separation and elevation angle, for the general conjunction. This closed-form solution is based on methods of projective geometry and is valid under the assumption of rectilinear motion approximation in the vicinity of a conjunction. It can be used to supplant the present method of ephemeris generation and subsequent comparison of the separation distance between the two orbiting objects at various instants of time near a conjunction.

Section 2.5 contained in-depth discussion of combined covariance for the general simplified model. Of special significance is the unstable behavior of the encounter coordinate system when the relative velocity is small. In an ultrasmall region, the coordinate axes change direction drastically and the elements of the combined covariance fluctuate violently. This radical behavior precludes the encounter system from being used for long-term encounters characterized by small relative velocities. This is the case with some infrequently observed pairs of GEOs that can spend an appreciable period of close to a day near each other.

In Section 2.6, the effects of correlation on the combined covariance were discussed. Insights were presented to explain why results of uncorrelated and correlated case studies do not differ much when the relative velocity is pointing along the major axis of the combined covariance ellipsoid or when it is pointing along the intermediate axis and the elevation angle is high.

In Section 2.7, examples were provided to illustrate that the point of closest approach is meaningful for short-term encounters and is meaningless for long-term encounters.

In Section 2.8, we concluded that two different methods must be used to study these two disparately different cases.

2.10 Reference

[2.1.] V. T. Coppola, J. Woodburn, and R. Hujsak, "Effects of Cross Correlated Covariance on Spacecraft Collision Probability," *AAS/AIAA Space Flight Mechanics Meeting* (Maui, HI, February 2004).

Chapter 3: The Encounter Region

We know that the trajectory of any object orbiting Earth is curved because of the effects of gravitational forces. Thus, in general, the relative motion of one object with respect to another can be represented by a curved line. However, if a spacecraft approaches, flies by, and then recedes from another, it may be unnecessary to account for the details of the nonlinear relative motion when computing the probability of collision between them. If we were to do so, we would introduce complications into the mathematical modeling, lengthen the computation times, and yet not see any of these nonlinear effects in the final numerical results.

Thus, in the vicinity of the point of closest approach, we assume that the two objects move along straight lines so that their relative motion is also described by a straight line. The question is: When can we make this assumption? Stated another way, what is the extent of this region for which the orbits can be considered to be straight lines, and how long can the two objects remain there? The objective of this chapter is to determine the extent of the encounter region and the transit time.

3.1 The Three-Dimensional Collision Integral

In Chapter 2, we derived the combined covariance C for the relative position of the orbiting objects. Let r_p denote the radius of the sphere that just circumscribes the primary spacecraft; the center of the sphere is located at the center of mass. Similarly, let r_s denote the radius of the circumscribing sphere of the secondary object. Let us now assume that both objects are spherical—first, because this simplifies the problem, and second, because we do not need to account for the orientation (attitude) of the secondary, which is usually not known. Then, if the secondary comes within a sphere with radius $r_A = r_p + r_s$ centered at the primary, there will be a collision.

Let $\mathbf{r} \equiv (x, y, z)$ denote the relative position of the primary with respect to the secondary. Then, the Gaussian probability density function (pdf) of this relative position in terms of the combined covariance C is given by[3.1]

$$f_3(x,y,z) = \frac{1}{\sqrt{(2\pi)^3 |C|}} e^{-\frac{1}{2} r^T C^{-1} r} \tag{3.1}$$

Therefore, the probability of collision is

$$P = \iiint_V f_3(x,y,z)\, dx\, dy\, dz \tag{3.2}$$

where V is the volume swept by the sphere of radius r_A centered at the primary as it moves through the space of random variables (x, y, z).

An assumption is usually made that in the vicinity of a conjunction, the objects' trajectories are straight lines. From a qualitative view, one argues that the orbiting velocities are of the order of several kilometers per second and the time spent in the encounter region is only a few seconds, so the effects of gravitational force are negligible. Also, the covariances of the primary and the secondary are essentially constant during the short time period the two orbiting objects are in the encounter region. Consequently, the combined covariance for the relative position is essentially constant. Thus, we can consider the variables (x, y, z) to be random variables for the collision probability.

Because the intrack standard deviation of the position covariance is a few kilometers, the objects' motion is therefore essentially rectilinear over a large region of several standard deviations in extent. Then, the volume swept out by the sphere of radius r_A is a long cylinder essentially extending along the y-direction from $-\infty$ to $+\infty$. Thus, a little consideration reveals that, instead of having to deal with a three-dimensional pdf, we need only consider the marginal two-dimensional pdf.

Section 3.5 of this chapter discusses this integration in detail. The outcome of this process is that, instead of having to deal with a cumbersome three-dimensional pdf, we now consider the corresponding marginal two-dimensional pdf. The volume integration over an infinitely long circular cylinder is replaced by the area integration over a circular cross section. We may view the situation as follows: At the instant of "nominal" closest approach, when the primary object nominally crosses the encounter (x, z)-plane defined in Chapter 2, its relative position uncertainty is described by the following bivariate Gaussian pdf:

$$f_2(x,z) = \frac{1}{2\pi\sigma_x\sigma_z\sqrt{1-\rho_{xz}^2}} e^{-\left[\left(\frac{x}{\sigma_x}\right)^2 - 2\rho_{xz}\left(\frac{x}{\sigma_x}\right)\left(\frac{z}{\sigma_z}\right)+\left(\frac{z}{\sigma_z}\right)^2\right] \Big/ 2\left(1-\rho_{xz}^2\right)} \tag{3.3}$$

The probability of collision is given by the two-dimensional integral

$$P = \iint_A f_2(x,z)\,dx\,dz \tag{3.4}$$

where A is the circular collision cross-sectional area of radius r_A centered at the primary.

The question now arises: When can this simplification—the use of Eq. (3.4) instead of (3.2)—be made, and how good is this approximation? The following three sections give quantitative conditions when this assumption may be invoked. These results should clarify the confusion between the assumption of rectilinear relative motion and the fact that the two spacecraft actually move in curved trajectories as governed by the laws of dynamics.

3.2 Requisite Path Length for Integration

In assuming that the three-dimensional integral in Eq. (3.2) can be integrated along the y-direction from $-\infty$ to $+\infty$ so that the three-dimensional integral (3.2) reduces to the two-dimensional integral (3.4), we need to investigate the integral I defined by

$$I = \frac{1}{\sqrt{2\pi}\sigma} \int_{-Y}^{+Y} e^{-y^2/2\sigma^2} dy \tag{3.5}$$

We know that when Y is equal to 3σ, the value of I is approximately 0.997. But this is an arbitrary criterion, for one can question why we do not choose some other multiple of σ. However, as will be discussed in Section 13.1 in Chapter 13, it is easily seen that when Y is approximately 8.5σ, the value of I differs from unity in the seventeenth decimal place, and this corresponds to the limits of accuracy in a computer using double-precision arithmetic. This means that if the path of the relative motion is essentially a straight line over a length of 17σ along the integration direction, then the transition from Eq. (3.2) to Eq. (3.4) is valid computationally. Any contribution beyond this integration limit will not appear in the displayed numerical results of the value of the integral I.

In practice, we may safely say that the standard deviation σ is approximately 5 km for low Earth orbits (LEOs) (15 km for geosynchronous orbits, GEOs). This means that we must have essentially rectilinear relative motion of 85 km for 17σ and 30 km for 6σ, depending on whether we have 15-digit or 2-digit accuracy for LEOs (255 km for 17σ and 90 km for 6σ respectively for GEOs).

Let ϕ be the approach angle between the velocity $\mathbf{v}_p$ of the primary object and that of the secondary, $\mathbf{v}_s$. Because the velocity of LEOs is approximately 7.5 km/sec, these distances are traversed in less than 11.3 and 4 sec respectively for the two requirements for $\phi \geq 60$ deg. (The velocity of GEOs is approximately 3.1 km/sec, and these transit times are less than 82.3 and 29 sec respectively.) If ϕ is very small, then the relative velocity $\mathbf{v}_{ps}$ is very small. In this case, the relative motion may not exhibit sufficient path length to meet the requirements of 17σ or even 6σ of straight path. Figure 3.1 illustrates the path of a spacecraft relative to another in the vicinity of the point of closest approach and also the requisite length of 17σ for the linear approximation to be valid. Note that this requirement is independent of the miss distance.

3.3 Rectilinear Motion Approximation

Now that we have derived the path length requirement of 85 km for 15-digit accuracy and 30 km for 2-digit accuracy for a LEO (255 km and 90 km respectively for a GEO), the next step is to investigate how accurately we can approximate a curved line by a straight line. Let us first consider two objects at the same altitude moving toward each other in circular orbits as illustrated in Fig. 3.2. Their paths form an isosceles spherical triangle. How accurately can we approximate this by an isosceles plane triangle?

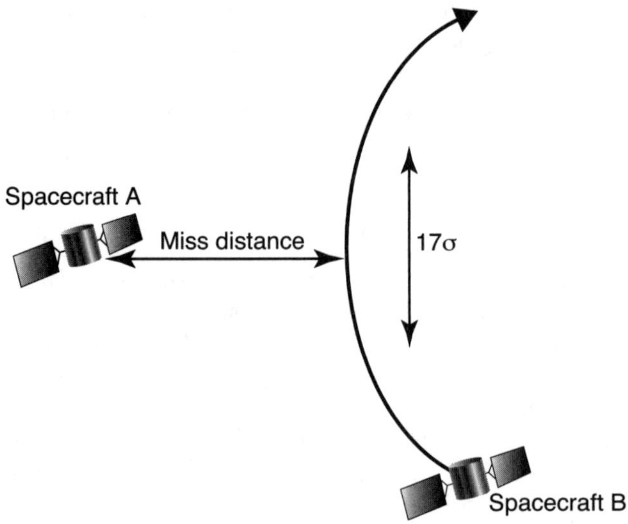

Figure 3.1. Requisite path length for integration. The length must be 17σ for the rectilinear approximation to be valid.

This figure depicts the relative configuration of the two circular trajectories (each of radius R) and their straight-line approximations. Let the two objects be separated by a distance S and let their velocities make an angle ϕ with each other. Let C

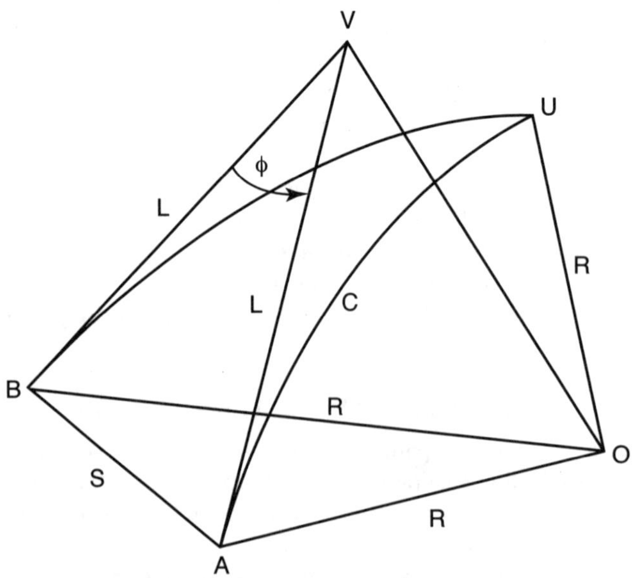

Figure 3.2. Rectilinear approximation of motion in encounter region. Two objects at the same altitude move toward each other in circular orbits.

denote the arc length from the point A to the intersection U. Similarly, let L denote the length of the straight line from A to the intersection V. It is easy to show that

$$L = \frac{S}{2\sin(\phi/2)} \tag{3.6}$$

$$C = R\tan^{-1}\left(\frac{L}{R}\right) \tag{3.7}$$

Let ε and δ respectively denote the accuracy of approximating C by L and approximating R by Q. Then, it can be shown that the relative errors are given by

$$\varepsilon = \frac{L}{C} - 1 \tag{3.8}$$

$$\delta = \frac{Q}{R} - 1 = \sqrt{\left[1 + \left(\frac{L}{R}\right)^2\right]} - 1 \tag{3.9}$$

But these relative errors are not a good indication of the approximation. This is because Eq. (3.9) is based on the difference between Q and R relative to R, which is a large number. If the mean radius of Earth is taken to be 6371 km, R is equal to 7151 km for a circular LEO at 780 km altitude (42,166 km for a GEO). To investigate the validity of our assumption of rectilinear motion in the encounter region, we need to obtain the radial difference $(Q - R)$. Related to this error is also the intrack difference $(L - C)$. Specifically, we use the notation

$$D \equiv Q - R \tag{3.10}$$

$$E \equiv L - C \tag{3.11}$$

Because OAV in Fig. 3.2 is a right triangle, therefore

$$Q^2 = R^2 + L^2 \tag{3.12}$$

From Eqs. (3.10) and (3.12), it follows that

$$L = \sqrt{D^2 + 2RD} \tag{3.13}$$

Thus, Eq. (3.13) gives the length of the approximating straight line L in terms of its departure D from the circular arc. Equation (3.6) is used to derive the distance S separating the two objects as they enter the encounter region with velocities at an angle ϕ. Equation (3.7) is used to compute the circular arc C. Equation (3.11) then yields the intrack error E associated with the radial error D. Finally, Eqs. (3.8) and (3.9) give the relative intrack and radial errors ε and δ.

Tables 3.1 and 3.2 show the values of L and E as functions of D, and the values of S as a function of D and ϕ. The value $R = 7151$ km is used for LEO (42,166 km for GEO) in the computations.

For the case of LEO, we derived the requirement of 85 km for approximating a straight-line path to achieve 15-digit accuracy in the Gaussian integral I in Eq. (3.5). Consider the case of the two objects approaching each other head-on (i.e., $\phi = 180$ deg). Let us take the ingress separation $S = 85$ km. From Table 3.1, it is seen that the radial error $D = 130$ m and the approximating line has length $L = 42.5$ km. Thus, the deflection angle $\alpha \equiv \tan^{-1}(D/L) = 0.18$ deg and it is sufficiently small so that the straight-line approximation is valid. Alternatively, if we relax the

Table 3.1. Rectilinear Approximations and Errors for Orbiting Objects in LEO

D (m)	L (km)	E (m)	S (km) $\phi = 5$ deg	S (km) $\phi = 10$ deg	S (km) $\phi = 30$ deg	S (km) $\phi = 60$ deg	S (km) $\phi = 90$ deg	S (km) $\phi = 180$ deg
10	11.96	0.01	1.04	2.08	6.19	11.96	16.91	23.92
20	16.91	0.03	1.48	2.95	8.75	16.91	23.92	33.83
30	20.71	0.06	1.81	3.61	10.72	20.71	29.29	41.43
40	23.92	0.09	2.09	4.17	12.38	23.92	33.83	47.84
50	26.74	0.12	2.33	4.66	13.84	26.74	37.82	53.48
60	29.29	0.16	2.56	5.11	15.16	29.29	41.43	58.59
70	31.64	0.21	2.76	5.52	16.38	31.64	44.75	63.28
80	33.83	0.25	2.95	5.90	17.51	33.83	47.84	67.65
90	35.88	0.30	3.13	6.25	18.57	35.88	50.74	71.75
100	37.82	0.35	3.30	6.59	19.58	37.82	53.48	75.64
200	53.48	1.00	4.67	9.32	27.68	53.48	75.64	106.97
300	65.50	1.83	5.71	11.42	33.91	65.50	92.64	131.01
400	75.64	2.82	6.60	13.18	39.15	75.64	106.97	151.27
500	84.57	3.94	7.38	14.74	43.77	84.57	119.59	169.13
600	92.64	5.18	8.08	16.15	47.95	92.64	131.01	185.27
700	100.06	6.53	8.73	17.44	51.79	100.06	141.51	200.12
800	106.97	7.98	9.33	18.65	55.37	106.97	151.28	213.94
900	113.46	9.52	9.90	19.78	58.73	113.46	160.45	226.92
1000	119.60	11.15	10.43	20.85	61.91	119.60	169.13	239.19

requirement to 2-digit accuracy by choosing the ingress separation S = 30 km, then D = 16 m, L = 15 km, and α = 0.06 deg.

For the case of GEO, we derived the requirement of 255 km for approximating a straight-line path to achieve 15-digit accuracy in the Gaussian integral I in Eq. (3.5). Consider the case of the two objects approaching each other at ϕ = 6 deg. Let us take the ingress separation S = 255 km. From Table 3.2, it is seen that the radial error D = 70.3 km and the approximating line has length L = 2435.7 km. Thus, the deflection angle α = 1.65 deg and is probably sufficiently small so that the straight-line approximation is valid. Alternatively, if we relax the requirement to 2-digit accuracy by choosing the ingress separation S = 90 km, then D = 8.8 km, L = 861.3 km, and α = 0.59 deg.

Tables 3.1 and 3.2 were constructed by specifying D and ϕ and then computing S. Therefore, when given S and ϕ, we need to perform interpolation to obtain D. However, we can also directly compute it by using Eqs. (3.6), (3.12), and (3.10) in sequence to obtain L, Q, and D. This procedure is more accurate and expedient than table look-up and interpolation.

Table 3.2. Rectilinear Approximations and Errors for Orbiting Objects in GEO

D (km)	L (km)	E (km)	S (km) ϕ = 1 deg	S (km) ϕ = 2 deg	S (km) ϕ = 3 deg	S (km) ϕ = 4 deg	S (km) ϕ = 5 deg	S (km) ϕ = 6 deg
1	290.40	0.00	5.07	10.14	15.20	20.27	25.33	30.40
2	410.69	0.01	7.17	14.34	21.50	28.67	35.83	42.99
3	503.00	0.02	8.78	17.56	26.33	35.11	43.88	52.65
4	580.81	0.04	10.14	20.27	30.41	40.54	50.67	60.79
5	649.37	0.05	11.33	22.67	34.00	45.33	56.65	67.97
6	711.36	0.07	12.42	24.83	37.24	49.65	62.06	74.46
7	768.36	0.09	13.41	26.82	40.23	53.63	67.03	80.43
8	821.41	0.10	14.34	28.67	43.00	57.33	71.66	85.98
9	871.25	0.12	15.21	30.41	45.61	60.81	76.01	91.19
10	918.38	0.15	16.03	32.06	48.08	64.10	80.12	96.13
20	1298.86	0.41	22.67	45.34	68.00	90.66	113.31	135.95
30	1590.87	0.75	27.77	55.53	83.29	111.04	138.79	166.52
40	1837.08	1.16	32.06	64.12	96.18	128.23	160.27	192.29
50	2054.04	1.62	35.85	71.70	107.54	143.37	179.19	215.00
60	2250.23	2.13	39.27	78.54	117.81	157.06	196.31	235.54
70	2430.67	2.69	42.42	84.84	127.25	169.66	212.05	254.42
80	2598.65	3.28	45.35	90.71	136.05	181.38	226.70	272.01
90	2756.44	3.92	48.11	96.21	144.31	192.40	240.47	288.52
100	2905.72	4.59	50.71	101.42	152.13	202.82	253.49	304.15

Finally, it must be pointed out that the relative motion is always nonlinear, but within the extent of the encounter region we may use the approximation of rectilinear motion to reduce Eq. (3.2) to Eq. (3.4). This should not be confused with the use of short-arc propagation to obtain an accurate representation of the point of closest approach. If the rectilinear motion approximation used is too far away from the conjunction, the relative velocity (being tangential to the path) will yield an erroneous value of the miss distance, as illustrated in Fig. 3.3. This can result in the collision probability being off by a few orders of magnitude. These two issues should not be treated as the same.

3.4 Extent of the Encounter Region

Consider the two isosceles triangles depicted in Fig. 3.4. It is seen that when $\phi <$ 60 deg, the largest side of the triangle is L; and when $\phi >$ 60 deg, the largest side of the triangle is S. When ϕ = 60 deg, all three sides are equal. The extent M of the encounter region is defined to be the largest side accordingly. That is,

$$\begin{array}{llll} \text{Case 1:} & M \equiv L & \text{for} & 0 < \phi < \pi/3 \\ \text{Case 2:} & M \equiv S & \text{for} & \pi/3 \leq \phi \leq \pi \end{array} \tag{3.14}$$

For case 1, the time T to traverse M is

$$T = \frac{L}{v} \quad \text{where} \quad v = v_p = v_s \tag{3.15}$$

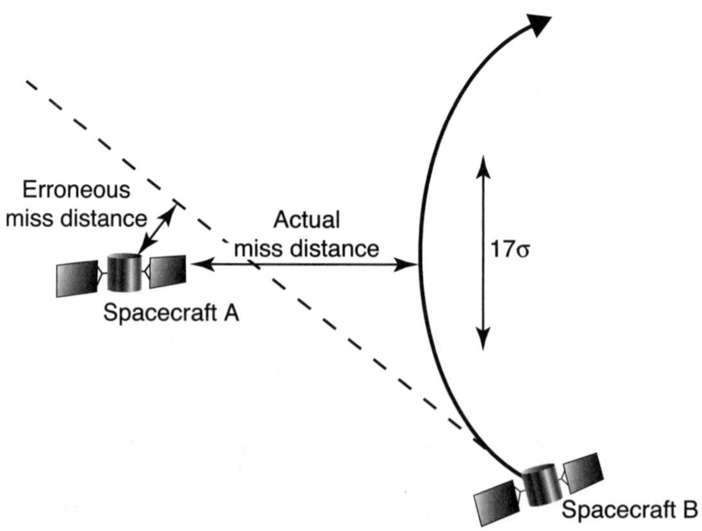

Figure 3.3. Premature linearization. In this case, approximation of rectilinear motion is too far from the conjunction, and the relative velocity yields an erroneous miss distance.

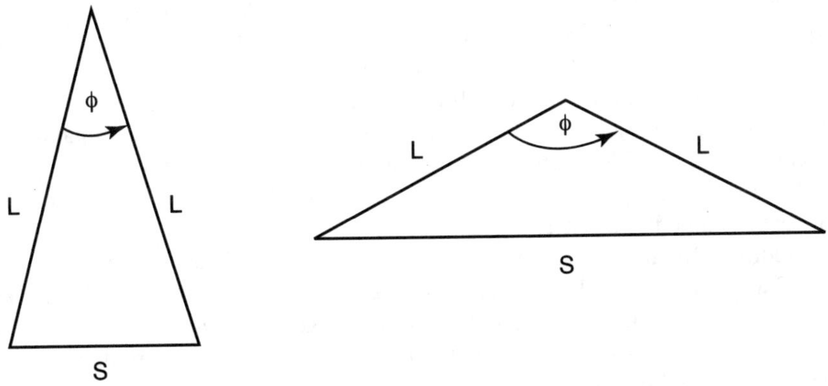

Figure 3.4. Two cases of the plane triangle that approximates the spherical triangle formed by the paths of two objects at the same altitude moving toward each other in circular orbits.

For case 2, the time T to traverse M is

$$T = \frac{S}{v_{ps}} \tag{3.16}$$

However, from Eq. (3.6) and the triangle for the addition of velocities, it follows that

$$S = 2L\sin(\phi/2) \quad \text{and} \quad v_{ps} = 2v\sin(\phi/2) \tag{3.17}$$

Hence, Eq. (3.16) becomes

$$T = \frac{L}{v} \tag{3.18}$$

which is precisely Eq. (3.15) of case 1.

For LEO, when $\phi = 2$ deg and $S = 85$ km for 15-digit accuracy, we use Eqs. (3.6), (3.12), and (3.10) to obtain $L = 2435.2$ km and $D = 403.3$ km. Thus, the deflection angle $\alpha = 9.4$ deg and the time T to traverse L is 324.7 sec = 5.4 min = 5% of the orbital period. This is an exceedingly large deflection angle and the transit time is too long. Consequently, the straight-line approximation is invalid. Even if we relax the requirement to 2-digit accuracy by choosing the ingress separation $S = 30$ km, then $L = 859.5$ km, $D = 51.5$ km, the deflection angle $\alpha = 3.4$ deg, and $T = 114.6$ sec = 1.9 min = 2% of the orbital period. This is probably on the verge of validity for the straight-line approximation.

For GEO, when $\phi = 2$ deg and $S = 255$ km for 15-digit accuracy, we obtain $L = 7305.6$ km and $D = 628.2$ km. Thus, the deflection angle $\alpha = 4.9$ deg and the time T to traverse L is 2356.6 sec = 39 min = 3% of the orbital period. Again, these figures are a little too much for the straight-line approximation to be valid. Even if we relax the requirement to 2-digit accuracy by choosing the ingress separation $S = 90$ km, then L = 2578.4 km, D = 78.8 km, the deflection angle $\alpha = 1.8$ deg, and $T = 831.7$ sec $\cong$ 13.9 min = 1% of the orbital period. The straight-line approximation is acceptable in this case.

Additionally, for GEO, when $\phi = 0.2$ deg and $S = 255$ km for 15-digit accuracy, if we formally use Eqs. (3.6), (3.12), and (3.10), we obtain $L = 73{,}052$ km and $D = 42{,}182$ km. Thus, the deflection angle $\alpha = 30$ deg and the time T to traverse L is 23,565 sec = 393 min = 6.5 h = 27% of the orbital period. Thus, it is absurd to invoke the straight-line approximation for this case. Even if we relax the requirement to 2-digit accuracy by choosing the ingress separation $S = 90$ km, then $L = 25{,}783$ km, $D = 7258$ km, the deflection angle $\alpha = 15.7$ deg, and $T = 8317$ sec = 139 min = 2.3 h = 10% of the orbital period. Again, it is ridiculous to use the straight-line approximation.

Hence, we observe once again that, when the approach angle is small so that the relative velocity is small, the extent of the encounter region is very large and we have trouble invoking the straight-line approximation for the relative motion. Consequently, we cannot make the transition from Eq. (3.2) to Eq. (3.4) to reduce the three-dimensional integral to a two-dimensional one. This is another manifestation of the problems inherently associated with small relative velocities that we have already observed (in Chapter 2).

3.5 Discussion

In Section 3.1, we omitted the details for integrating the collision probability given by Eq. (3.2) with respect to the variable y from $-\infty$ to $+\infty$. We shall take up this task in this section.

In the (x, y, z) coordinate system, let the combined covariance C describing the relative position uncertainties be defined by

$$C = \begin{bmatrix} \sigma_x^{\,2} & \rho_{xy}\sigma_x\sigma_y & \rho_{xz}\sigma_x\sigma_z \\ \rho_{xy}\sigma_x\sigma_y & \sigma_y^{\,2} & \rho_{yz}\sigma_y\sigma_z \\ \rho_{xz}\sigma_x\sigma_z & \rho_{yz}\sigma_y\sigma_z & \sigma_z^{\,2} \end{bmatrix} \tag{3.19}$$

From this, we obtain the inverse matrix C^{-1} and the determinant $|C|$. Then, we substitute into (3.1) to obtain

$$f_3(x,y,z)=A\exp\left\{-\frac{1}{2R}\left[\begin{array}{l}\dfrac{(1-\rho_{yz}{}^2)x^2}{\sigma_x{}^2}+\dfrac{(1-\rho_{xz}{}^2)y^2}{\sigma_y{}^2}+\dfrac{(1-\rho_{xy}{}^2)z^2}{\sigma_z{}^2}\\ -\dfrac{2(\rho_{xy}-\rho_{xz}\rho_{yz})xy}{\sigma_x\sigma_y}-\dfrac{2(\rho_{yz}-\rho_{xy}\rho_{xz})yz}{\sigma_y\sigma_z}-\dfrac{2(\rho_{xz}-\rho_{xy}\rho_{yz})xz}{\sigma_x\sigma_z}\end{array}\right]\right\} \tag{3.20}$$

where A and R are given by

$$\begin{aligned} A&=\frac{1}{Q}\\ Q&=\sqrt{(2\pi)^3 R\sigma_x\sigma_y\sigma_z}\\ R&=\left(1+2\rho_{xy}\rho_{yz}\rho_{xz}-\rho_{xy}{}^2-\rho_{yz}{}^2-\rho_{xz}{}^2\right)\end{aligned} \tag{3.21}$$

For convenience, we rewrite Eq. (3.20) as

$$f_3(x,y,z)=Ae^{-(ay^2-2by+c)/2R}=Ae^{-\frac{1}{2R}\left[a\left(y-\frac{b}{a}\right)^2+c-\frac{b^2}{a}\right]} \tag{3.22}$$

where

$$\begin{aligned} a&=\frac{(1-\rho_{xz}{}^2)}{\sigma_y{}^2}\\ b&=\frac{(\rho_{xy}-\rho_{xz}\rho_{yz})x}{\sigma_x\sigma_y}+\frac{(\rho_{yz}-\rho_{xy}\rho_{xz})z}{\sigma_y\sigma_z}\\ c&=\frac{(1-\rho_{yz}{}^2)x^2}{\sigma_x{}^2}+\frac{(1-\rho_{xy}{}^2)z^2}{\sigma_z{}^2}-\frac{2(\rho_{xz}-\rho_{xy}\rho_{yz})xz}{\sigma_x\sigma_z}.\end{aligned} \tag{3.23}$$

After algebraic simplification, we obtain

$$c-\frac{b^2}{a}=\frac{R}{\left(1-\rho_{xz}{}^2\right)}\left(\frac{x^2}{\sigma_x{}^2}-\frac{2\rho_{xz}xz}{\sigma_x\sigma_z}+\frac{z^2}{\sigma_z{}^2}\right) \tag{3.24}$$

If we integrate $f_3(x, y, z)$ with respect to y from $-\infty$ to $+\infty$, we obtain

$$\int_{-\infty}^{+\infty} f_3(x,y,z)\,dy = ABe^{-\left(\frac{x^2}{\sigma_x{}^2} - \frac{2\rho_{xz}xz}{\sigma_x\sigma_z} + \frac{z^2}{\sigma_z{}^2}\right)\Big/2\left(1-\rho_{xz}{}^2\right)} \tag{3.25}$$

where

$$B \equiv \int_{-\infty}^{+\infty} e^{-\frac{a}{2R}\left(y-\frac{b}{a}\right)^2} dy \tag{3.26}$$

Let us introduce a new variable η defined by

$$\eta = \sqrt{\frac{a}{R}}\sigma_y\left(y - \frac{b}{a}\right) \tag{3.27}$$

Then, we have

$$B = \sqrt{\frac{R}{a}}\frac{1}{\sigma_y}\int_{-\infty}^{+\infty} e^{-\eta^2/2\sigma_y{}^2} d\eta = \sqrt{\frac{2\pi R}{a}}\left[\frac{1}{\sqrt{2\pi}\sigma_y}\int_{-\infty}^{+\infty} e^{-\eta^2/2\sigma_y{}^2} d\eta\right] \tag{3.28}$$

We note that the integral in the square brackets is identically equal to unity because it is the one-dimensional Gaussian pdf integrated from $-\infty$ to $+\infty$. Hence,

$$B = \sqrt{\frac{2\pi R}{a}} \tag{3.29}$$

By substituting Eqs. (3.21), (3.23), and (3.29) for A, a, and B into Eq. (3.25), we obtain

$$\int_{-\infty}^{+\infty} f_3(x,y,z)\,dy = \frac{1}{2\pi\sigma_x\sigma_z\sqrt{1-\rho_{xz}{}^2}} e^{-\left(\frac{x^2}{\sigma_x{}^2} - \frac{2\rho_{xz}xz}{\sigma_x\sigma_z} + \frac{z^2}{\sigma_z{}^2}\right)\Big/2\left(1-\rho_{xz}{}^2\right)} \tag{3.30}$$

By integrating the general three-dimensional pdf of Eq. (3.1) with respect to the variable y from $-\infty$ to $+\infty$, we have obtained the general marginal two-dimensional pdf in (3.3). This approach is along the lines of reasoning given by Papoulis,[3.2] who considered the case of integrating a general two-dimensional bivariate Gaussian pdf over the same range to obtain a one-dimensional marginal pdf.

The term "marginal" pdf usually applies to one variable as defined by Papoulis, who also noted that if two random variables are jointly Gaussian, then they are also marginally Gaussian but the converse is not necessarily true. Here, we shall use the term "marginal" to include the case of a proper subset of the given set of variables (see Anderson[3.3]). In the derivation given here, we obtained the two-dimensional marginal pdfs starting from three-dimensional Gaussian pdfs. This result was obtained by Chan[3.4] in an unpublished work. In the same way, by completing squares with respect to the integration variable in the exponent, we obtain the following rule of thumb concerning marginal Gaussian pdfs. For the case of the marginal pdf of a joint Gaussian distribution of n random variables, no tedious explicit integral evaluation need be performed as demanded with a direct approach. We make a slice of the pdf through the origin by merely setting the particular integration variable to zero in the n-dimensional pdf. We also set any of its correlation coefficients to zero because it has nothing more to do with the other variables. We then change the coefficient to be commensurate with the $(n - 1)$-dimensional Gaussian pdf because the $(n - 1)$-dimensional pdf, when integrated over the whole $(n - 1)$-dimensional space, has to be unity. This process circumvents an exorbitant amount of algebraic manipulations that eventually comes to naught.

In the discussion given here, we went through great length to integrate the variable y from $-\infty$ to $+\infty$ in order to obtain the two-dimensional integral in Eq. (3.4) from the three-dimensional integral in (3.2). Foster[3.5] obtained the same integral but he did not start with any three-dimensional integral. He erroneously stated that "the problem is deterministic along the relative velocity vector since there is no position uncertainty in that direction." (*Note*: We know that the covariance is a three-dimensional ellipsoid as a function of time and certainly does not flatten into a two-dimensional elliptic disc at any instant of time.) Moreover, he assumed that "nominal" position of an object is the same as the "actual" position, whatever the latter might be. (*Note*: We know that the pdf, centered at the nominal position, gives the uncertainty of the actual position. This is the crux of the whole concept of the pdf.) Furthermore, he perturbed an object from its nominal position and then assumed that the time of closest approach, which is also the transit time across the encounter plane, is the same for all perturbations in his construction of the 3×3 covariance matrix. (*Note*: We can talk about the transit time of the nominal and there is no uncertainty associated with it. However, we do not know the transit time of the actual object for if we do, there will be absolute certainty in the motion along the relative velocity direction.)

The end result is that Foster obtained a 2×2 submatrix to be used in Eq. (3.4) that is correct for short-term encounters for the wrong reasons. An innocuously innocent explanation is the following: When the actual object crosses the encounter plane, its positional uncertainty in the (x, z)-plane is given by the two-dimensional Gaussian pdf of Eq. (3.3), and the collision probability is given by the integral in (3.4) over the circular area A. That this reasoning is incorrect is borne out by the fact that infinitely many different nonrectilinear relative motions as well as rectilinear relative motion can have the same encounter plane and the same point of closest approach and yet each has a different collision probability. (See Chapter 9 for short-term vs. long-term encounters.)

Furthermore, Klinkrad[3.6] based his argument only at the point of closest approach and failed to note that collision can occur at other points. He went on to state that, at the time of closest approach, the collision probability is given by the volume integral with integrand pdf of Eq. (3.1) over the sphere of the combined radius, and this volume integral can be reduced to an area integral with integrand pdf of (3.3) over the projected circular cross section of the same radius. This statement is obviously incorrect. We can demonstrate this by performing numerical integration for a particular example. Better still, all we need do is give a counter-example for a simple case. Consider the case of a three-dimensional pdf with all three standard deviations equal to σ and a distance of approach equal to zero. It is easy to show that the integral over a sphere of radius R is given by the following exact expression:

$$P = erf\left(\frac{R}{\sqrt{2}\sigma}\right) - \sqrt{\frac{2}{\pi}}\frac{R}{\sigma}e^{-R^2/2\sigma^2} \tag{3.31}$$

However, the corresponding area integral is given by the exact expression

$$P = 1 - e^{-R^2/2\sigma^2} \tag{3.32}$$

which is a contradiction. More concretely, we can specifically let $R = 1$ and $\sigma = 1$ to show that the two numerical values are not equal.

3.6 Conclusion

The transition from Eq. (3.2) to Eq. (3.4) is the result of integrating the variable y from $-\infty$ to $+\infty$. This integration is in accordance with the rectilinear relative motion modeling, nothing more and nothing less. In the vernacular of statistics, it is the process of obtaining a general two-dimensional marginal Gaussian pdf from a general three-dimensional Gaussian pdf.

3.7 Summary

In this chapter, we obtained the collision integral from the relative position covariance. It is a three-dimensional integral that is conceptually very difficult to evaluate.

In Section 3.1, we discussed the possibility of simplifying the task by replacing this integral with a two-dimensional one. We raised the question of under what circumstances this can be done.

In Section 3.2, we discussed what would be the requisite path length for 15-digit accuracy so that this procedure would be valid. Any contribution beyond this integration limit will not appear in the displayed numerical results of the integral value. We derived a requirement of 17σ for the approximating straight-line path to achieve this accuracy. We also derived a requirement of 6σ for the approximating straight-line path to achieve a 2-digit accuracy.

In Section 3.3, we studied the geometry of two conjoining objects with circular orbits having the same radius. We approximated the curved motion by rectilinear motion in a region containing the point of closest approach. In this process, we obtained the length of the straight line approximating the curved trajectory and also the associated radial and intrack errors when given the approach angle and the separation distance between the two objects.

In Section 3.4, we defined the extent of the encounter region to be the largest side of the plane triangle used in the rectilinear motion. We computed the time to traverse the encounter region. For large angles of approach, the transit time is relatively small so that the approximation becomes valid. However, for small approach angles, the relative velocity of transit is very small and the transit time is very large. Consequently, the approximation is invalid and it is not possible to reduce the three-dimensional collision integral to a two-dimensional one.

In Section 3.5, we discussed the details of obtaining Eq. (3.4) from Eq. (3.2) through the process of integrating the variable y from $-\infty$ to $+\infty$. We also clarified how this transition is accomplished.

In Section 3.6, we concluded that this transition results solely from the integration in accordance with the assumption of rectilinear motion in the modeling of short-term encounters.

3.8 References

3.1. P. S. Maybeck, *Stochastic Models, Estimation, and Control, Vol. 1* (Academic Press, New York, 1979), p. 102.

3.2. A. Papoulis, *Probability, Random Variables, and Stochastic Processes*, 3rd ed. (McGraw-Hill, New York, 1991), pp. 127–128.

3.3. T. W. Anderson, *An Introduction to Multivariate Statistical Analysis* (John Wiley, New York, 1984), pp. 9–10.

3.4. F. K. Chan, "Integration of the Probability Density Function over the Variable y," Unpublished work performed in 1995 for the Iridium Program at Motorola Inc. in Chandler, Arizona. Work now appears as Section 3.5 of this chapter.

3.5. J. L. Foster and H. S. Estes, "A Parametric Analysis of Orbital Debris Collision Probability and Maneuver Rate for Space Vehicles," NASA/JSC-25898 (August 1992), pp. 7, C1, and C-2.

3.6. H. Klinkrad, *Space Debris Models and Risk Analysis* (Springer Praxis Publishing, Chichester, UK, 2006), pp. 222–224.

Chapter 4: The Isotropic Problem

In Chapter 3, we derived the conditions for considering the two-dimensional collision integral in Eq. (3.4) with the corresponding bivariate Gaussian probability density function (pdf) given by Eq. (3.3). There is no known closed-form solution even to this problem. In a quest for an analytical solution, some simplifying assumption is usually made. For instance, if the circular cross section of radius r_A is "small" so that the integrand does not vary much over it, then we may replace the integrand by its value at the center (x_e, 0). Then, the collision probability is approximately given by

$$P = \frac{r_A^2}{2\sigma_x \sigma_z \sqrt{1-\rho_{xz}^2}} e^{-x_e^2/2\sigma_x^2(1-\rho_{xz}^2)} \tag{4.1}$$

This expression may be used in some cases and should be used with extreme caution, because it can yield a result an order (or several orders) of magnitude different from the correct value. The problem with most analytical expressions is that we do not know when they fail until we have tested them over a range of input collision parameters. As an example, if we let $\rho_{xz} = 0$, $\sigma_x = 100$ m, $\sigma_z = 10$ m, $x_e = 100$ m, and $r_A = 60$ m in Eq. (4.1), we obtain the absurd answer of $P \cong 1.09$.

For more general cases, we need to develop expressions that are not dependent on such oversimplifying assumptions. It is imperative to find an approach that yields an accurate answer over a fairly wide range of representative input parameters. Even if it involves an approximation, it must be justifiable and sufficiently accurate with small error bounds that, preferably, can be expressed analytically. To illustrate this point, we shall consider in this chapter the isotropic case for which the two standard deviations σ_x and σ_z are equal. Though this case may seem somewhat limited in applicability, nevertheless, it proves to be a stepping-stone to handling the general bivariate Gaussian problem.

4.1 The Rician Distribution

The pdf and the probability integral are respectively

$$f(x,z) = \frac{1}{2\pi\sigma^2} e^{-(x^2+z^2)/2\sigma^2} \tag{4.2}$$

$$P = \frac{1}{2\pi\sigma^2} \iint_A e^{-(x^2+z^2)/2\sigma^2} dxdz \tag{4.3}$$

The lines of constant pdf are concentric circles with centers at the origin of the (x, z)-plane and the cross-sectional area is an offset circle A of radius r_A with its center at the point $(x_e, 0)$. Obviously, Eq. (4.3) may be reformulated as

$$P = \frac{1}{2\pi\sigma^2} \iint_{A_0} e^{-[(x-x_e)^2+z^2]/2\sigma^2} \, dxdz \tag{4.4}$$

for which the lines of constant pdf are concentric circles with centers at the point $(x_e, 0)$ and the cross-sectional area is a circle A_0 of radius r_A with its center at the origin. These two configurations are depicted in Figs. 4.1 and 4.2.

It may be shown[4.1] that the integral (4.4) in two variables x and z may be written exactly in terms of the following integral in only one variable r:

$$f(r) = \frac{r}{\sigma^2} e^{-(r^2+x_e^2)/2\sigma^2} I_0\left(\frac{rx_e}{\sigma^2}\right) \tag{4.5}$$

$$P = \int_0^{r_A} f(r)\, dr \tag{4.6}$$

The integrand is known as the Rician pdf. This pdf arises frequently in the detection of signals in the presence of noise. The transformation was obtained in 1944 by Rice,[4.2] who studied the case of a sine wave plus random noise and obtained asymptotic expressions for the integral under some simplifying assumptions. The Rician pdf also arises in studies of target detection by pulsed radar, noncoherent detection of band-passed binary signals, accuracy of unguided ballistic bombs hitting their targets, artillery effectiveness of fragmentation bombs, and presently in collisions of spacecraft with space debris.

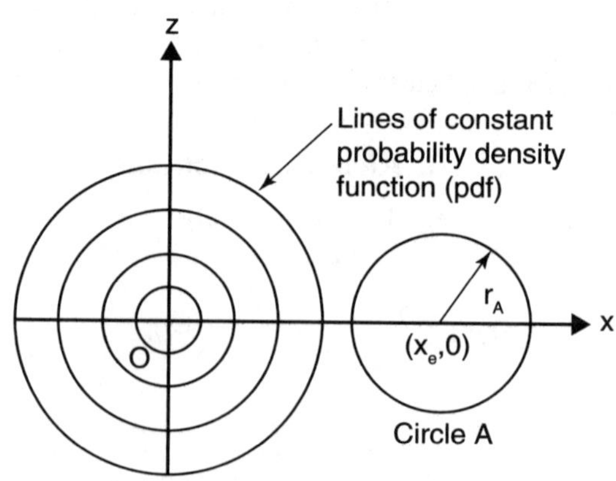

Figure 4.1. Circle of integration offset from origin.

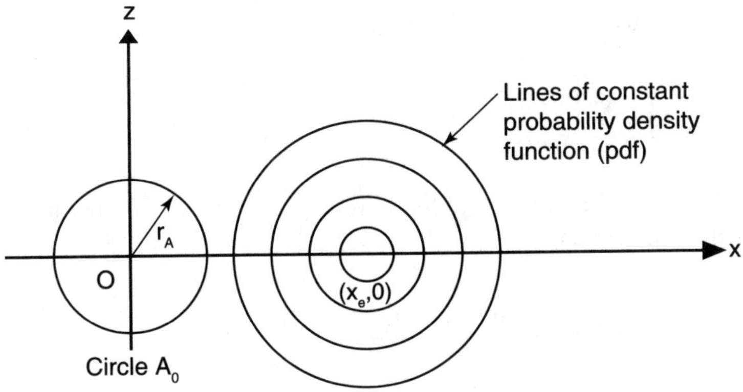

Figure 4.2. Lines of constant pdf offset from origin.

This pdf has the following properties: When the displacement of the circular cross section is equal to zero, it is precisely the Rayleigh pdf. If it is large, the pdf tends to be symmetrical in the interval of several units of standard deviation containing the maximum point and resembles the Gaussian pdf in this interval (keep in mind that it is defined from 0 to ∞, whereas the latter is defined from −∞ to +∞). Computer programs are presently used for the numerical evaluation of this integral. However, an analytical solution in the form of an infinite series that is convergent for all values of the relevant parameters and expressions with error bounds has been obtained.[4.3] Figure 4.3 illustrates the shapes of the Rician pdf as a function of r for $\lambda \equiv x_e/\sigma$ in the range from 0 to 6. Note that when $\lambda \geq 6$, the Rician curve resembles the symmetrical Gaussian pdf.

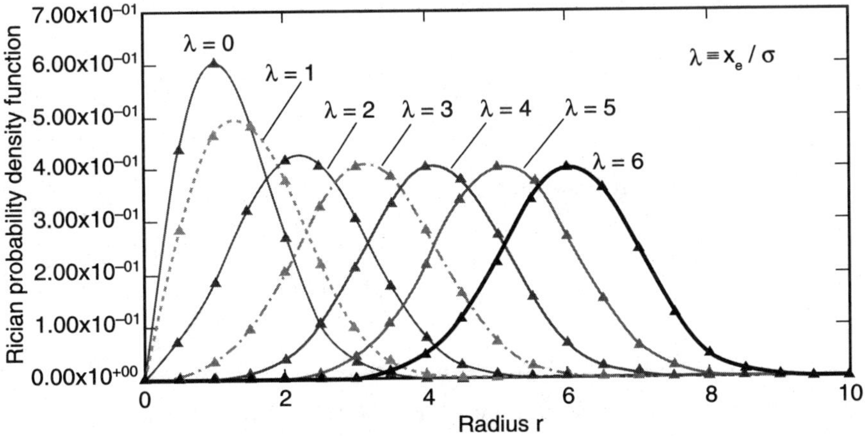

Figure 4.3. The Rician distribution.

The function $I_0(\cdot)$ in Eq. (4.5) denotes the modified Bessel function of the first kind of order zero. It is given by the following infinite series:

$$I_0\left(\sqrt{\eta}\right)=\sum_{m=0}^{\infty}\frac{(\eta/4)^m}{(m!)^2}=1+\frac{(\eta/4)}{(1!)^2}+\frac{(\eta/4)^2}{(2!)^2}+\frac{(\eta/4)^3}{(3!)^2}+\cdots \tag{4.7}$$

We know that it is convergent for all values of η because it is dominated termwise by the exponential series

$$e^{\eta/4}=1+\frac{(\eta/4)}{1!}+\frac{(\eta/4)^2}{2!}+\frac{(\eta/4)^3}{3!}+\cdots \tag{4.8}$$

which converges for all values of η.

For convenience, let us introduce the notation

$$\eta\equiv\left(\frac{rx_e}{\sigma^2}\right)^2>0 \tag{4.9}$$

$$\eta_A\equiv\left(\frac{r_A x_e}{\sigma^2}\right)^2>0 \tag{4.10}$$

$$u\equiv\left(\frac{r_A}{\sigma}\right)^2>0 \tag{4.11}$$

$$v\equiv\left(\frac{x_e}{\sigma}\right)^2>0 \tag{4.12}$$

Equation (4.6) may be written as

$$P=\frac{1}{2v}e^{-v/2}\int_0^{\eta_A}e^{-\eta/2v}I_0\left(\sqrt{\eta}\right)d\eta \tag{4.13}$$

4.2 Analytical Expressions for the Rician Integral

If we substitute the convergent infinite series (4.7) into Eq. (4.13) and then justifiably interchange the order of integration and summation, we obtain

$$P = \frac{1}{2v} e^{-v/2} \sum_{m=0}^{\infty} \frac{1}{4^m (m!)^2} \int_0^{\eta_A} \eta^m e^{-\eta/2v} d\eta \tag{4.14}$$

For convenience, let us define

$$J_m \equiv \int_0^{\eta_A} \eta^m e^{-\eta/2v} d\eta \tag{4.15}$$

Then, from integral tables, it may be shown[4.4] that

$$J_m = m!(2v)^{m+1} \left(1 - e^{-u/2} \sum_{k=0}^{m} \frac{u^k}{2^k k!} \right) \tag{4.16}$$

By substituting Eq. (4.16) into (4.14), we find that

$$P = e^{-v/2} \sum_{m=0}^{\infty} \frac{v^m}{2^m m!} \left(1 - e^{-u/2} \sum_{k=0}^{m} \frac{u^k}{2^k k!} \right) \tag{4.17}$$

This is an analytical expression for the collision probability P and is an infinite series convergent for all values of the relevant collision parameters. This is the preferred form for use. An alternative form obtained by regrouping terms is the following:

$$P = 1 - e^{-(u+v)/2} \sum_{m=0}^{\infty} \frac{v^m}{2^m m!} \sum_{k=0}^{m} \frac{u^k}{2^k k!} \tag{4.18}$$

If only the first term in the series is retained ($m = 0$), then we have the extremely simple expression

$$P = e^{-v/2} \left(1 - e^{-u/2} \right) + T_1 \tag{4.19}$$

where T_1 denotes the truncation error after the first term. If the first two terms in the series are retained ($m = 0$ and 1), then the expression becomes somewhat more complicated but still manageable:

$$P = e^{-v/2} \left\{ \left(1 - e^{-u/2} \right) + \frac{v}{2} \left[1 - \left(1 + \frac{u}{2} \right) e^{-u/2} \right] \right\} + T_2 \tag{4.20}$$

where T_2 denotes the truncation error after the second term. In the next section, we shall derive error bounds for these two truncation errors.

Finally, note that every term in the infinite series (4.7) is positive. Therefore, truncation after any number of terms and subsequent substitution into Eqs. (4.5) and (4.6) will yield an analytical expression of the collision probability that can never theoretically (and rarely computationally) exceed unity for any set of input parameters.

4.3 Error Bounds

In Eq. (4.7), let R_m denote all the (infinite) remaining terms after the first m terms of the series. That is,

$$I_0\left(\sqrt{\eta}\right) = 1 + R_1(\eta) \tag{4.21}$$

$$I_0\left(\sqrt{\eta}\right) = 1 + \frac{\eta}{4} + R_2(\eta) \tag{4.22}$$

We note that

$$0 < R_1(\eta) < \frac{\eta}{4}\left[1 + \frac{(\eta/4)}{1!} + \frac{(\eta/4)^2}{2!} + \cdots\right] \tag{4.23}$$

$$0 < R_2(\eta) < \frac{\eta^2}{64}\left[1 + \frac{(\eta/4)}{1!} + \frac{(\eta/4)^2}{2!} + \cdots\right] \tag{4.24}$$

Hence,

$$0 < R_1(\eta) < \frac{\eta}{4} e^{\eta/4} \tag{4.25}$$

$$0 < R_2(\eta) < \frac{\eta^2}{64} e^{\eta/4} \tag{4.26}$$

From Eqs. (4.13) and (4.21), it follows that

$$\begin{aligned} T_1 &= \frac{1}{2v} e^{-v/2} \int_0^{\eta_A} e^{-\eta/2v} R_1(\eta) d\eta \\ &< \frac{1}{2v} e^{-v/2} \int_0^{\eta_A} \frac{\eta}{4} e^{\eta/4} d\eta \\ &< \frac{1}{2v} e^{-v/2} \int_0^{\eta_A} \frac{\eta_A}{4} e^{\eta_A/4} d\eta = \frac{\eta_A^2}{8v} e^{-v/2} e^{\eta_A/4} \end{aligned} \tag{4.27}$$

Because, by Eqs. (4.10) through (4.12),

$$\eta_A = uv \tag{4.28}$$

therefore

$$T_1 < \frac{1}{8} u^2 v e^{-v/2} e^{uv/4} \tag{4.29}$$

In the same way, from Eqs. (4.13) and (4.22), we obtain

$$T_2 < \frac{1}{128} u^3 v^2 e^{-v/2} e^{uv/4} \tag{4.30}$$

Even though we may not know what the exact answer is, the use of error bounds gives us an indication of how many significant figures the collision probability is accurate to.

As an example, let $r = 5$ m, $x = 10$ m, and $\sigma = 50$ m. From Eqs. (4.11), (4.12), (4.19), (4.20), (4.29), and (4.30), we obtain the following values:

$$u = 1 \times 10^{-2}, \qquad v = 4 \times 10^{-2}$$

$$P = 4.8887612784 \times 10^{-3} + T_1$$

$$T_1 < 4.90148349 \times 10^{-7}$$

$$P = 4.8890055128 \times 10^{-3} + T_2$$

$$T_2 < 1.225370873 \times 10^{-11}$$

From this example, we see that the zeroth-order approximation ($m = 0$) in the series in Eq. (4.17) yields an error in the fifth significant digit. Thus, we know that the collision probability P is accurate to four significant figures. That is, $P = 4.889 \times 10^{-3}$. Moreover, the first-order approximation ($m = 1$) in the series in Eq. (4.17) yields an error in the ninth significant digit. Thus, we know that the collision probability P is accurate to eight significant figures. That is, $P = 4.8890055 \times 10^{-3}$. These two values are mutually consistent. In this example, it is fortuitous that we attain such high accuracy. For more general input collision parameters, we can show that the second-order approximation ($m = 2$) will generally yield two- or three-place accuracy for the collision probability in spacecraft encounters over a wide range of input collision parameters for most present-day applications. (See Table 4.2.)

4.4 Recursive Algorithms for Computing the Rician Distribution

We have just seen that for spacecraft encounters, the collision parameters are such that only the first term is sufficient for computing the probability of collision. However, in the detection of signals in the presence of noise, the amplitude of the signal, the standard deviation of the Gaussian noise, and the threshold of detection have a much wider range of variation. Consequently, it is not possible to retain just the first few terms of the series. For most applications, it may be necessary to include as many as 25 terms just to ensure adequate accuracies of 15 significant digits in evaluating the modified Bessel function or the Rician integral. Because the expression on the right-hand side (RHS) of Eqs. (4.7) and (4.17) contains factorials, it is not feasible or judicious to perform a simple direct method of term-by-term computation. To circumvent the evaluation of large factorials and the loss of significant digits when subtracting two large numbers, the terms on the RHS are evaluated by using appropriate recursive relations. This approach is very efficient and accurate.

We begin first by developing a recursive algorithm for computing the modified Bessel function $I_0(\sqrt{\eta})$. Let us define the initial values

$$a_0 = 1, \qquad A_0 = 1 \tag{4.31}$$

and the recursive relations

$$a_m = \frac{(\eta/4)}{m^2} a_{m-1}, \qquad A_m = A_{m-1} + a_m \qquad m = 1, 2, 3, \cdots \tag{4.32}$$

We note that

$$I_0\left(\sqrt{\eta}\right) = \lim_{m \to \infty} A_m \tag{4.33}$$

The variable η is defined by Eq. (4.9). This is the recursive algorithm for computing the Rician pdf (4.5) in Fig. 4.3.

One way of formulating a recursive algorithm for computing the Rician integral is to write Eq. (4.17) as

$$P = e^{-v/2} \sum_{m=0}^{\infty} t_m - e^{-(u+v)/2} \sum_{m=0}^{\infty} t_m S_m \tag{4.34}$$

$$t_m \equiv \frac{v^m}{2^m m!} \tag{4.35}$$

$$s_m \equiv \frac{u^m}{2^m m!} \tag{4.36}$$

$$S_m \equiv \sum_{k=0}^{m} \frac{u^k}{2^k k!} \tag{4.37}$$

The iteration uses the initial values

$$t_0 = 1, \qquad s_0 = 1, \qquad S_0 = 1 \tag{4.38}$$

and the recursive relations

$$t_m = \frac{v}{2m} t_{m-1}, \qquad s_m = \frac{u}{2m} s_{m-1}, \qquad S_m = S_{m-1} + s_m \qquad m = 1, 2, 3, \cdots \tag{4.39}$$

The variables u and v are defined by Eqs. (4.11) and (4.12). This is the recursive algorithm for computing the Rician integral (4.13) in signal fading. In that application, it is necessary to compute the probability over a very wide range of input parameters.

4.5 Discussion

In Chapter 2, we stated that (for most of our applications) the intrack, crosstrack, and radial standard deviations can be taken to be in the ratio 10:2:1. In Chapter 3, we stated that (for most of our applications) the intrack standard deviation is approximately 5 km for low Earth orbits (LEOs) and 15 km for geosynchronous orbits. Thus, for LEOs, the largest σ of the combined covariance is $\sqrt{(5^2 + 5^2)} \cong$ 7 km. Similarly, the smallest σ is $\sqrt{(0.5^2 + 0.5^2)} \cong 0.7$ km. Therefore, for simplicity, we shall take σ to be between 1 km and 10 km for LEOs. For most spacecraft dimensions, we can safely take the radius r_A up to 100 m. (Most large spacecraft are at most 40 m, so that r_A is 20 m; the largest dimension of the International Space Station is approximately 140 m—see Section 6.10 of Chapter 6—so that r_A is 70 m.) For encounters between two orbiting objects, we can take the miss distance x_e up to 100 km, which is more than we really need to consider. Hence, we can establish the following present limits for our collision parameters:

$$0 < \left(\frac{r_A}{\sigma}\right) \leq 10^{-1} \quad \text{and} \quad 0 \leq \left(\frac{x_e}{\sigma}\right) \leq 100 \tag{4.40}$$

For some future systems, we may have very accurate orbit determinations and thus σ may lie between 10 m and 100 m. Accordingly, we may consider miss distance up to 100 m. Therefore, the future limits become

$$0 < \left(\frac{r_A}{\sigma}\right) \leq 10 \qquad \text{and} \qquad 0 \leq \left(\frac{x_e}{\sigma}\right) \leq 10 \tag{4.41}$$

If we depict these two regions on a plane of the collision parameter ratios (r_A/σ) and (x_e/σ), we see that the present range is a narrow vertical strip of width 10^{-1} and height 100. The future range is a square of side 10. Table 4.1 shows the probability as a function of the two ratios (r_A/σ) and (x_e/σ). The probabilities are accurate to five significant figures and are obtained by high-precision numerical computation using Eq. (5.30) of Chapter 5. It is formulated in (r, θ) coordinates with 0.5 deg angular step size and $r_A/240$ radial step size. The present range of applicability is shown by the table's first three columns, which depict values of the probability for (r_A/σ) up to 10^{-1} and (x_e/σ) up to 100. The future range of applicability is shown by the first seven rows, which depict values of the probability for (r_A/σ) up to 10 and (x_e/σ) up to 10. There are no entries in the table cells that fall outside these regions, because they are not applicable and, more important, we encounter cases with numerical truncation problems when the ratios we are working with are large.

Table 4.2 shows the order of approximation m in Eq.(4.17) used in the computation to attain an accuracy of 1% or less in the probabilities. In the present range of applicability, we observe that the zeroth order ($m = 0$) is sufficient to achieve the desired accuracy over most of the range where (r_A/σ) and/or (x_e/σ) is small. However, the first order ($m = 1$) and second order ($m = 2$) are needed where $(r_A/\sigma) = 0.1$ and (x_e/σ) exceeds 2. In the future range of applicability, we observe that we need much higher orders of approximation to achieve the desired accuracy. Because of truncation problems, the entry marked with an asterisk is the best we can achieve in the approximation process.

Table 4.1. Probability as a Function of (r_A/σ) and (x_e/σ)

	(r_A/σ)					
(x_e/σ)	0.001	0.01	0.1	1	5	10
0	5.00×10^{-07}	5.00×10^{-05}	4.99×10^{-03}	3.93×10^{-01}	$1.00 \times 10^{+00}$	$1.00 \times 10^{+00}$
1	3.03×10^{-07}	3.03×10^{-05}	3.03×10^{-03}	2.67×10^{-01}	$1.00 \times 10^{+00}$	$1.00 \times 10^{+00}$
2	6.77×10^{-08}	6.77×10^{-06}	6.78×10^{-04}	8.19×10^{-02}	9.98×10^{-01}	$1.00 \times 10^{+00}$
3	5.55×10^{-09}	5.55×10^{-07}	5.60×10^{-05}	1.08×10^{-02}	9.69×10^{-01}	$1.00 \times 10^{+00}$
4	1.68×10^{-10}	1.68×10^{-08}	1.71×10^{-06}	5.90×10^{-04}	8.13×10^{-01}	$1.00 \times 10^{+00}$
5	1.86×10^{-12}	1.86×10^{-10}	1.92×10^{-08}	1.28×10^{-05}	4.60×10^{-01}	9.99×10^{-01}
10	9.64×10^{-29}	9.66×10^{-27}	1.09×10^{-24}	3.42×10^{-20}	2.14×10^{-07}	4.79×10^{-01}
15	6.93×10^{-56}	6.95×10^{-54}	9.05×10^{-52}			
20	6.92×10^{-94}	6.95×10^{-92}	1.10×10^{-89}			
100	$0.00 \times 10^{+00}$	$0.00 \times 10^{+00}$	$0.00 \times 10^{+00}$			

Table 4.2. Lowest Order of Approximation for Accuracy of 1% or Less

	(r_A/σ)					
(x_e/σ)	0.001	0.01	0.1	1	5	10
0	0	0	0	0	0	0
1	0	0	0	1	3	3
2	0	0	0	2	6	6
3	0	0	1	3	10	10
4	0	0	1	4	13	15
5	0	0	1	5	17	21
10	0	0	1	8	35*	59
15	0	0	2			
20	0	0	2			
100	0	0	0			

Table 4.3 shows the percentage error in the probabilities incurred using the orders of approximation depicted in Table 4.2. The values are 1% or less because the orders of approximation were chosen to achieve this outcome. Because of truncation error problems, the entry marked with an asterisk is the best we can achieve in the approximation process.

4.6 Conclusion

If we recall the definitions of u and v given by Eqs. (4.11) and (4.12) as being the squares of the parameter ratios, an examination of Table 4.2 reveals that for most

Table 4.3. Percent Error in Approximating Probability

	(r_A/σ)					
(x_e/σ)	0.001	0.01	0.1	1	5	10
0	0.00	0.00	0.00	0.00	0.00	0.00
1	0.00	0.00	–0.12	–0.42	–0.17	–0.18
2	0.00	0.00	–0.50	–0.41	–0.41	–0.45
3	0.00	–0.01	0.00	–0.33	–0.37	–0.67
4	0.00	–0.02	–0.01	–0.24	–0.89	–0.82
5	0.00	–0.03	–0.03	–0.18	–0.57	–0.88
10	0.00	–0.12	–0.47	–0.86	–6.84*	–0.65
15	0.00	–0.28	–0.10			
20	0.00	–0.50	–0.46			
100	0.00	0.00	0.00			

present and future applications, we may use the following expression to compute collision probabilities accurate to within 1% error when the standard deviation is specified.

$$P = e^{-v/2} \sum_{m=0}^{M} \frac{v^m}{2^m m!} \left(1 - e^{-u/2} \sum_{k=0}^{m} \frac{u^k}{2^k k!} \right)$$

$$\begin{aligned} &M = 3 \text{ for } u \le 0.01 \text{ or } v \le 1, \\ &M = 10 \text{ for } 0.01 < u \le 1 \text{ or } 1 < v \le 9, \\ &M = 20 \text{ for } 1 < u \le 25 \text{ or } 9 < v \le 25, \\ &M = 60 \text{ otherwise} \end{aligned} \tag{4.42}$$

This analytical expression yields results with sufficient accuracy over a wide range of input collision parameters, given that the standard deviations are probably known to no less than 5%.

Note: Even though the infinite series in Eq. (4.17) is a convergent one, we should not replace M in Eq. (4.42) by a large number like 1000 to cover the whole parameter space (u, v). This is because computational instability manifests itself in the recursive algorithm defined by Eqs. (4.34) through (4.37) for certain combinations of u and v. This is evident for the case of $u = 25$ and $v = 100$ in Table 4.3.

4.7 Summary

In this chapter, we considered the isotropic case for which the two standard deviations σ_x and σ_z are equal in the two-dimensional Gaussian pdf used in computing the collision probability.

In Section 4.1, we related this collision integral to the Rician integral frequently used in signal detection. This latter integral involves only one variable.

In Section 4.2, we derived an analytical expression for the Rician integral in the form of an infinite series that is convergent for all values of the input parameters. We also obtained explicitly one-term and two-term truncated expressions.

In Section 4.3, we obtained error bounds for these truncated solutions and showed in an illustrative example the accuracies of these two expressions for use in computing spacecraft collision probability.

In Section 4.4, we devised a recursive algorithm for computing the general series solution up to any desired number of terms. For most applications in signal detection, it suffices to include up to 25 terms for accuracy up to 15 significant digits.

In Section 4.5, we derived the present limits of the collision parameter ratios based on generally available values of the standard deviations. We also discussed the future limits based on anticipated values of the standard deviation. We showed that the first three orders of approximation are sufficient to compute the present regime of collision parameter ratios but that substantially higher orders are needed for the future regime of parameter ratios.

In Section 4.6, we concluded that for most present-day applications (combined object radius less than one-tenth the standard deviation), the zeroth-order and first-order approximations provide collision probabilities accurate to within 1% error.

4.8 References

4.1. A. Papoulis, *Probability, Random Variables, and Stochastic Processes* (McGraw-Hill, New York, 1965), pp. 195–196.

4.2. S. O. Rice, "Mathematical Analysis of Random Noise," *Bell System Tech. J.* **23**, 282–332 (1944) and **24**, 46–156 (1945).

4.3. F. K. Chan, "Improved Analytical Expressions for Computing Spacecraft Collision Probabilities," Paper AAS 03-184, *AAS/AIAA Space Flight Mechanics Meeting* (Ponce, Puerto Rico, February 2003).

4.4. I. S. Gradshteyn and I. W. Ryzhik, *Tables of Integrals, Series and Products* (Academic Press, New York, 1965), p. 310.

Chapter 5: Analytical Expressions for Short-Term Encounters

In the last chapter, we laid the groundwork for considering the probability of a spacecraft colliding with another orbiting object. We considered an isotropic Gaussian probability density function (pdf) in the encounter (x, z)-plane even though the three-dimensional covariance might not necessarily be isotropic. We obtained analytic expressions by relating the collision integral to the Rician integral that primarily arises in signal detection. The expressions were derived after retaining only the first or second terms in a convergent infinite series. They were very simple and accurate for spacecraft collision probability computations.

5.1 Nonisotropic Probability Density Function

In this chapter, we consider the more general case of a nonisotropic pdf. In Chapter 2, we showed that at the instant of "nominal" closest approach when the primary object in the collision nominally crosses the encounter (x, z)-plane, its position uncertainty relative to the secondary is described by the following bivariate Gaussian pdf:

$$f_2(x,z) = \frac{1}{2\pi\sigma_x\sigma_z\sqrt{1-\rho_{xz}^2}} e^{-\left[\left(\frac{x}{\sigma_x}\right)^2 - 2\rho_{xz}\left(\frac{x}{\sigma_x}\right)\left(\frac{z}{\sigma_z}\right) + \left(\frac{z}{\sigma_z}\right)^2\right] \Big/ 2\left(1-\rho_{xz}^2\right)} \tag{5.1}$$

Hence, the probability of collision is given by the two-dimensional integral

$$P = \iint_A f_2(x,z)\,dxdz \tag{5.2}$$

where A is the collision cross-sectional area, which is a circle with radius r_A centered at the primary.

Corresponding to this is the covariance C defined by

$$C = \begin{bmatrix} \sigma_x^2 & \rho_{xz}\sigma_x\sigma_z \\ \rho_{xz}\sigma_x\sigma_z & \sigma_z^2 \end{bmatrix} \tag{5.3}$$

In general, Eq. (5.3) contains an undesirable diagonal term when the correlation coefficient ρ_{xz} is not zero. To simplify analysis, we rotate the coordinate system (x, z) to a new coordinate system (x', z') such that the off-diagonal terms no longer appear in the pdf. In this new coordinate system, the major and minor axes of the ellipse associated with the covariance matrix C will be along the coordinate axes, which are the principal directions.

Rotation of coordinates to principal directions yields the covariance matrix C' given by

$$C' = \begin{bmatrix} \sigma_{x'}^{2} & 0 \\ 0 & \sigma_{z'}^{2} \end{bmatrix} \tag{5.4}$$

Then, we may show that the requisite rotational angle θ is given by

$$\theta = \frac{1}{2}\tan^{-1}\left[\frac{2\rho_{xz}\sigma_x\sigma_z}{\left(\sigma_x^{2} - \sigma_z^{2}\right)}\right] \tag{5.5}$$

For the case of $\sigma_x \neq \sigma_z$, Eq. (5.5) yields two values of the rotational angle θ from the x-axis to the x'-axis corresponding to the two noncollinear eigenvectors. We may take one of these to be in the first quadrant and the other in the fourth quadrant. If we wish to assign $\sigma_{x'} \geq \sigma_{z'}$, then we choose θ to be in the first or fourth quadrant according to the correlation coefficient $\rho_{xz} > 0$ or < 0. This is shown in Fig. 5.1.

For the case of $\sigma_x = \sigma_z$, the right-hand side (RHS) of Eq. (5.5) is undefined. A little consideration reveals that we choose θ to be $\pm\pi/4$ depending on the sign of ρ_{xz}. However, in general, Eq. (5.5) applies to rotation to either one of the two principal axes x' or z' without requiring that $\sigma_{x'} \geq \sigma_{z'}$.

Because the determinant remains invariant under a rotation, therefore, from Eqs. (5.3) and (5.4),

$$\sigma_{x'}\sigma_{z'} = \sqrt{1-\rho_{xz}^{2}}\,\sigma_x\sigma_z \tag{5.6}$$

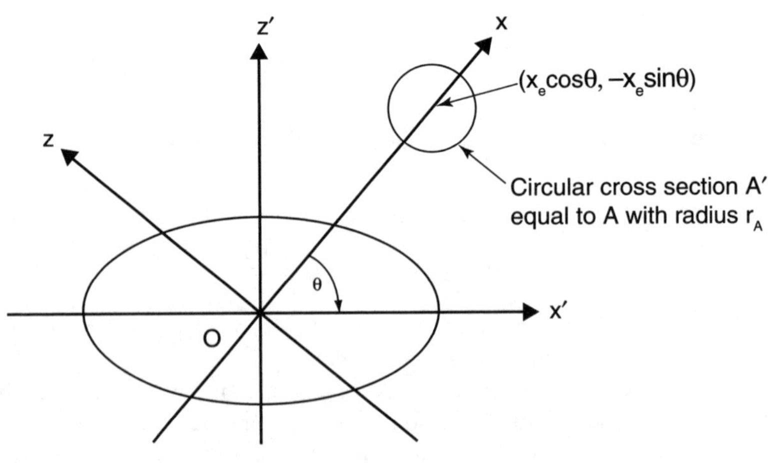

Figure 5.1. Rotation to principal axes.

In the (x', z') system, the pdf (5.1) becomes

$$f(x',z') = \frac{1}{2\ \sigma_{x'}\sigma_{z'}} e^{-\frac{1}{2}\left[\left(\frac{x'}{\sigma_{x'}}\right)^2 + \left(\frac{z'}{\sigma_{z'}}\right)^2\right]} \tag{5.7}$$

and the collision probability (5.2) is given by

$$P = \frac{1}{2\ \sigma_{x'}\sigma_{z'}} \iint_{A'} e^{-\frac{1}{2}\left[\left(\frac{x'}{\sigma_{x'}}\right)^2 + \left(\frac{z'}{\sigma_{z'}}\right)^2\right]} dx'dz' \tag{5.8}$$

where A' is the circular cross section with radius r_A' centered at the primary. Let (x_p', z_p') denote the coordinates of the center of mass of the primary in the (x', z') system. Therefore, we have

$$A' = A, \qquad r_{A'} = r_A, \qquad x_p' = x_e \cos\theta, \qquad z_p' = -x_e \sin\theta \tag{5.9}$$

where x_e is the nominal distance of closest approach.

5.2 Transformation to an Isotropic Density Function

We next wish to map the ellipses of constant pdf

$$\frac{x'^2}{\sigma_{x'}^2} + \frac{z'^2}{\sigma_{z'}^2} = k^2 \tag{5.10}$$

into circles of constant pdf having the equation

$$\frac{x''^2}{\sigma_{z'}^2} + \frac{z''^2}{\sigma_{z'}^2} = k^2 \tag{5.11}$$

The constant k is a label for the corresponding ellipse or circle. This mapping is accomplished by the following transformation:

$$x'' = \frac{\sigma_{z'}}{\sigma_{x'}} x', \qquad z'' = z' \tag{5.12}$$

In the (x'', z'') system, the pdf of Eq. (5.7) becomes isotropic, viz.,

$$f(x', z') = \frac{1}{2\pi\, \sigma_{z'}^{\,2}}\, e^{-\left(x''^2 + z''^2\right)/2\sigma_{z'}^{\,2}} \tag{5.13}$$

and the collision probability of Eq. (5.8) is equivalently given by

$$P = \frac{1}{2\pi\, \sigma_{z'}^{\,2}} \iint_{A''} e^{-\left(x''^2 + z''^2\right)/2\sigma_{z'}^{\,2}}\, dx''\, dz'' \tag{5.14}$$

where A'' is the elliptical cross-sectional area with semimajor axis a and semiminor axis b, respectively defined to be along the z'' and x'' axes. Let (x_p'', z_p'') denote the coordinates of the center of mass of the primary in the (x'', z'') system. Therefore, we have

$$A'' = \frac{\sigma_{z'}}{\sigma_{x'}} A', \qquad a = r_{A'}, \qquad b = \frac{\sigma_{z'}}{\sigma_{x'}} r_{A'}, \qquad x_p'' = \frac{\sigma_{z'}}{\sigma_{x'}} x_p', \qquad z_p'' = z_p' \tag{5.15}$$

5.3 Approximation of Cross Section by a Circle

Up to this step, we have not made any approximations. Suppose we now approximate the elliptical cross section A'' with a circular cross section A''' of the same area with radius $r_{A'''}$. This is illustrated in Fig. 5.2.

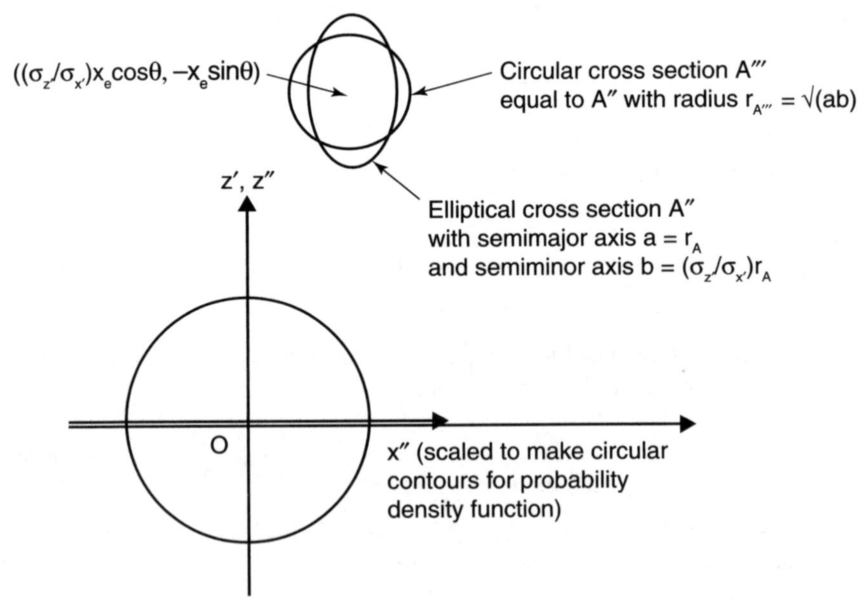

Figure 5.2. Approximation of elliptical cross section by a circular cross section.

Let r_p'' denote the distance of the primary from the origin in the (x'', z'') system. Then, we have

$$A''' = \pi r_{A'''}^{\,2}, \qquad r_{A'''} = \sqrt{ab} = \sqrt{\frac{\sigma_{z'}}{\sigma_{x'}}}\, r_{A'}, \qquad r_p''^{\,2} = x_p''^{\,2} + z_p''^{\,2} \tag{5.16}$$

Thus, the collision probability (5.14) is approximated by

$$P = \frac{1}{2\pi\,\sigma_{z'}^{\,2}} \iint_{A'''} e^{-\left(x''^2 + z''^2\right)/2\sigma_{z'}^{\,2}}\, dx''\, dz'' \tag{5.17}$$

By using Eqs. (5.9), (5.15), and (5.16), we may easily show that the distance r_p'' of the primary from the origin in the (x'', z'') system is given by the following two equivalent forms:

$$r_p''^{\,2} = x_e^{\,2}\left\{1 + \left[\left(\frac{\sigma_{z'}}{\sigma_{x'}}\right)^2 - 1\right]\cos^2\theta\right\} \tag{5.18}$$

$$r_p''^{\,2} = x_e^{\,2}\left\{1 + \left[\left(\frac{\sigma_{z'}}{\sigma_{x'}}\right)^2 - 1\right]\left(\frac{x_p'^{\,2}}{x_p'^{\,2} + z_p'^{\,2}}\right)\right\} \tag{5.19}$$

5.4 Improved Analytical Expressions

A benefit from the previous approximation is that, as shown in Chapter 4, the two-dimensional isotropic Gaussian pdf with standard deviation $\sigma_{z'}$ in Eq. (5.17) integrated over a circle of radius $r_{A'''}$ displaced a distance r_p'' from the origin can be transformed into the following one-dimensional Rician pdf integrated from 0 to $r_{A'''}$:

$$P = \int_0^{r_{A'''}} \frac{r}{\sigma_{z'}^{\,2}}\, e^{-\left(r^2 + r_p''^{\,2}\right)/2\sigma_{z'}^{\,2}}\, I_o\!\left(\frac{r\, r_p''}{\sigma_{z'}^{\,2}}\right) dr \tag{5.20}$$

In this equation, $I_0(\cdot)$ denotes the modified Bessel function of the first kind of order zero. An analytical solution in the form of an infinite series that is convergent for all values of the relevant parameters is

$$P = e^{-v/2} \sum_{m=0}^{\infty} \frac{v^m}{2^m\, m!}\left[1 - e^{-u/2} \sum_{k=0}^{m} \frac{u^k}{2^k\, k!}\right] \tag{5.21}$$

where, by using Eqs. (5.16) through (5.20), it is convenient to introduce the dimensionless variables u and v (see Chapter 4), which are now defined in terms of the mean standard deviation σ, the companion standard deviation σ^*, the miss distance x_e, and the radius r_A of collision cross-sectional integration by

$$u \equiv \left(\frac{r_{A'''}}{\sigma_{z'}}\right)^2 = \left(\frac{r_A^{\,2}}{\sigma_{x'}\sigma_{z'}}\right) = \left(\frac{r_A}{\sigma}\right)^2 > 0 \tag{5.22}$$

$$v \equiv \left(\frac{r''_p}{\sigma_{z'}}\right)^2 = x_e^{\,2}\left\{1+\left[\left(\frac{\sigma_{z'}}{\sigma_{x'}}\right)^2 - 1\right]\left(\frac{x'^{2}_p}{x'^{2}_p + z'^{2}_p}\right)\right\}\Big/\sigma_{z'}^{\,2} = \left(\frac{x_e}{\sigma^*}\right)^2 > 0 \tag{5.23}$$

where

$$\sigma^2 \equiv \sigma_{x'}\sigma_{z'} \qquad \text{and} \qquad \sigma^{*2} \equiv \sigma_{z'}^{\,2}\left\{1+\left[\left(\frac{\sigma_{z'}}{\sigma_{x'}}\right)^2 - 1\right]\left(\frac{x'^{2}_p}{x'^{2}_p + z'^{2}_p}\right)\right\}^{-1} \tag{5.24}$$

Note that Eqs. (5.22) and (5.23) are the immediate generalizations of Eqs. (4.11) and (4.12) in Chapter 4, because they are expressed explicitly in terms of dimensionless ratios with respect to the standard deviations σ and σ^*. However, in view of Eqs. (5.15) and (5.16), it is more convenient to write Eq. (5.23) devoid of the nonessential singularity at $x'_p = 0$ and $z'_p = 0$ as simply

$$v = \frac{x'^{2}_p}{\sigma_{x'}^{\,2}} + \frac{z'^{2}_p}{\sigma_{z'}^{\,2}} \tag{5.25}$$

If only the first term in the series is retained ($m = 0$ in Eq. [5.21]), it is proved that this collision integral may be expressed analytically as

$$P = e^{-v/2}(1 - e^{-u/2}) + T_1 \tag{5.26}$$

where T_1 satisfies the inequality

$$T_1 < \frac{1}{8}u^2 v e^{-v/2} e^{uv/4} \tag{5.27}$$

We may refer to T_1 as the truncation error after the first term. Unlike signal detection with different parameter ranges in its applications, it turns out that, for most spacecraft encounters considered in Section 5.5 of this chapter, this truncation after the first term yields an error that appears in the third significant digit. Thus, it suffices to retain only the explicit terms in Eq. (5.26). For a wider range of applications, we would truncate after the second term ($m = 1$ in Eq. [5.21]) and use the explicit terms in the following equation:

$$P = e^{-v/2}\left\{\left(1 - e^{-u/2}\right) + \frac{v}{2}\left[1 - \left(1 + \frac{u}{2}\right)e^{-u/2}\right]\right\} + T_2 \tag{5.28}$$

where T_2 satisfies the inequality

$$T_2 < \frac{1}{128}u^3 v^2 e^{-v/2} e^{uv/4} \tag{5.29}$$

As noted in Chapter 4, if the cross-sectional radius and the miss distance are approximately greater than the standard deviations, we may need to retain more terms in Eq. (5.21). In addition, we made an approximation in representing the elliptical cross section by a circular cross section in the transition from Eq. (5.14) to (5.17). This second approximation ultimately determines the accuracy of using the Rician pdf in our modeling.

5.5 Comparison with Other Models

As mentioned before, the analytical expressions in Eqs. (5.26) and (5.28) yield results that agree extremely well with those of other formulations. In 1992, Foster analyzed the case of the International Space Station (ISS) in a circular orbit encountering space debris also in circular orbits. He "derived" the two-dimensional NASA model[5.1] and obtained the collision probability by numerically integrating the following integral:

$$P = \frac{1}{2\pi\sigma_{x'}\sigma_{z'}} e^{-\frac{1}{2}x_e^2\left[\left(\frac{\sin\varphi}{\sigma_{x'}}\right)^2 + \left(\frac{\cos\varphi}{\sigma_{z'}}\right)^2\right]} \int_0^{r_A} r \int_0^{2\pi} e^{-\frac{1}{2}r^2\left[\left(\frac{\sin\theta}{\sigma_{x'}}\right)^2 + \left(\frac{\cos\theta}{\sigma_{z'}}\right)^2\right] + r x_e\left[\left(\frac{\sin\theta\sin\varphi}{\sigma_{x'}^2}\right) + \left(\frac{\cos\theta\cos\varphi}{\sigma_{z'}^2}\right)\right]} d\theta\, dr \tag{5.30}$$

where ϕ is the angle of the primary object from the z'-axis. In the implementation, the angle step size is 0.5 deg and the radius step size is $r_A/12$.

In 1995, Chan[5.2] reduced the two-dimensional integral to the following one-dimensional integral in the (x, z)-encounter plane:

$$P = \frac{1}{\sqrt{2\pi}\sigma_x} \int_{x_e - r_A}^{x_e + r_A} e^{-x^2/2\sigma_x^2} \frac{1}{2}\left[erf\left(\frac{\lambda + m}{\sqrt{2}\sigma'}\right) + erf\left(\frac{\lambda - m}{\sqrt{2}\sigma'}\right)\right] dx \tag{5.31}$$

where

$$\frac{\lambda \pm m}{\sqrt{2}\sigma'} \equiv \frac{\sqrt{r_A - (x - x_e)^2} \pm \left(\frac{\rho_{xz}\sigma_z}{\sqrt{2}\sigma'}\right)}{\sqrt{2}\sigma_z\sqrt{1 - \rho_{xz}^2}} \tag{5.32}$$

The integrand involves the error function, which is difficult to deal with analytically, especially if the argument is large. Thus, the collision probability has to be computed by numerically evaluating the error function using standard algorithms. For this reason, this formulation was not pursued further.

In 2000, Patera[5.3] derived the following mathematically equivalent model, which is a one-dimensional "line" integral:

$$P = -\frac{1}{2\pi} \oint_{\text{Ellipse}} e^{-\alpha r^2} d\theta \tag{5.33}$$

if origin of encounter lies outside elliptical cross section;

$$P = 1 - \frac{1}{2\pi} \oint_{\text{Ellipse}} e^{-\alpha r^2} d\theta \tag{5.34}$$

if origin of encounter lies inside elliptical cross section.

The expression for α appearing in the exponent of the integrand is extremely complicated and depends on expressions involving elements of the transformation matrix from the three-dimensional encounter system to the three-dimensional principal axes system and also on the standard deviations in the diagonal covariance matrix. The integration is performed numerically around a circuit in the counterclockwise direction.

In 2002, Alfano[5.4] obtained the integral of Eq. (5.31) but expressed it in the (x', z')-encounter plane in which the pdf has only diagonal terms:

$$P = \frac{1}{2\sqrt{2\pi}\sigma_{x'}} \int_{x'_p - r_A}^{x'_p + r_A} e^{-\frac{x'^2}{2\sigma_{x'}^2}} \left\{ erf\left[\frac{z'_p + \left(r_A^2 - (x' - x'_p)^2\right)^{1/2}}{\sqrt{2}\sigma_{z'}}\right] + erf\left[\frac{-z'_p + \left(r_A^2 - (x' - x'_p)^2\right)^{1/2}}{\sqrt{2}\sigma_{z'}}\right]\right\} dx' \tag{5.35}$$

where (x'_p, z'_p) denotes the center of mass of the primary. Even though the integrand is simpler, the evaluation of this integral has still to be performed numerically. Again, when the argument exceeds approximately 6 (approximately 8.5 standard deviations), it is difficult to accurately evaluate the error function numerically even by the use of recursion relations because of truncation errors. The value of 6 corresponds to the limits of computing the error function using double precision. All the above formulations rely strictly on numerical integration for implementation. However, Alfano also used the algebraic-series–processing algorithms in Mathcad to expand the integrand and then integrate termwise the RHS of Eq. (5.8) to obtain the following expression:

$$P = \left(1 + P_1 + P_2 + P_3 + P_4 + P_5 + P_6\right)\frac{1}{2\sigma_{x'}\sigma_{z'}}e^{-\frac{1}{2}\left[\left(\frac{x'_p}{\sigma_{x'}}\right)^2+\left(\frac{z'_p}{\sigma_{z'}}\right)^2\right]} \tag{5.36}$$

The polynomials P_i are very complicated expressions involving the diagonal standard deviations, the coordinates of the primary in the (x',z')-encounter plane, and the radius of the circular cross section. This expression yields results that agree to at least four significant digits in comparison with the more accurate numerical integration models. Thus, in essence, Eqs. (5.26), (5.28), and (5.36) are the only analytical models that are applicable over a fairly large range of parameters for spacecraft collision probability computations.

The above four formulations (NASA, Chan, Patera, and Alfano), described by Eqs. (5.30), (5.26), (5.33), and (5.35), were coded and investigations were performed to study their comparative accuracies. The tables on the following pages show results comparing Eqs. (5.26) and (5.28) with the NASA, Patera, and Alfano formulations. For convenience, we shall refer to the formulations as "models" even though they are not truly different models but are all traceable to the same original three-dimensional Gaussian pdf. (In common usage, the term "model" usually involves mathematical assumptions entering into the description of a physical problem.)

The NASA model is used as a basis of comparison for all the other models. To replicate the exact NASA model, we retain the same number of integration steps ($12 \times 720 = 8640$). Because there are two trigonometric evaluations and one exponential evaluation in the inner loop, there are approximately 25,921 evaluations (abbreviated as evals) in the integration. For the Patera model, 1000 steps were used. Because each step involves one exponential evaluation and one inverse sine function evaluation (for $d\theta$), therefore there are 2000 evals in the integration. For the Alfano model, 1000 steps were used. Because each step involves one exponential and two error function evaluations, therefore there are 3000 evals in the integration. Finally, only two exponential evaluations for both the one-term and the two-term Chan models are required to compute the collision probability.

5.5.1 Extremely Close Encounters

Table 5.1 shows comparisons for the case of extremely close encounters between a small spacecraft and space debris with a combined cross-sectional radius of 5 m. The nominal miss distance is 10 m. In the first two columns, their standard deviations in the encounter plane are described by ellipses with aspect ratios of 2:1 and are 50 and 25 m respectively. This does not necessarily mean that their three-dimensional covariances are small because they could be approaching head-on with a much larger standard deviation in the intrack direction (maybe 10 times larger).

The first data column is for the case of the primary on the major axis of the error ellipse while the second column is for the primary on the minor axis. In the first column, the collision probability is 9.74×10^{-3} computed by the numerical NASA, Patera, and Alfano models. The analytical Chan model yields 9.75×10^{-3}. In the last two columns, the standard deviations in the encounter plane are described by ellipses with aspect ratios of 3:1 and are 75 and 25 m respectively. The third column is for the case of the primary on the major axis of the error ellipse while the fourth column is for the primary on the minor axis. The above general observations hold for the numerical results. The only difference is that the collision probability has decreased by one-third when the aspect ratio of the error ellipses changes from 2:1 to 3:1.

Table 5.1. Comparison for Extremely Close Encounters with Small Covariance[a]

	Input Variables			
$\sigma_{x'}$ (km)	0.05	0.05	0.075	0.075
$\sigma_{z'}$ (km)	0.025	0.025	0.025	0.025
Collision Cross Section Radius r_A (km)	0.005	0.005	0.005	0.005
x'_p (km)	0.01	0	0.01	0
z'_p (km)	0	0.01	0	0.01
	Output: Collision Probability for Each Model Discussed			
NASA	9.742×10^{-03}	9.181×10^{-03}	6.571×10^{-03}	6.125×10^{-03}
Patera	9.741×10^{-03}	9.181×10^{-03}	6.571×10^{-03}	6.125×10^{-03}
Error (%)	0.00	0.00	0.00	0.00
Alfano	9.741×10^{-03}	9.181×10^{-03}	6.571×10^{-03}	6.125×10^{-03}
Error (%)	0.00	0.00	0.00	0.00
Chan (One Term)	9.753×10^{-03}	9.185×10^{-03}	6.586×10^{-03}	6.134×10^{-03}
Error (%)	0.12	0.04	0.22	0.14
Chan (Two Terms)	9.754×10^{-03}	9.189×10^{-03}	6.586×10^{-03}	6.135×10^{-03}
Error (%)	0.13	0.08	0.22	0.17

[a]This table compares the probability of collision for the NASA, Patera, Alfano, and Chan models using the NASA model as the basis of comparison. The collision cross section is a circle.

5.5.2 Close and Distant Encounters

The first two data columns of Table 5.2 show comparisons for the case of close encounters between two small spacecraft or a slightly larger spacecraft and space debris with a combined cross-sectional radius of 10 m. The nominal miss distance is 1 km. In the first two columns, their standard deviations in the encounter plane are described by ellipses with aspect ratios of 3:1 and are 3 and 1 km respectively. In the first two columns, the collision probability is 1.577×10^{-5} and 1.011×10^{-5} respectively for the cases of the primary on the major and the minor axes. These numbers were obtained using the numerical NASA, Patera, and Alfano models as well as the two analytical Chan models. The last two columns are for distant encounters with the nominal miss distance being 10 km and everything else unchanged.

These general observations hold for the collision probabilities that are 6.443 $\times 10^{-8}$ and 3.22×10^{-27} (the latter being essentially zero). The Alfano model was implemented on Mathcad, which gives an output of 0.00×10^{0} for very small numbers. This is the reason for the misleading 100% error as recorded for that that inconsequentially insignificant case. Numerous cases were run by keeping all parameters the same but increasing the aspect ratio of the error ellipse in the

Table 5.2. Comparison for Close and Distant Encounters with Moderate Covariance[a]

Input Variables				
	Close Encounters		Distant Encounters	
$\sigma_{x'}$ (km)	3	3	3	3
$\sigma_{z'}$ (km)	1	1	1	1
Collision Cross Section Radius r_A (km)	0.01	0.01	0.01	0.01
x'_p (km)	1	0	10	0
z'_p (km)	0	1	0	10
Output: Collision Probability for Each Model Discussed				
NASA	1.577×10^{-05}	1.011×10^{-05}	6.443×10^{-08}	3.219×10^{-27}
Patera	1.577×10^{-05}	1.011×10^{-05}	6.443×10^{-08}	3.219×10^{-27}
Error (%)	0.00	0.00	0.00	0.00
Alfano	1.577×10^{-05}	1.011×10^{-05}	6.443×10^{-08}	$0.000 \times 10^{+00}$
Error (%)	0.00	0.00	0.00	−100.00
Chan (One Term)	1.577×10^{-05}	1.011×10^{-05}	6.443×10^{-08}	3.215×10^{-27}
Error (%)	0.00	0.00	0.00	−0.12
Chan (Two Terms)	1.577×10^{-05}	1.011×10^{-05}	6.443×10^{-08}	3.216×10^{-27}
Error (%)	0.00	0.00	0.00	−0.08

[a]This table compares the probability of collision for the NASA, Patera, Alfano, and Chan models using the NASA model as the basis of comparison. The collision cross section is a circle.

encounter plane from 3:1 progressively to 10:1. These results are not shown here because the general trends of consistency among the four models were observed (i.e., they agree to three or four significant figures).

5.5.3 Distant Encounters for Large Spacecraft

The first two data columns of Table 5.3 show comparisons for the case of distant encounters between two space-orbiting objects with a combined cross-sectional radius of 10 m. The nominal miss distance is 10 km. In the first two columns, their standard deviations in the encounter plane are described by ellipses with aspect ratios of 10:1 and are 10 and 1 km respectively. The four models yield collision probabilities of 3.03×10^{-6} and 9.65×10^{-28} respectively for the cases of the primary on the major and the minor axes. In the third column, we consider encounters of debris with an extremely large spacecraft, such as the ISS, of dimensions of $2 \times 50 = 100$ m. The standard deviations in the encounter plane are described by ellipses with aspect ratios of 3:1 and are 3 and 1 km respectively. The nominal miss distance of the debris is 5 km. The third column is for the case of the ISS on the major axis of the error ellipse. All four models yield collision probability of 1.04×10^{-4}. The

Table 5.3. Comparison for Distant Encounters for Large Spacecraft[a]

Input Variables				
	Encounters with Large Covariance		Encounters with Moderate Covariance for Large Collision Cross Section	
$\sigma_{x'}$ (km)	10	10	3	3
$\sigma_{z'}$ (km)	1	1	1	1
Collision Cross Section Radius r_A (km)	0.01	0.01	0.05	0.05
x'_p (km)	10	0	5	0
z'_p (km)	0	10	0	5
Output: Collision Probability for Each Model Discussed				
NASA	3.033×10^{-06}	9.656×10^{-28}	1.039×10^{-04}	1.564×10^{-09}
Patera	3.033×10^{-06}	9.656×10^{-28}	1.039×10^{-04}	1.564×10^{-09}
Error (%)	0.00	0.00	0.00	0.00
Alfano	3.033×10^{-06}	$0.000 \times 10^{+00}$	1.039×10^{-04}	1.564×10^{-09}
Error (%)	0.00	−100.00	0.00	−100.00
Chan (One Term)	3.033×10^{-06}	9.644×10^{-28}	1.039×10^{-04}	1.552×10^{-09}
Error (%)	0.00	−0.12	0.00	−0.76
Chan (Two Terms)	3.033×10^{-06}	9.645×10^{-28}	1.039×10^{-04}	1.556×10^{-09}
Error (%)	0.00	−0.11	0.00	−0.50

[a]This table compares the probability of collision for the NASA, Patera, Alfano, and Chan models using the NASA model as the basis of comparison. The collision cross section is a circle.

fourth column is for the case of the primary on the minor axis of the error ellipse. The three numerical models yield collision probability of 1.564×10^{-9}. The Chan results are off by 0.76% and 0.5% respectively for the one-term and the two-term model. From the three tables given thus far, we observe not much significant difference between all these models for the wide range of cases studied.

From the standpoint of the number of trigonometric, exponential, and error function evaluations, either Chan model is still much faster because it requires only one-thousandth of the time taken by the Patera (2000 evals) and the Alfano (3000 evals) models and approximately one-ten-thousandth the time taken by the NASA model (26,000 evals). If collision probability is used in screening thousands of pairs of orbiting objects that are candidates for potential collision, this difference in computation speed is an important factor to be considered.

5.6 Generalization to More Complex Cross Sections

Up to this point, the analysis has been based on modeling the primary and secondary spacecraft by spheres of radii r_p and r_s centered at their respective centers of mass. The approximation of the secondary by a sphere is usually justified because the attitude is not known in general. However, the approximation of the primary by a sphere does not yield accurate results because the spacecraft comprises many components that may be modeled as spheres, cylinders, cones, or circular, rectangular, and triangular plates, etc. These components may also eclipse one another depending on the projection onto the encounter plane.

Thus, the collision cross section can be very complicated to describe. Even if the outline of the cross section is available, the method of integrating using radial and angular variables as in the NASA model is not applicable because that formulation is strictly based on a circular collision cross section. One using that model would have to perform an extremely time-consuming two-dimensional integration, most likely in Cartesian coordinates.

The methods of Patera and Alfano may be extended to spacecraft structures more complicated than a sphere. The collision probability of a tethered satellite colliding with a secondary has been formulated by Patera.[5.5] For this case, the collision cross section is a ribbon of width equal to $2r_s$ with its centerline coinciding with the tether. To be precisely correct, the ends of this ribbon should be two semicircles, but Patera implicitly simplified them to be straight lines. For practical reasons, this simplification does not introduce substantial errors.

If we consider very complex spacecraft structures, even this method of "line" integration does not prove feasible because it relies on knowing the analytical description of the various components, and this knowledge explicitly depends on the detailed projection on the encounter plane even for the case of no self-shadowing.

In investigative studies, the following method of equivalent cross section areas (MECSA) may be fruitfully applied to compute the collision probability for the case of complex spacecraft structures. Basically, it simply involves the cosine of the angle between the unit normal vector $\mathbf{n}_{comp}$ of the particular component and the relative velocity vector $\mathbf{v}_{ps}$ so that the projected area A on the encounter plane is given in terms of the area A_{comp} by the relation

$$A = \left| \mathbf{n}_{comp} \cdot \mathbf{v}_{ps} / v_{ps} \right| A_{comp} \tag{5.37}$$

This is substituted into Eqs. (5.9) and (5.15) to obtain in succession the cross sections A' and A''. Finally, A″ is converted into an equivalent circular cross section A''' of radius r_A''' having the same area as A''. The center of A''' is chosen to be at the centroid of A'', which also corresponds to the centroids of A' and A because the transformations between the various coordinates are affine. (Affine transformations include rotation, dilation, contraction, shear, and translation.) This is another salient feature of MECSA.

The justification (but not proof) of this method lies in the fact that if the cross-sectional dimensions are small compared to the standard deviations or the miss distance, then the pdf does not vary much within the cross-sectional area. Under these conditions, the collision integral (5.14) is essentially given by the value of the integrand at the centroid multiplied by the area. This is not a simple straightforward multiplication of a function value by the area to obtain the integral. We still invoke the Rician integral (5.20) with a circular area A''' equal to the noncircular area A''.

The question that remains to be answered is the merit of this method if the cross-sectional dimensions are not small compared to the standard deviations or the miss distance. The subject of this applicability is taken up in the following case studies. To illustrate the accuracy of this method, we first consider the case of A being a square.

5.6.1 Encounters for Square Cross Sections

Table 5.4 shows the comparison between the numerical integration and MECSA for extremely close encounters with small covariance similar to the parameters in Table 5.1. The numerical integration uses Eq. (5.33) with 400 integration steps. The approximation of a square by an equivalent circle gives very accurate collision probabilities, less than 0.4% for the cases studied. Other cases involving rectangles with aspect ratios up to 10:1 have been studied with comparably small errors introduced. (This will be shown in Table 5.8.)

Table 5.5 shows the comparison between the numerical integration and MECSA for close encounters and distant encounters with moderate covariance similar to the parameters in Table 5.2. Again, the numerical integration uses Eq. (5.33) with 400 integration steps. The approximation of a square by an equivalent circle gives very accurate collision probabilities, less than 0.2% for the cases studied. Other cases involving rectangles with aspect ratios up to 10:1 have been studied with comparable resulting accuracies. (This will also be shown in Table 5.8.)

Table 5.4. Comparison for Extremely Close Encounters for Squares with Small Covariance[a]

Input Variables				
$\sigma_{x'}$ (km)	0.05	0.05	0.075	0.075
$\sigma_{z'}$ (km)	0.025	0.025	0.025	0.025
Base of Rectangle (km)	0.01	0.01	0.01	0.01
Height of Rectangle (km)	0.01	0.01	0.01	0.01
x'_p (km)	0.01	0	0.01	0
z'_p (km)	0	0.01	0	0.01
Output: Collision Probability for Each Model Discussed				
Patera	1.238×10^{-02}	1.167×10^{-02}	8.351×10^{-03}	7.786×10^{-03}
Alfano	1.238×10^{-02}	1.167×10^{-02}	8.351×10^{-03}	7.786×10^{-03}
Error (%)	0.00	0.00	0.00	0.00
Chan (One Term)	1.240×10^{-02}	1.168×10^{-02}	8.378×10^{-03}	7.802×10^{-03}
Error (%)	0.19	0.09	0.32	0.21
Chan (Two Terms)	1.240×10^{-02}	1.168×10^{-02}	8.378×10^{-03}	7.805×10^{-03}
Error (%)	0.20	0.14	0.32	0.24

[a]This table compares the probability of collision for the Patera, Alfano, and Chan models using the Patera model as the basis of comparison. The collision cross section is a square.

5.6.2 Encounters for Triangular Cross Sections

To illustrate the accuracy of MECSA, we next consider the case of A being an isosceles triangle. Table 5.6 shows the comparison between the numerical integration and MECSA for extremely close encounters with small covariance similar to the parameters in Tables 5.1 and 5.4. The approximation of an isosceles triangle by an equivalent circle gives very accurate collision probabilities, less than 0.2% for the cases studied. Other cases involving general triangles with aspect ratios up to 10:1 have been studied with comparable results. (See Table 5.8.)

Table 5.7 shows the comparison between the numerical integration and MECSA for close encounters and distant encounters with moderate covariance similar to the parameters in Tables 5.2 and 5.5. The approximation of an isosceles triangle by an equivalent circle gives very accurate collision probabilities, less than 0.2% for the cases studied. Other cases involving general triangles with aspect ratios up to 10:1 have been studied, yielding results of comparable accuracies. (See Table 5.8.)

5.6.3 Encounters for Elongated Rectangular and Triangular Cross Sections

Table 5.8 shows the comparison between the numerical integration and MECSA for close encounters with moderate covariance similar to the parameters in Tables

Table 5.5. Comparison for Close and Distant Encounters for Squares with Moderate Covariance[a]

Input Variables				
	Close Encounters		Distant Encounters	
$\sigma_{x'}$ (km)	3	3	3	3
$\sigma_{z'}$ (km)	1	1	1	1
Base of Rectangle (km)	0.02	0.02	0.02	0.02
Height of Rectangle (km)	0.02	0.02	0.02	0.02
x'_p (km)	1	0	10	0
z'_p (km)	0	1	0	10
Output: Collision Probability for Each Model Discussed				
Patera	2.007×10^{-05}	1.287×10^{-05}	8.204×10^{-08}	4.100×10^{-27}
Alfano	2.007×10^{-05}	1.287×10^{-05}	8.204×10^{-08}	$0.000 \times 10^{+00}$
Error (%)	0.00	0.00	0.00	–100.00
Chan (One Term)	2.007×10^{-05}	1.287×10^{-05}	8.204×10^{-08}	4.093×10^{-27}
Error (%)	0.00	0.00	0.00	–0.17
Chan (Two Terms)	2.007×10^{-05}	1.287×10^{-05}	8.204×10^{-08}	4.095×10^{-27}
Error (%)	0.00	0.00	0.00	–0.11

[a]This table compares the probability of collision for the Patera, Alfano, and Chan models using the Patera model as the basis of comparison. The collision cross section is a square.

5.2, 5.5, and 5.7. For convenience, the pdf is chosen to be isotropic. The first two columns are for the case of elongated rectangles having aspect ratios of 10:1 oriented parallel or perpendicular to the axes respectively. Similarly, the last two columns are for the case of elongated triangles. The corresponding approximations by an equivalent circle give very accurate collision probabilities, less than 0.2% for the cases studied, even for large linear dimensions of 200 m. The cases for which the pdf is bivariate Gaussian may be reduced to the case of isotropic pdf by changing the aspect ratio of the rectangle or triangle. It is quite remarkable that the MECSA computations have such high fidelity.

5.7 Discussion

Tables 5.1, 5.4, and 5.6 show cases of extremely good agreement for which the collision cross-sectional dimensions are of the order of the standard deviations and the miss distance. A sufficient (but not necessary) condition for the Chan model to apply is that the collision cross-sectional dimensions are small compared to the standard deviations as shown in Table 4.2 of Chapter 4. This sufficient condition holds for most problems because the standard deviations are hundreds of

Table 5.6. Comparison for Extremely Close Encounters for Triangles with Small Covariance[a]

Input Variables				
$\sigma_{x'}$ (km)	0.05	0.05	0.075	0.075
$\sigma_{z'}$ (km)	0.025	0.025	0.025	0.025
Base of Triangle (km)	0.01	0.01	0.01	0.01
Height of Triangle (km)	0.01	0.01	0.01	0.01
x'_p (km)	0.01	0	0.01	0
z'_p (km)	0	0.01	0	0.01
Output: Collision Probability for Each Model Discussed				
Patera	1.239×10^{-02}	1.167×10^{-02}	8.364×10^{-03}	7.796×10^{-03}
Alfano	1.239×10^{-02}	1.167×10^{-02}	8.364×10^{-03}	7.795×10^{-03}
Error (%)	0.00	0.00	0.00	0.00
Chan (One Term)	1.240×10^{-02}	1.168×10^{-02}	8.378×10^{-03}	7.802×10^{-03}
Error (%)	0.13	0.07	0.17	0.09
Chan (Two Terms)	1.240×10^{-02}	1.168×10^{-02}	8.378×10^{-03}	7.805×10^{-03}
Error (%)	0.14	0.12	0.17	0.12

[a]This table compares the probability of collision for the Patera, Alfano, and Chan models using the Patera model as the basis of comparison. The collision cross section is an isosceles triangle.

meters to a few kilometers whereas the collision cross-sectional dimensions are of the order of tens of meters. It is possible to assign values to these parameters such that this model yields poor approximations. For these cases, it is permissible to break up the cross section into a number of smaller pieces such that the sufficient condition holds and the Chan model will then apply.

We next consider how various components in a complex spacecraft structure will project onto the encounter plane. For simplicity, we shall ignore the eclipsing of one spacecraft component by another. We know that a sphere will project as a circle. A cylinder will project as a parallelogram plus two semiellipses. A cone will generally project as a triangle plus a segment of an ellipse or in some cases as an ellipse. A circular plate will project as an ellipse. A rectangle will project as a parallelogram. A triangle will project as a triangle.

For each of these components, we know the centroid in the spacecraft body frame. We may easily obtain the centroid of the projection of each component in the encounter plane. The area of the projected cross section is determined using Eq. (5.37). Thus, we may now use Eqs. (5.22) through (5.29) to compute accurate collision probabilities with approximately 0.4% error for the cases considered.

Table 5.7. Comparison for Close and Distant Encounters for Triangles with Moderate Covariance[a]

Input Variables				
	Close Encounters		Distant Encounters	
$\sigma_{x'}$ (km)	3	3	3	3
$\sigma_{z'}$ (km)	1	1	1	1
Base of Triangle (km)	0.04	0.04	0.04	0.04
Height of Triangle (km)	0.02	0.02	0.02	0.02
x'_p (km)	1	0	10	0
z'_p (km)	0	1	0	10
Output: Collision Probability for Each Model Discussed				
Patera	2.007×10^{-05}	1.287×10^{-05}	8.204×10^{-08}	4.097×10^{-27}
Alfano	2.007×10^{-05}	1.287×10^{-05}	8.204×10^{-08}	$0.000 \times 10^{+00}$
Error (%)	0.00	0.00	0.00	–100.00
Chan (One Term)	2.007×10^{-05}	1.287×10^{-05}	8.204×10^{-08}	4.093×10^{-27}
Error (%)	0.00	0.00	0.00	–0.11
Chan (Two Terms)	2.007×10^{-05}	1.287×10^{-05}	8.204×10^{-08}	4.095×10^{-27}
Error (%)	0.00	0.00	0.00	–0.06

[a]This table compares the probability of collision for the Patera, Alfano, and Chan models using the Patera model as the basis of comparison. The collision cross section is an isosceles triangle.

Finally, in MECSA, we recall that we convert A'' into an equal-area circular cross section A''' of radius $r_{A'''}$ for use in Eq. (5.22). Because of the affine transformations between A, A', A'', and A''', a little consideration of Eqs. (5.9), (5.15), and (5.16) reveals that we can also convert the area A into an equal-area circle, thus simplifying the computations. That is, we may immediately obtain the radius r_A for use in Eq. (5.22) by simply setting at the start

$$A = \pi r_A^{\,2} \tag{5.38}$$

When there is no substantial self-shadowing, MECSA may be applied to rapidly and accurately compute the collision probability for the case of complex spacecraft structures. It does not rely on a detailed analytical description of the various components on the encounter plane. Rather, it depends only on the angle between the unit normal spacecraft component vector and the relative velocity vector. The key step is the conversion of the component into an equivalent circle of the same area centered at the centroid. It is hoped that MECSA will be used for efficiently computing the collision probabilities of the ISS when it encounters other orbiting objects. This subject is the central point of Chapter 6.

Table 5.8. Comparison for Close Encounters for Elongated Rectangular and Triangular Cross Sections with 10:1 Aspect Ratio[a]

Input Variables				
	Rectangles		Triangles	
$\sigma_{x'}$ (km)	1	1	1	1
$\sigma_{z'}$ (km)	1	1	1	1
Base of Rectangle or Triangle (km)	0.2	0.2	0.2	0.2
Height of Rectangle or Triangle (km)	0.02	0.02	0.02	0.02
x'_p (km)	1	0	1	0
z'_p (km)	0	1	0	1
Output: Collision Probability for Each Model Discussed				
Patera	3.861×10^{-04}	3.855×10^{-04}	1.931×10^{-04}	1.929×10^{-04}
Chan (One Term)	3.860×10^{-04}	3.860×10^{-04}	1.930×10^{-04}	1.930×10^{-04}
Error (%)	–0.03	0.13	–0.01	0.07
Chan (Two Terms)	3.861×10^{-04}	3.861×10^{-04}	1.930×10^{-04}	1.930×10^{-04}
Error (%)	–0.01	0.15	–0.01	0.08

[a]This table compares the probability of collision for the Patera and Chan models using the Patera model as the basis of comparison. The collision cross section is a rectangle or triangle as indicated.

5.8 Conclusion

The results obtained here show that it suffices to use the zeroth-order approximation for an extremely wide range of encounter parameters, including standard deviations in the encounter plane described by elongated ellipses with aspect ratios up to 10 and possibly beyond. (Note that in Section 2 of Chapter 2, we demonstrated that for most short-term encounters, the aspect ratio of the ellipse in the encounter plane is less than 7. Moreover, in Section 4.5 of Chapter 4, we showed that for most present-day applications the zeroth- and first-order approximations provide collision probabilities accurate to within 1%.)

The four models—NASA, Patera, Alfano, and Chan—yield collision probabilities in agreement to three or four significant figures for the case of circular collision cross section. The NASA model is strictly applicable to the case of circular cross section, whereas the other three may be extended in principle to noncircular areas; however, the Patera and Alfano models are not easily extendable to complex shapes because they rely on the detailed analytical description of the boundary so that the numerical integration may be performed. The Chan model is easily generalized to include these general shapes because it is based only on areas.

5.9 Summary

In this chapter, we considered the nonisotropic case for which the two standard deviations σ_x and σ_z are not equal in the two-dimensional Gaussian pdf used in computing the collision probability. The covariance C, in general, contains an off-diagonal term with a nonzero correlation coefficient ρ_{xz}.

In Section 5.1, we rotated the (x, z)-coordinate axes to new (x', z')-coordinate axes so that the new covariance C' has only diagonal terms $\sigma_{x'}$ and $\sigma_{z'}$.

In Section 5.2, we transformed the (x', z')-coordinate axes to new (x'', z'')-coordinate axes so that the new covariance C'' has diagonal terms $\sigma_{x''}$ and $\sigma_{z''}$, which are equal. In this process, the circular cross section becomes an elliptical cross-sectional area of integration.

In Section 5.3, we approximated this elliptical cross section by an equivalent circular one having the same area and the same centroid; thus, we converted the probability problem into the one already solved in Chapter 4.

In Section 5.4, we derived improved analytical expressions that involved two standard deviations, the mean standard deviation σ and the auxiliary standard deviation σ^*, for use in the Rician integral. We also obtained explicitly one-term and two-term truncated expressions.

In Section 5.5, we described four other well-known formulations for use in computing spacecraft collision probability: These are the Foster (used by NASA), Chan, Patera, and Alfano "models." We compared the numerical results over a very wide range of input collision parameters: miss distance x_e, cross-sectional radius r_A, and standard deviations $\sigma_{x'}$ and $\sigma_{z'}$. The four models yield collision probabilities that agree to three or four significant digits for the case of circular collision cross section. The NASA model is strictly applicable to the case of circular cross section, whereas the other three may be extended in principle to noncircular areas.

In Section 5.6, we compared the collision probabilities for triangles and rectangles using the Chan, Patera, and Alfano formulations. Again, the numerical results agree to two or three significant digits.

In Section 5.7, we discussed how to compute the collision probabilities for complex spacecraft structures having geometrical components such as plates, discs, spheres, ellipsoids, cylinders, cones, and parallelepipeds if self-shadowing is ignored. The approach is to obtain the centroid of the projection of each component in the encounter plane and convert the projection to an equivalent circle having the same area and the same centroid.

In Section 5.8, we concluded that, for a wide range of present-day encounter parameters (object radius less than one-tenth the standard deviation and encounter plane elliptic aspect ratios up to 10), we may use the analytical expression for computing collision probability.

5.10 References

[5.1.] J. L. Foster and H. S. Estes, "A Parametric Analysis of Orbital Debris Collision Probability and Maneuver Rate for Space Vehicles," NASA/JSC-25898 (August 1992).

[5.2.] F. K. Chan, "Collision Probability Analyses for Earth-Orbiting Satellites," *Proceedings of the 7th International Space Conference of Pacific Basin Societies* (Nagasaki, Japan, July 1997). (Work performed in Iridium program, 1995.)

[5.3.] R. P. Patera, "A General Method for Calculating Satellite Collision Probability," *AAS/AIAA Space Flight Mechanics Meeting* (Clearwater, FL, January 2000).

[5.4.] S. Alfano, "Aerospace Support to Space Situation Awareness," *MIT Lincoln Laboratory Satellite Operations and Safety Workshop* (Haystack Observatory, Chelmsford, MA, October 2002).

[5.5.] R. P. Patera, "A Method for Calculating Collision Probability between a Satellite and a Space Tether," *AAS/AIAA Space Flight Mechanics Meeting* (Santa Barbara, CA, February 2001).

Chapter 6: International Space Station Collision Probability

Most spacecraft have complex geometrical shapes. It would not be appropriate to model them simplistically as spheres under all circumstances. Instead, we need to model them in a way that takes their complexity into account. This chapter considers the specific case of the International Space Station (ISS) and how it can best be modeled for computing its collision probability.

In Chapter 5, we outlined a general approach for using the method of equivalent cross section area (MECSA) to compute the probability of collision. This method does not rely on the detailed analytical description of the various components of the spacecraft. The key step of the method is to obtain the collision cross section of each component and convert it to an equivalent circle having the same area and the same centroid. In this chapter, we shall use MECSA to compute the collision probability of the ISS when it encounters orbiting objects.

6.1 The Method of Equivalent Cross Section Area

The geometrical components of many spacecraft may be modeled as spheres; cylinders; cones; circular, rectangular, and triangular plates; etc. The position and orientation of these components are usually well defined in the spacecraft body frame. They may eclipse one another depending on the direction of view. For simplicity, we shall assume that there is no occultation of one component by another when the spacecraft geometry is very complicated. However, we account for obvious exclusions, as in scenarios where cylindrical (or cuboidal) components of essentially the same cross section are connected in series so that their common interfaces are not visible.

Moreover, we shall confine our analysis to the case of short-term encounters. Suppose a secondary object encounters a large spacecraft of complex structure. It is possible that the nominal miss distance will be comparable to or smaller than the dimensions of the spacecraft. In this case, we may need to consider many encounter planes, one for each component. Thus, each component is regarded as a primary object. This is why, in Chapter 2, we chose to define the origin of the combined covariance to be at the secondary so as to have only one origin, thus avoiding undue complications.

Next, let us consider parallel projection of geometric solids in three-dimensional space onto a plane orthogonal to the projecting rays. Such projections are called orthogonal projections; the following assertions about them are easily verified.

(1) A sphere will project as a circle in any direction.

(2) A right circular cylinder will project as a circle along its axis of symmetry, as a rectangle in any direction orthogonal to this axis, and as a parallelogram plus two semiellipses in any other direction.

(3) A right circular cone will project as a circle along its axis of symmetry, as a triangle in any direction orthogonal to this axis, as an ellipse in any direction within the cone angle, and as a triangle plus a segment of an ellipse in any other direction.

(4) A circular plate will project as a circle along its normal, and as an ellipse in any other direction not orthogonal to its normal.

(5) A rectangular plate will project as a rectangle along its normal or in any direction orthogonal to any of its sides, and as a parallelogram in any other direction not orthogonal to its normal.

(6) A triangular plate will project as a triangle in any direction not orthogonal to its normal.

Consider a component in the form of a flat plate of any shape. Let A_i denote the area of the ith component and let $\mathbf{R}_i$ and $\hat{\mathbf{N}}_i$ respectively denote the geometrical centroid and the unit normal of that particular component in the spacecraft body frame. Let $\mathbf{v}_{ps}$ denote the relative velocity of the spacecraft with respect to the secondary. The encounter plane is perpendicular to $\mathbf{v}_{ps}$. Let $\hat{\mathbf{n}}_i$ be the unit normal $\hat{\mathbf{N}}_i$ expressed in the encounter coordinate system. (Vectors in the encounter system are indicated here by lowercase characters; those in the spacecraft body system, by uppercase characters.)

Then, the projected area A on the encounter plane is given by the relation

$$A = \left| \widehat{\mathbf{n}_i} \cdot \widehat{\mathbf{v}_{ps}} \right| A_i \tag{6.1}$$

If the component is not a plate but is a geometric solid such as a sphere, cylinder, cone, or truncated cone (conical frustum), then we use property (1), (2), or (3) from the list of orthogonal projections given previously to determine its projection A on the encounter plane. For the cases of a sphere and a cylinder, the orthogonal projections are simple, and the centroids of these two-dimensional projections are also the projections of the centroids of the three-dimensional solids.

For a sphere of radius r, the orthogonal projection is a circle of the same radius and the centroid is the center of the circle. That is, we have

$$A = \pi r^2 \tag{6.2}$$

For a right circular cylinder of radius r and height h, the general orthogonal projection is a parallelogram plus two semiellipses. The centroid is the point of symmetry of this geometric figure. Let ψ be the angle between the velocity $\mathbf{v}_{ps}$ and the axis of the cylinder. Then, we have

$$A = 2hr\left|\sin\psi\right| + \pi r^2\left|\cos\psi\right| \tag{6.3}$$

According to Eq. (6.3), when $\psi = \pi/2$ we have a rectangle of area $A = 2hr$, and when $\psi = 0$ we have a circle of area $A = \pi r^2$. These results are consistent with geometrical expectations.

As mentioned earlier, if we have a series of cylindrical components of essentially the same cross section connected together, then their obliterated common interfaces are not included in the computation of the projected area. In this case, the projected area of each cylindrical component is

$$A = 2hr\left|\sin\psi\right| \tag{6.4}$$

From Eq. (6.4), the projected area of the curved cylindrical surface (without the subsumed common elliptical interface) is respectively $A = 2hr$ and $A = 0$ for the cases of $\psi = \pi/2$ and $\psi = 0$.

It is easy to verify (by using the principle of area, centroids, and moments) that the centroid lies on the line of symmetry at a distance d from the center of the concealed common elliptical interface where

$$d = \frac{1}{2}h\left|\sin\psi\right| + \frac{\pi r}{4}\left|\cos\psi\right| \tag{6.5}$$

According to Eq. (6.5), when $\psi = \pi/2$ we have $d = h/2$ and when $\psi = 0$ we have $d = \pi r/4$. The result $d = h/2$ in the case of $\psi = \pi/2$ is consistent with geometrical expectation, whereas the other result cannot be derived from geometrical considerations but may also be derived using calculus for small h.

Thus far, we have discussed orthogonal projections of right circular cylinders in great detail. For the cases of a cone and a conical frustum, the orthogonal projections are more complicated and they require much analysis. Moreover, the centroids of these two-dimensional projections are not necessarily the projections of the centroids of the three-dimensional solids. As an example, the centroid of a conical solid is one-quarter of the height of the cone measured from the base, whereas the centroid of the projection in a direction orthogonal to the conical axis is one-third of the height of the projected triangle measured from the base.

Once A is obtained, it is substituted into Eqs. (5.9) and (5.15) of Chapter 5 to obtain in succession the cross sections A' and A''. Because the component with area A_i can be of any shape, it appears that we also have to obtain the shapes of A' and A'', and that can involve substantial work. For instance, if A_i is triangular, then we also have to obtain the triangles A, A', and A''. Because the transformations between A, A', and A'' are affine, their centroids map into each other.[6.1] This is another salient feature of MECSA. (Affine transformations, which are nonsingular, include translation, rotation, dilation, contraction, shear, and reflection or any combination of these transformations. If there is no translation, affine transformations are linear; otherwise, they are not.) Finally, the cross section A'' is converted into an equivalent circular cross section A''' having the same area and the same centroid. (Note that the transformation $A_i \to A$ is not affine because it is not invertible. Also, the transformation $A'' \to A'''$ is not affine because the two coordinate systems are the same, only the collision cross section is changed.)

A little consideration reveals that we need only Eq. (6.1) to obtain A from A_i. Then, we can bypass the sequence of transformations $A \to A' \to A''$ and simplify the computations by first converting A into an equivalent circular cross section of radius r_A having the same area and centroid as A. That is, we may immediately obtain the radius r_A by simply setting at the start $r_A{}^2 = A/\pi$ for use in Eq. (5.22) of Chapter 5 to compute the dimensionless parameter u. Thus, we have

$$u = \frac{r_A{}^2}{\sigma_{x'}\sigma_{z'}} = \frac{A}{\pi\sigma_{x'}\sigma_{z'}} \tag{6.6}$$

The other dimensionless parameter, v, is given by Eq. (5.25) of Chapter 5:

$$v = \frac{x'^2_p}{\sigma_{x'}^2} + \frac{z'^2_p}{\sigma_{z'}^2} \tag{6.7}$$

In Eqs. (6.6) and (6.7), $\sigma_{x'}{}^2$ and $\sigma_{z'}{}^2$ are the diagonal terms when the combined covariance matrix C' is expressed in its principal axes (x'_p, z'_p)-system (see Eq. [5.4] of Chapter 5). This combined covariance depends only on the covariance of the spacecraft and that of the secondary object (see Chapter 2). Therefore, it is the same for all the components of the spacecraft even if each is considered as a primary for our purpose. In Eqs. (6.6) and (6.7), we need r_A, x'_p, and z'_p as the only inputs for each component. Thus, u and v depend on the component of interest. Once they are obtained, we proceed to compute the collision probability for each component in the spacecraft by Eq. (4.19), (4.20), or (4.42) of Chapter 4:

$$P_0 = e^{-v/2}\left(1 - e^{-u/2}\right) \tag{6.8}$$

$$P_1 = e^{-v/2}\left\{\left(1 - e^{-u/2}\right) + \frac{v}{2}\left[1 - \left(1 + \frac{u}{2}\right)e^{-u/2}\right]\right\} \tag{6.9}$$

$$P_M = e^{-v/2} \sum_{m=0}^{M} \frac{v^m}{2^m m!} \left(1 - e^{-u/2} \sum_{k=0}^{m} \frac{u^k}{2^k k!} \right)$$

$$\begin{aligned} &M = 3 \; for \; u \leq 0.01 \; or \; v \leq 1, \\ &M = 10 \; for \; 0.01 < u \leq 1 \; or \; 1 < v \leq 9, \\ &M = 20 \; for \; 1 < u \leq 25 \; or \; 9 < v \leq 25, \\ &M = 60 \; otherwise. \end{aligned} \tag{6.10}$$

Henceforth, we shall identify the ISS specifically as the spacecraft with complex structure. Figures 6.1 and 6.2 are frontal views (artist's conceptions) of the ISS as it will appear upon completion according to present plans. As of this writing, in mid-2007, approximately half the anticipated components have already been assembled and are orbiting Earth. The configuration of most modules will remain intact, but the solar panels will be repositioned as appropriate.

In the ISS body system, the ith component, if it is a *plate*, is identified by its area A_i, centroid vector $\mathbf{R}_i$, $\equiv (X_i, Y_i, Z_i)$, and unit normal vector $\hat{\mathbf{N}}_i \equiv (U_i, V_i, W_i)$. The ISS dynamical body system has its origin at its center of mass. It is the motion of the center of mass that is described in the relative motion with respect to the

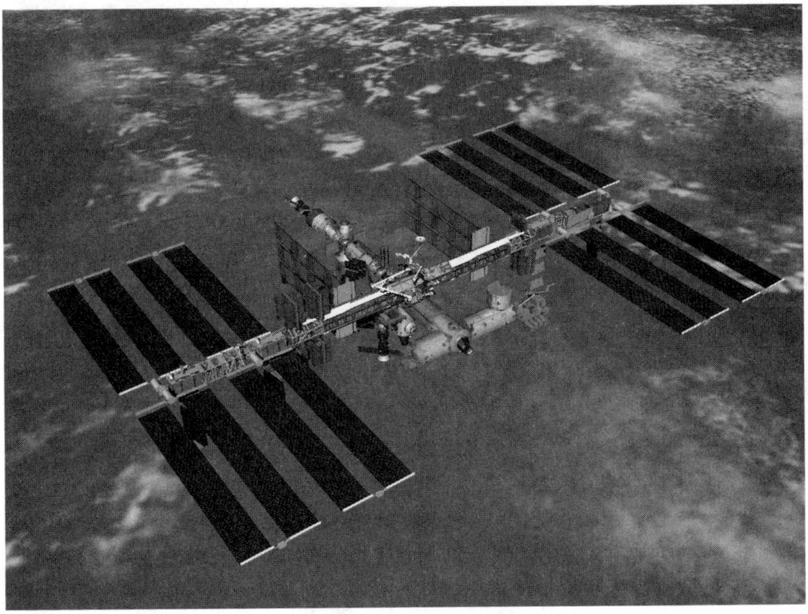

Figure 6.1. Artist's conception of the starboard frontal view of the ISS. (Courtesy NASA)

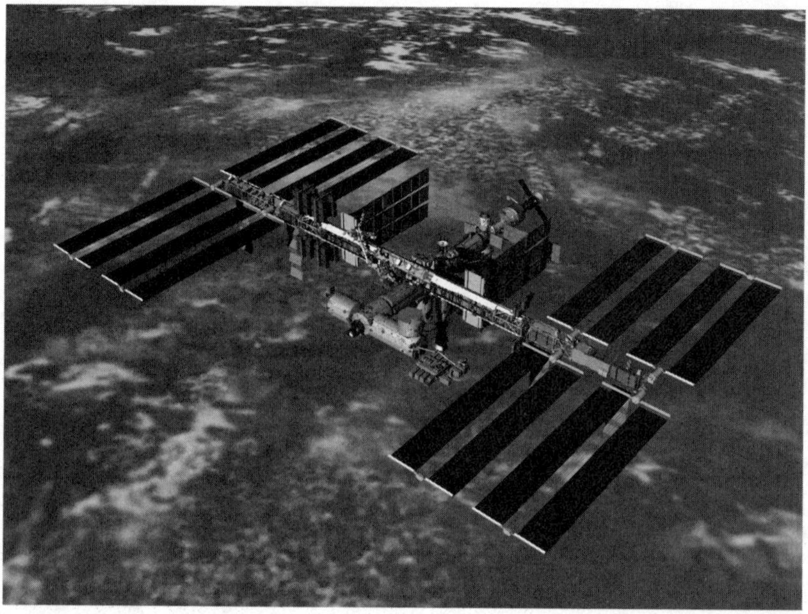

Figure 6.2. Artist's conception of the port frontal view of the ISS. (Courtesy NASA)

secondary object. The unit vectors $(\hat{\mathbf{X}}, \hat{\mathbf{Y}}, \hat{\mathbf{Z}})$ defining the body system with respect to an inertial frame can be taken from the spacecraft orbit and attitude data.

In Chapter 2, we defined the encounter system $(\hat{\mathbf{x}}, \hat{\mathbf{y}}, \hat{\mathbf{z}})$. The unit vector $\hat{\mathbf{y}}$ is defined along the relative vector $\mathbf{v}_{ps}$. That is, $\hat{\mathbf{y}} \equiv \hat{\mathbf{v}}_{ps}$. The unit vector $\hat{\mathbf{x}}$ is defined such that the center of mass of the ISS is nominally at the point $(x_e, 0, 0)$ at the instant of "nominal" closest approach, say $t = t_{\mathrm{ISS}}$. The unit $\hat{\mathbf{z}}$ vector completes the right-handed triad. Figure 6.3 illustrates the relation between the $(\hat{\mathbf{X}}, \hat{\mathbf{Y}}, \hat{\mathbf{Z}})$ system and the $(\hat{\mathbf{x}}, \hat{\mathbf{y}}, \hat{\mathbf{z}})$ system.

Let $\mathbf{r}_i \equiv (x_i, y_i, z_i)$ and $\mathbf{n}_i \equiv (u_i, v_i, w_i)$ respectively denote the centroid vector and the normal vector of the ith component in the encounter system. Then, we have

$$\mathbf{n}_i = S\mathbf{N}_i \tag{6.11}$$

$$\mathbf{r}_i = x_e\hat{\mathbf{x}} + S\mathbf{R}_i \tag{6.12}$$

where the transformation matrix S is given by

$$S = \begin{bmatrix} \hat{\mathbf{X}}\cdot\hat{\mathbf{x}} & \hat{\mathbf{Y}}\cdot\hat{\mathbf{x}} & \hat{\mathbf{Z}}\cdot\hat{\mathbf{x}} \\ \hat{\mathbf{X}}\cdot\hat{\mathbf{y}} & \hat{\mathbf{Y}}\cdot\hat{\mathbf{y}} & \hat{\mathbf{Z}}\cdot\hat{\mathbf{y}} \\ \hat{\mathbf{X}}\cdot\hat{\mathbf{z}} & \hat{\mathbf{Y}}\cdot\hat{\mathbf{z}} & \hat{\mathbf{Z}}\cdot\hat{\mathbf{z}} \end{bmatrix} \tag{6.13}$$

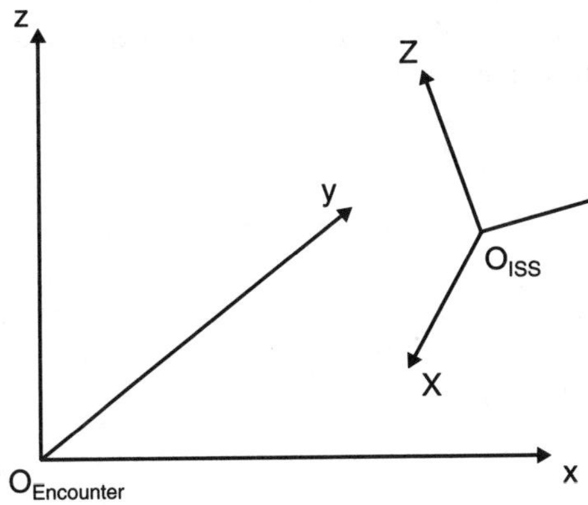

Figure 6.3. Relation between the ISS body system $(\hat{\mathbf{X}}, \hat{\mathbf{Y}}, \hat{\mathbf{Z}})$ and the spacecraft encounter coordinate system $(\hat{\mathbf{x}}, \hat{\mathbf{y}}, \hat{\mathbf{z}})$.

Written explicitly, Eqs. (6.9) and (6.10) are

$$
\begin{aligned}
u_i &= (\widehat{\mathbf{X}}\cdot\widehat{\mathbf{x}})U_i + (\widehat{\mathbf{Y}}\cdot\widehat{\mathbf{x}})V_i + (\widehat{\mathbf{Z}}\cdot\widehat{\mathbf{x}})W_i \\
v_i &= (\widehat{\mathbf{X}}\cdot\widehat{\mathbf{y}})U_i + (\widehat{\mathbf{Y}}\cdot\widehat{\mathbf{y}})V_i + (\widehat{\mathbf{Z}}\cdot\widehat{\mathbf{y}})W_i \\
w_i &= (\widehat{\mathbf{X}}\cdot\widehat{\mathbf{z}})U_i + (\widehat{\mathbf{Y}}\cdot\widehat{\mathbf{z}})V_i + (\widehat{\mathbf{Z}}\cdot\widehat{\mathbf{z}})W_i
\end{aligned}
\tag{6.14}
$$

$$
\begin{aligned}
x_i &= x_e + (\widehat{\mathbf{X}}\cdot\widehat{\mathbf{x}})X_i + (\widehat{\mathbf{Y}}\cdot\widehat{\mathbf{x}})Y_i + (\widehat{\mathbf{Z}}\cdot\widehat{\mathbf{x}})Z_i \\
y_i &= (\widehat{\mathbf{X}}\cdot\widehat{\mathbf{y}})X_i + (\widehat{\mathbf{Y}}\cdot\widehat{\mathbf{y}})Y_i + (\widehat{\mathbf{Z}}\cdot\widehat{\mathbf{y}})Z_i \\
z_i &= (\widehat{\mathbf{X}}\cdot\widehat{\mathbf{z}})X_i + (\widehat{\mathbf{Y}}\cdot\widehat{\mathbf{z}})Y_i + (\widehat{\mathbf{Z}}\cdot\widehat{\mathbf{z}})Z_i\,.
\end{aligned}
\tag{6.15}
$$

At time t_{ISS} the ith component may not necessarily be at its nominal closest point of approach with respect to the secondary object. However, its closest point of approach occurs at time $t = t_i$, given by

$$
t_i = t_{ISS} - y_i / v_{ps} \tag{6.16}
$$

If we substitute Eq. (6.12) into (6.1), we obtain

$$
A = \left|\widehat{\mathbf{n}}_i \cdot \widehat{\mathbf{y}}\right| A_i = \left|(\widehat{\mathbf{X}}\cdot\widehat{\mathbf{y}})U_i + (\widehat{\mathbf{Y}}\cdot\widehat{\mathbf{y}})V_i + (\widehat{\mathbf{Z}}\cdot\widehat{\mathbf{y}})W_i\right| A_i \tag{6.17}
$$

Let the encounter (x, z)-plane of the ISS be rotated through an angle θ to the (x', z')-plane so that the combined covariance C' is diagonal (see Chapter 5).

Therefore, at time t_i when the ith component passes through its own encounter plane, it will be at an angle $(\gamma - \theta)$ with the x'-axis where the additional rotation angle γ is determined from the equation

$$\tan\gamma = \frac{z_i}{x_i} \tag{6.18}$$

Figure 6.4 illustrates the relation between the ith component encounter system and the (x', z')-system. Hence, the nominal miss distance $x_{e,i}$ of the ith component in its own encounter plane is

$$x_{e,i} = \sqrt{(x_i^2 + z_i^2)} \tag{6.19}$$

Therefore, the coordinates of the centroid of the ith component in its own encounter plane are

$$\begin{aligned} x_p' &= x_{e,i}\cos(\gamma - \theta) \\ z_p' &= x_{e,i}\sin(\gamma - \theta) \end{aligned} \tag{6.20}$$

Thus, for the ith component we have now obtained u and v for computing the collision probability by Eqs. (6.6) and (6.7).

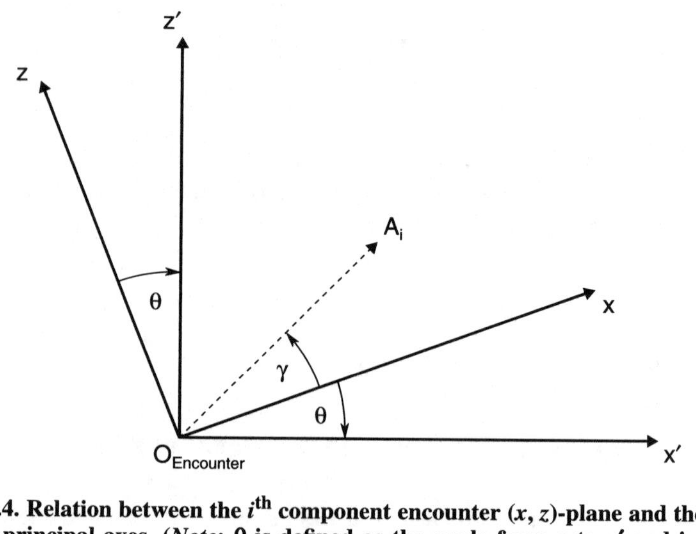

Figure 6.4. Relation between the ith component encounter (x, z)-plane and the (x', z')-plane of principal axes. (*Note*: θ is defined as the angle from x to x' and is positive counterclockwise.)

We know that the orbital motions of the ISS and the secondary object yield the unit vectors $(\hat{\mathbf{x}}, \hat{\mathbf{y}}, \hat{\mathbf{z}})$ defining the encounter system. Specifically, $\hat{\mathbf{y}}$ is defined to be the unit-relative velocity vector $\hat{\mathbf{v}}_{ps}$ of the ISS with respect to the secondary object, $\hat{\mathbf{x}}$ is defined to point from the secondary object to the ISS at the instant of "nominal" closest approach, and $\hat{\mathbf{z}}$ is defined by

$$\hat{\mathbf{z}} = \hat{\mathbf{x}} \times \hat{\mathbf{y}} \tag{6.21}$$

Thus, we can obtain the transformation matrix S in Eq. (6.13) from orbit and attitude data under actual flight conditions.

However, for the purpose of investigating the collision probability with the secondary object from various approach directions, it is more convenient to recast the input data slightly differently. Let α_x, δ_x, α_y, and δ_y respectively denote the right ascension and declination of $\hat{\mathbf{x}}$ and $\hat{\mathbf{y}}$ in the $(\hat{\mathbf{X}}, \hat{\mathbf{Y}}, \hat{\mathbf{Z}})$ system. Then, we have

$$\hat{\mathbf{x}} = \cos\alpha_x \cos\delta_x \hat{\mathbf{X}} + \sin\alpha_x \cos\delta_x \hat{\mathbf{Y}} + \sin\delta_x \hat{\mathbf{Z}} \tag{6.22}$$

$$\hat{\mathbf{y}} = \cos\alpha_y \cos\delta_y \hat{\mathbf{X}} + \sin\alpha_y \cos\delta_y \hat{\mathbf{Y}} + \sin\delta_y \hat{\mathbf{Z}} \tag{6.23}$$

$$\begin{aligned} \hat{\mathbf{z}} &= \left(\sin\alpha_x \cos\delta_x \sin\delta_y - \sin\alpha_y \cos\delta_y \sin\delta_x\right)\hat{\mathbf{X}} \\ &+ \left(\sin\delta_x \cos\alpha_y \cos\delta_y - \sin\delta_y \cos\alpha_x \cos\delta_x\right)\hat{\mathbf{Y}} \\ &+ \left(\cos\alpha_x \cos\delta_x \sin\alpha_y \cos\delta_y - \cos\alpha_y \cos\delta_y \sin\alpha_x \cos\delta_x\right)\hat{\mathbf{Z}} \end{aligned} \tag{6.24}$$

Therefore, the elements of the transformation matrix S in Eq. (6.13) are given by

$$\begin{aligned} &S_{11} = \cos\alpha_x \cos\delta_x, \quad S_{12} = \sin\alpha_x \cos\delta_x, \quad S_{13} = \sin\delta_x, \\ &S_{21} = \cos\alpha_y \cos\delta_y, \quad S_{22} = \sin\alpha_y \cos\delta_y, \quad S_{23} = \sin\delta_y, \\ &S_{31} = \left(\sin\alpha_x \cos\delta_x \sin\delta_y - \sin\delta_x \sin\alpha_y \cos\delta_y\right), \\ &S_{32}\left(\sin\delta_x \cos\alpha_y \cos\delta_y - \cos\alpha_x \cos\delta_x \sin\delta_y\right), \\ &S_{33} = \left(\cos\alpha_x \cos\delta_x \sin\alpha_y \cos\delta_y - \sin\alpha_x \cos\delta_x \cos\alpha_y \cos\delta_y\right) \end{aligned} \tag{6.25}$$

We have now completed the formulation of an algorithm to compute the probability of collision between the ISS and an oncoming secondary object. In addition to the area A_i, unit normal $\hat{\mathbf{N}}_i$, and centroid location $\mathbf{R}_i$, there are five input parameters (α_x, δ_x , α_y, δ_y, and x_e) in Eqs. (6.9) and (6.10) for the transformation of the ISS body system $(\hat{\mathbf{X}}, \hat{\mathbf{Y}}, \hat{\mathbf{Z}})$ to the encounter system $(\hat{\mathbf{x}}, \hat{\mathbf{y}}, \hat{\mathbf{z}})$. There are two more parameters ($\sigma_{x'}$ and $\sigma_{z'}$) in Eqs. (6.7) and (6.8) for the computation of the collision probability given by Eq. (6.9) or (6.10).

In Sections 6.7, 6.8, and 6.9 of this chapter, we shall examine three special cases of approach directions of the secondary object (head-on, broadside, and overhead) to illustrate the differences in collision probabilities that we can expect. Before we can proceed with these computations, however, we need to obtain the dimensions and locations of various components of the ISS.

6.2 Geometric Specifications of the ISS

This section summarizes the dimensions of the main components of the ISS. The data have been gleaned from the NASA Web site. The structures page[6.2] provides the NASA specifications in feet as well as in meters. The scale model page[6.3] gives details of a NASA model in a scale of 1:100 inches, component by component, and also supplies an exploded view. For comparison, all dimensions have been converted to meters. The two sets of data agree to within 0.2 m except for four cases: the lengths of the U.S. Node 2, the European Space Agency laboratory, the Japanese experiment laboratory, and the Russian docking compartment 1.

The information in the ISS structure description is periodically updated and is considered more current. This information takes precedence over that in the scale model drawings, which were done many years ago. Sometimes the specifications for a particular component are not completely given in the ISS structure description. In those cases, the scale model information provides the missing data. Figure 6.5 is an exploded view of the major ISS components used for collision probability computations.

For convenience, each component is modeled as the simplified geometric solid or plate that it resembles. The centroid of the component is given in the ISS *geometrical* body system $(\hat{\mathbf{X}}, \hat{\mathbf{Y}}, \hat{\mathbf{Z}})$, the origin being at the center of the S0 truss. The X-axis is in the direction of the ISS velocity vector (roll axis), the Y-axis is along the starboard trusses (pitch axis), and the Z-axis points toward Earth (yaw axis). In general, the center of mass of the ISS does not coincide with the origin of the geometrical body system.

For clarity, we will not introduce another notation to distinguish between the ISS dynamical and geometrical body systems, but we should include a displacement vector to account for this difference in our computations. Note that the origin of the geometrical body system is defined to be a constant. However, the center of mass changes with the inclusion of new components, the relocation of current components, or the reorientation of any particular component. In this chapter, this displacement vector is temporarily set equal to zero for the sake of simplicity and (more important) because of the lack of knowledge.

Tables 6.1 and 6.2 summarize the geometric specifications of the ISS.

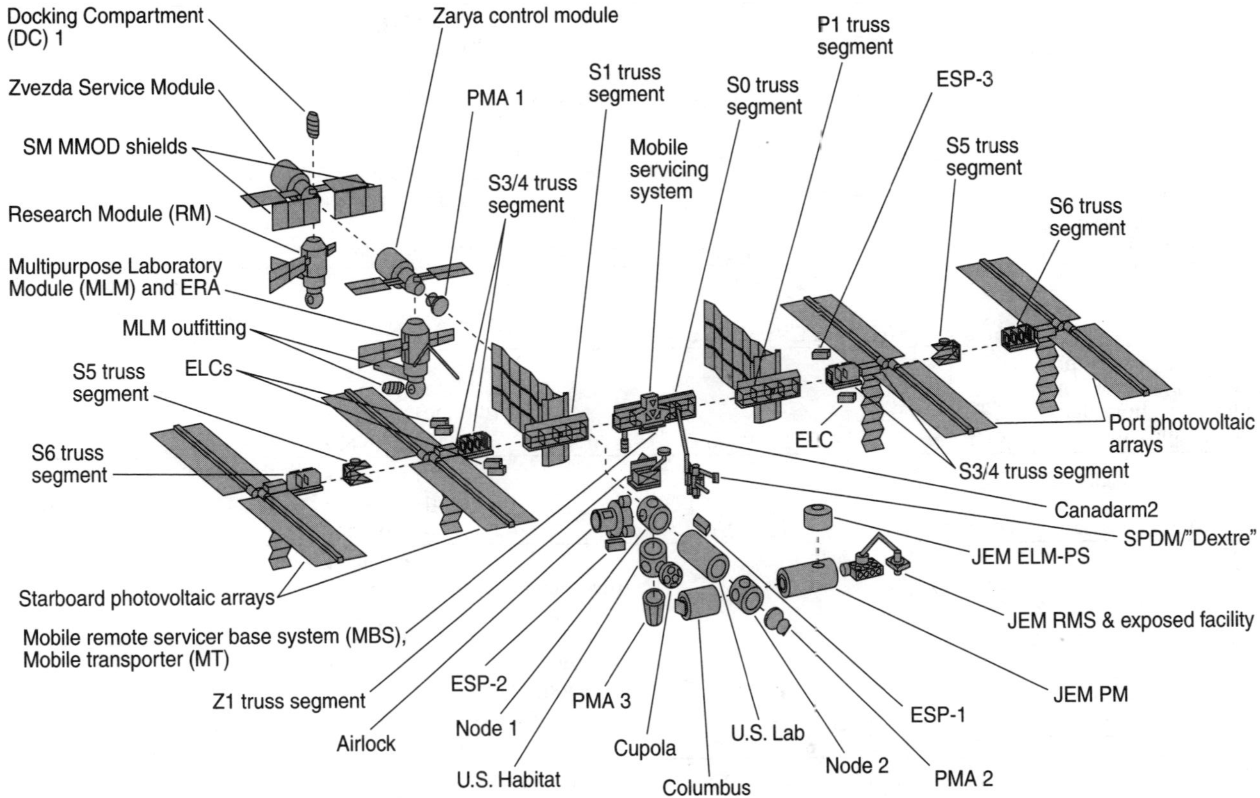

Figure 6.5. Exploded view of the ISS major components.

Table 6.1. Modules on the International Space Station[a]

Module	Location on ISS	Attachments (Location on Module)	Centroid	Length (m)	Diameter (m)	Comment
Node 1 (also Unity)	Not applicable (NA)	• Z1 Truss (top) • US Destiny Lab (front) • US Habitat Module (bottom) • Russian Zarya (rear) through pressurized mating adaptor (PMA) 1 • Quest joint airlock (starboard) • Cupola (port)	–4.42, 0, 4.28	5.49	4.57	This was the second ISS module sent up.
US Lab (also Destiny)	NA	• S0 truss (top) • Node 2 (front) • Node 1 (rear)	0, 0, 4.28	8.53	4.27	NA
US Habitat	NA	• Node 1 (top) • PMA 3 (bottom)	–3.90, 0, 10.96	8.79	4.45	Has oven, fridge/freezer, trash compactor, water supply, hand washer, and bathroom with shower.
PMA 3	Attached to the bottom of US Habitat module.	NA	–3.90, 0, 16.37	2.03	2.79	NA
Node 2 (also Harmony)	NA	• Centrifuge accommodation module (CAM) (top) • PMA 2 (front) • Mini pressurized logistics module (MPLM) (bottom) • US Destiny Lab (rear) • European Space Agency (ESA) lab (starboard) • Japanese Experiment Module (JEM) (port)	10.45, 0, 4.28	7.19	4.42	Provides passageway between three experiment facilities: US, Japanese, and European.

Table 6.1. Modules on the International Space Station[a] *(Continued)*

Module	Location on ISS	Attachments (Location on Module)	Centroid	Length (m)	Diameter (m)	Comment
CAM	Attached to top of Node 2.	NA	11.83, 0, –2.34	8.79	4.45	NA
PMA 2	Attached to front of Node 2.	NA	15.07, 0, 4.28	2.03	2.79	NA
MPLM	Attached to bottom of Node 2.	NA	11.83, 0, 9.73	6.45	4.45	NA
ESA Lab (also Columbus Orbital Facility, COF)	Attached to starboard of Node 2.	NA	11.83, 5.72, 4.28	7.01	4.57	NA
Japanese Experiment Module Pressurized Module (JEM-PM) (also Kibo)	NA	• JEM Experiment Logistics Module (ELM) Pressurized Section (PS) (top) • JEM Exposed Facility (EF) (port) • JEM Remote Manipulator System (RMS) (port)	11.85, –7.81, 4.28	11.2	4.4	NA
JEM-ELM-PS	Attached to the port top of JEM-PM.	NA	11.85, –11.21, 0.13	3.9	4.4	Used for stowage of experiment materials, maintenance tools, and supplies.
JEM-EF	NA	• JEM-PM (starboard) • JEM-ELM-ES (port)	11.85, –15.41, 8.98	4.0	NA	5.0 m height, 5.6 m width. Can hold up to 10 experiment payloads.
JEM-ELM-ES	Attached to the port-side of JEM-EF.	NA	9.05, –19.51, 8.98	4.2	NA	2.2 m height, 4.9 m width. Can hold up to 3 experiment payloads.

Table 6.1. Modules on the International Space Station[a] *(Continued)*

Module	Location on ISS	Attachments (Location on Module)	Centroid	Length (m)	Diameter (m)	Comment
JEM remote manipulator system (RMS)	Attached to the port-side of JEM-PM.	NA	11.85, –18.90, 3.18	10.97	0.33	Astronauts inside the JEM-PM use the JEM-RMS to exchange experiment payloads located on the JEM-EF and the JEM-ELM-ES.
Space Station RMS (SSRMS) (also Canadarm2)	Attached to the mobile servicing system (MSS) that moves along the truss.	NA	0, Y, 0[b]	17.60	0.41	Astronauts inside the ISS use it for heavy-duty functions around the space station. It has a special purpose dexterous manipulator (SPDM) with two 2 m arms.
Quest joint airlock	Attached to the starboard of Node 1.	NA	–3.66, 5.03, 4.28	5.49	3.96	This is the primary entry and departure for ISS space walks by astronauts using US space suits. It can also support space walks by cosmonauts using Russian Orlan space suits.
Cupola	Attached to the port of Node 1.	NA	–2.86, 1.58, 4.28	1.42	2.36	It has windows for observation.
Zarya (also Functional Cargo Block, FGB)	NA	• Node 1 through PMA 1 (front) • Docking and stowage module (DSM) (bottom) • Zvezda (rear) • Two solar arrays (one each on starboard and port)	–14.48, 0, 4.28	12.6	4.1	This was the first ISS module sent up. It was originally used for providing propulsion and power. It is now used for stowage.
PMA 1	Attached to the rear of Node 1 and to the front of Zarya.	NA	–8.18, 0, 4.28	2.03	2.79	NA

Table 6.1. Modules on the International Space Station[a] *(Continued)*

Module	Location on ISS	Attachments (Location on Module)	Centroid	Length (m)	Diameter (m)	Comment
Zarya solar arrays	Two arrays attached to the starboard and port of Zarya.	NA	–13.22, 0, 4.28 (for the pair)	10.7	NA	Specifications are for each solar array. Array width is 3.4 m.
DSM	NA	• Zarya (top) • Sometimes Soyuz to transport crew or supplies or parked to serve as lifecraft (bottom)	–9.63, 0, 10.37	8.08	2.9	NA
Zvezda Service Module	NA	• Science Power Platform (SPP) (top) • Zarya (front) • Universal Docking Module (UDM) (bottom, front end) • Two solar arrays (one each on starboard and port) • Sometimes Progress to transport supplies (rear)	–27.33, 0, 4.28	13.1	3.5	This was the third ISS module sent up. It was modeled after the Mir core module and would have been the core module for Mir 2, which was never built. It provides living quarters and some life support systems to the ISS.
Zvezda solar arrays	Two arrays attached to the starboard and port of Zvezda.	NA	–24.05, 0, 4.28 (for the pair)	13.16	NA	Specifications are for each solar array. Array width is 3.86 m.
UDM	NA	• Zvezda (top) • Docking compartment 1 (DC 1) (starboard/rear) • Research module (RM) 1 (starboard/front) • RM 2 (port/front) • Two life support modules (port/rear)	–22.76, 0, 12.32	12.57	3.96	Serves as docking port for transport and cargo vehicles.

Table 6.1. Modules on the International Space Station[a] *(Continued)*

Module	Location on ISS	Attachments (Location on Module)	Centroid	Length (m)	Diameter (m)	Comment
DC 1 (also Pirs)	In the earlier stages of the ISS, it was attached to the front end bottom of the Zvezda. In the later stages, it was attached to the starboard/rear of the UDM after the latter was integrated into the ISS.	NA	–25.90, 3.14, 17.33	4.91	2.55	In the earlier stages of the ISS, it served as docking port for transport and cargo vehicles and also for spacewalks by cosmonauts using Russian Orlan space suits.
RM 1	Attached to the starboard/front of the UDM.	NA	–18.50, 4.26, 17.16	8.08	2.90	NA
RM 2	Attached to the portside/front of the UDM.	NA	–18.50, –4.26, 17.16	8.08	2.90	NA
Life Support Module (LSM) 1	Attached to the portside/rear of the UDM.	NA	–26.07, –3.31, 17.16	5.41	2.90	NA
LSM 2	Attached to the rear of LSM 1	NA	–29.90, –7.14, 17.16	5.41	2.90	NA
Science Power Platform (SPP) Core	NA	• A pair of SPP photovoltaic arrays (top) • Zvezda (bottom) • SPP radiator (port)	–21.80, 0, –7.31	19.69	2.03	NA
Two SPP photovoltaic arrays (SPP-PVA)	Attached to the top of the SPP Core.	NA	–21.80, 0, –17.16	19.08	NA	Specifications are for each solar array. Average array width is 14.05 m.

Table 6.1. Modules on the International Space Station[a] *(Continued)*

Module	Location on ISS	Attachments (Location on Module)	Centroid	Length (m)	Diameter (m)	Comment
SPP radiator	Attached to the port of the SPP core.	NA	–21.80, –10.99, 2.53	19.94	NA	Width is 3.76 m.
Soyuz spacecraft (piloted)	NA	NA	NA	7.01	2.69	Sometimes docks at the bottom of the DSM or the UDM for transport of crew and also serves as lifecraft.
Progress (unpiloted)	NA	NA	NA	7.24	2.77	Sometimes docks at the rear of Zvezda for transport of supplies.

[a] In the descriptions, if the component resembles a cuboid, the convention used is: Length is measured along the *Y*-axis, height along the *Z*-axis, and width along the *X*-axis. If the component resembles a plate or a cylinder, length denotes the dimension along the axis that makes obvious sense according to the layout in the exploded view. The geometrical centroid of each component is obtained by geometrically assembling the ISS components according to the exploded view and then computing the location. Finally, in the following descriptions of components, the term "starboard" refers to the right and "port" refers to the left if one faces the same direction as the velocity of the ISS.

[b] Y is variable and is dependent on the position of the MSS on the track of the trusses. The extreme values of Y are given by the edge of the S3 Truss + 0.5 × extended SSRMS robot arm length and similarly by the edge of the P3 Truss + 0.5 ×extended SSRMS robot arm length. Hence, we have $-36.08 \le Y \le +36.08$.

Table 6.2. Trusses[a] and Attached Components on the International Space Station

Truss	ISS Location	Centroid	Length (m)	Height (m)	Width (m)	Attached Component			
						Name	Length/Width (m)	Centroid	Axis
S0	Center	0, 0, 0	13.41	4.57	3.35	NA	NA	NA	NA
S1	Starboard	0, 13.56, 0	13.72	4.57	1.83	Thermal power system radiators[b]	23.04/11.53	–12.43, 13.56, 0	NA
S3	Starboard	0, 23.85, 0	6.86	4.29	3.35	NA	NA	NA	NA
S4	Starboard	0, 31.40, 0	8.23	2.82	2.24	Photovoltaic arrays - US[c]	72.19/11.68	0, 33.90, 0	6.62 m from S3/S4 truss interface (I/F)
						Electrical power system radiators[d]	13.69/3.40	0, 29.78, 8.26	2.50 m from S3/S4 truss I/F
S5	Starboard	0, 39.52, 0	8.03	2.82	2.24	NA	NA	NA	NA
S6	Starboard	0, 47.04, 0	7.01	2.82	2.24	Photovoltaic arrays - US[c]	72.19/11.68	0, 49.54, 0	6.01 m from S5/S6 truss I/F
						Electrical power system radiators[d]	13.69/3.40	0, 46.04, 8.26	2.50 m from S5/S6 truss I/F
P1	Port	0, –13.56, 0	13.72	4.57	1.83	Thermal power system radiators[b]	23.04/11.53	–12.43, –13.56, 0	NA

Table 6.2. Trusses[a] and Attached Components on the International Space Station *(Continued)*

						Attached Component			
Truss	ISS Location	Centroid	Length (m)	Height (m)	Width (m)	Name	Length/Width (m)	Centroid	Axis
P3	Port	0, –23.85, 0	6.86	4.29	3.35	NA	NA	NA	NA
P4	Port	0, –31.40, 0	8.23	2.82	2.24	Photovoltaic arrays - US[c]	72.19/11.68	0, –33.90, 0	6.62 m from P3/P4 truss I/F
						Electrical power system radiators[d]	13.69/3.40	0, –29.78, 8.26	2.50 m from P3/P4 truss I/F
P5	Port	0, –39.52, 0	8.03	2.82	2.24	NA	NA	NA	NA
P6	Port	0, –47.04, 0	7.01	2.82	2.24	Photovoltaic arrays - US[c]	72.19/11.68	0, –49.54, 0	6.01 m from S5/S6 truss I/F
						Electrical power system radiators[d]	13.69/3.40	0, –46.04, 8.26	2.50 m from P5/P6 truss I/F
Z1[e]	Top of Unity	–2.82, 0, 0.52	4.50	2.95	2.29	NA	NA	NA	NA

[a] Some truss components have hexagonal cross sections. However, for simplicity, we shall assume these cross sections to be rectangular so that we shall characterize the truss components by length, width, and height.

[b] There are two radiators, one each attached to the rear of S1 and P1 trusses. The specifications are for each radiator.

[c] One inch thick. There are four arrays, one each attached to S4, S6, P4, and P6 trusses. The specifications are for each array.

[d] There are four radiators, one each attached to the bottom of S4, S6, P4, and P6 trusses. The specifications are for each radiator.

[e] Temporarily installed on Unity for mounting US solar array to provide power supply during early stages of ISS assembly.

6.3 Transformation from Inertial to ISS Body System

In this section, we shall derive the equations that transform a point in the inertial system (X_I,Y_I,Z_I) to the corresponding point in the ISS body system (X, Y, Z). The inertial system has its origin at Earth's center, with the X_I-axis in the direction of the vernal equinox, the Z_I-axis perpendicular to the Earth's equator, and the Y_I-axis completing the right-handed triad. The ISS body system was described in Section 6.2. Let Ω denote the longitude of the ascending node, i the inclination, and u the argument of latitude of the ISS. That is, we have

$$u = \omega + \nu \tag{6.26}$$

where ω is the argument of perigee and ν is the true anomaly.

Let the prime system (X', Y', Z') be obtained from the inertial system by a rotation through an angle Ω about the Z_I-axis. Next, let the double-prime system (X'', Y'', Z'') be obtained from the prime system by a rotation through an angle i about the X′-axis. Furthermore, let the triple-prime system (X''', Y''', Z''') be obtained from the double-prime system by a rotation through an angle u about the Z''-axis. All three systems (prime, double-prime, and triple-prime) have their origins at the center of Earth. The three Euler angles (Ω, i, u) and the sequence of rotations 3-1-3 are well known in rigid-body dynamics.[6.4]

Let $\mathbf{R}_I$ denote any vector in the inertial system, and let $\mathbf{R}'''$ denote the corresponding vector in the triple-prime system. Then, we have

$$\mathbf{R}''' = T\mathbf{R}_I \tag{6.27}$$

where the transformation matrix T is given by

$$\begin{aligned} T &= \begin{bmatrix} c_u & s_u & 0 \\ -s_u & c_u & 0 \\ 0 & 0 & 1 \end{bmatrix} \begin{bmatrix} 1 & 0 & 0 \\ 0 & c_i & s_i \\ 0 & -s_i & c_i \end{bmatrix} \begin{bmatrix} c_\Omega & s_\Omega & 0 \\ -s_\Omega & c_\Omega & 0 \\ 0 & 0 & 1 \end{bmatrix} \\ &= \begin{bmatrix} (c_\Omega c_u - s_\Omega c_i s_u) & (s_\Omega c_u + c_\Omega c_i s_u) & (s_i s_u) \\ (-c_\Omega s_u - s_\Omega c_i c_u) & (-s_\Omega s_u + c_\Omega c_i c_u) & (s_i c_u) \\ (s_\Omega s_i) & (-c_\Omega s_i) & (c_i) \end{bmatrix} \end{aligned} \tag{6.28}$$

In Eq. (6.28), we have used the widely accepted notation to denote the sine and cosine functions by the abbreviations s and c, and denote their arguments by subscripts.

The ISS is three-axis-stabilized and always Earth-pointing and, moreover, the eccentricity of the orbit is very small ($e \approx 0.002$). Thus, there is a relation between the triple-prime system and the ISS body system (**X**, **Y**, **Z**). This is illustrated in Fig. 6.6, from which we obtain

$$\widehat{\mathbf{X}'''} = -\widehat{\mathbf{Z}}, \qquad \widehat{\mathbf{Y}'''} = \widehat{\mathbf{X}}, \qquad \widehat{\mathbf{Z}'''} = -\widehat{\mathbf{Y}} \tag{6.29}$$

We had stated in Section 6.1 that we can use the spacecraft orbit and attitude data to obtain the unit vectors ($\hat{\mathbf{X}}, \hat{\mathbf{Y}}, \hat{\mathbf{Z}}$) defining the ISS body system with respect to an inertial frame. Now, we have simplified the requirements to just the orbit data.

From Eq. (6.29), we obtain

$$\begin{bmatrix} \widehat{\mathbf{X}'''}\cdot\widehat{\mathbf{X}} & \widehat{\mathbf{Y}'''}\cdot\widehat{\mathbf{X}} & \widehat{\mathbf{Z}'''}\cdot\widehat{\mathbf{X}} \\ \widehat{\mathbf{X}'''}\cdot\widehat{\mathbf{Y}} & \widehat{\mathbf{Y}'''}\cdot\widehat{\mathbf{Y}} & \widehat{\mathbf{Z}'''}\cdot\widehat{\mathbf{Y}} \\ \widehat{\mathbf{X}'''}\cdot\widehat{\mathbf{Z}} & \widehat{\mathbf{Y}'''}\cdot\widehat{\mathbf{Z}} & \widehat{\mathbf{Z}'''}\cdot\widehat{\mathbf{Z}} \end{bmatrix} = \begin{bmatrix} 0 & 1 & 0 \\ 0 & 0 & -1 \\ -1 & 0 & 0 \end{bmatrix} \tag{6.30}$$

Let $\mathbf{R}_I$ denote any vector in the inertial system (with origin at the center of Earth), and let **R** denote the corresponding vector in the ISS body system (with origin at the center of mass of the ISS). Let $\mathbf{R}_{ISS}$ denote the orbital position of the ISS in the inertial system. It follows from Eqs. (6.27) through (6.30) that

$$\mathbf{R} = Q\left(\mathbf{R}_I - \mathbf{R}_{ISS}\right) \tag{6.31}$$

where the transformation matrix Q is given by

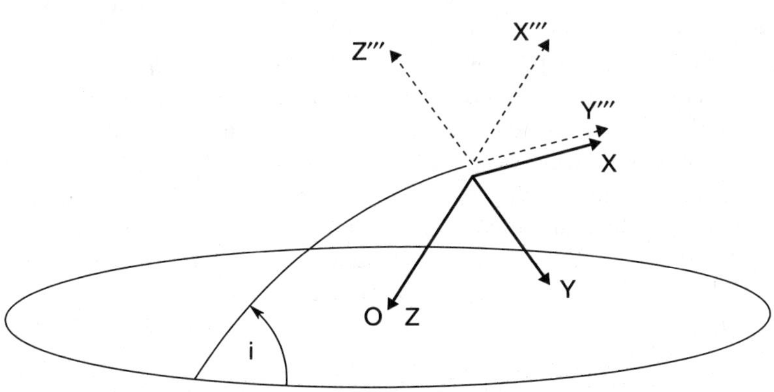

Figure 6.6. Relation between the triple-prime system and the ISS body system.

$$Q=\begin{bmatrix} 0 & 1 & 0 \\ 0 & 0 & -1 \\ -1 & 0 & 0 \end{bmatrix}\begin{bmatrix} (c_\Omega c_u - s_\Omega c_i s_u) & (s_\Omega c_u + c_\Omega c_i s_u) & (s_i s_u) \\ (-c_\Omega s_u - s_\Omega c_i c_u) & (-s_\Omega s_u + c_\Omega c_i c_u) & (s_i c_u) \\ (s_\Omega s_i) & (-c_\Omega s_i) & (c_i) \end{bmatrix}$$

$$=\begin{bmatrix} (-c_\Omega s_u - s_\Omega c_i c_u) & (-s_\Omega s_u + c_\Omega c_i c_u) & (s_i c_u) \\ (-s_\Omega s_i) & (c_\Omega s_i) & (-c_i) \\ (-c_\Omega c_u + s_\Omega c_i s_u) & (-s_\Omega c_u - c_\Omega c_i s_u) & (-s_i s_u) \end{bmatrix}. \tag{6.32}$$

In particular, suppose the vector $\mathbf{R}_I$ in the inertial system is the sun vector $\mathbf{R}_{\text{Sun}}$. Its magnitude is approximately 1.5×10^8 km. For the ISS, the magnitude of $\mathbf{R}_{\text{ISS}}$ is approximately 6.72×10^3 km. Thus, the direction of $(\mathbf{R}_{\text{Sun}} - \mathbf{R}_{\text{ISS}})$ is essentially the same as that of $\mathbf{R}_{\text{Sun}}$. It follows from Eq. (6.32) that the unit sun vector $\hat{\mathbf{R}}$ as seen from the ISS is essentially given by

$$\hat{\mathbf{R}} = Q\widehat{\mathbf{R}_{Sun}} \tag{6.33}$$

The apparent right ascension α and declination δ of the sun are given yearly in tabular form in the *Astronomical Almanac*[6.5] and are accurate to approximately 4×10^{-5} deg. However, they are available only on integral days. At other times, it is necessary to resort to table lookup and interpolation. Equations may be used to compute the values at any particular time, but these formulas are rather complicated and cumbersome to use in-line within a standalone computer program. A relatively compact algorithm is given in the *Almanac for Computers,*[6.6] but it yields results accurate to approximately 3×10^{-1} deg. Another algorithm given in the *Astronomical Almanac*[6.5] is accurate to 1×10^{-2} deg, but the answer is expressed in a mean J2000 system.

The next section of this chapter presents a simple method for computing right ascension and declination accurate to approximately 3×10^{-3} deg. For simulation studies to compute the probability of collision of the ISS with orbiting debris, it is important to compute the unit sun vector easily and accurately in-line because the huge sun-pointing solar panels present a major contribution to the collision integral. In actual flight, the pointing of solar panels to track the sun is accomplished with a gimbal system. There are errors in the sun-pointing of the solar panels so that their normals are not perfectly aligned in the direction of the sun vector.

6.4 Computation of the Sun Vector

The orbit of Earth around the sun varies slightly from year to year because of forces from planets and other sources. Thus, the sun vector (the vector from Earth to the sun) varies likewise. If we concentrate on a particular year, we may perform a Fourier decomposition of the true longitude θ of the sun as follows:

$$\theta - \phi \equiv f(\phi) = \frac{1}{2}a_0 + a_1 \cos\phi + a_2 \cos 2\phi + \cdots \\ + b_1 \sin\phi + b_2 \sin 2\phi + \cdots \tag{6.34}$$

where

$$\begin{aligned} \phi &\equiv \varpi\left(t - t_{VE}\right) \\ a_0 &= \frac{1}{\pi}\int_{-\pi}^{+\pi} f(\phi)\,d\phi \\ a_n &= \frac{1}{\pi}\int_{-\pi}^{+\pi} f(\phi)\cos n\phi\,d\phi \qquad n = 1,2,\cdots \\ b_n &= \frac{1}{\pi}\int_{-\pi}^{+\pi} f(\phi)\sin n\phi\,d\phi \qquad n = 1,2,\cdots \end{aligned} \tag{6.35}$$

In Eqs. (6.34) and (6.35), the period is the tropical year from equinox to equinox, t_{VE} is the universal time (UT) of vernal equinox in the year of interest, and ϖ is the rate of daily change of the geometric mean longitude of the sun (0.985647359 deg per 24 h). However, if we proceed exactly as described above, we need to obtain the longitude θ of the sun as a function of time and then perform lengthy computations to evaluate the integrals to obtain the coefficients a_n and b_n. These are then substituted into Eq. (6.34) so as to obtain θ for computing the right ascension and declination of the sun. The logic of the whole scheme is circuitous!

However, Chan,[6.7] retaining some of these concepts, has bypassed the process described here and developed a novel compact algorithm that can be used to compute the sun vector over a long period, say 100 years. The details are given in Appendix A. The main results of the computation of the sun vector are summarized here.

6.4.1 Results of Computing the Sun Vector

Let θ be written in the form

$$\begin{aligned} \theta = \phi &- A'\left[\left(1 - B'\right) - \cos\left(\phi - C'\right)\right] \\ &- A''\left[\left(1 - B''\right) - \cos\left(\phi - C''\right)\right] \\ &+ A'''\cos 2\left(\phi - C'''\right) + \cdots \end{aligned} \tag{6.36}$$

(1) Retention of only the first term ϕ in Eq. (6.36) typically leads to results with errors less than 3.5 deg in the right ascension and declination of the sun vector throughout the entire year.

(2) The coefficients A', B', and C' are constant from year to year and are respectively set equal to 1.8, 0.0285, and 15 deg. Inclusion of the A', B', and C' terms typically leads to results with errors less than 0.25 deg in the right ascension and declination of the sun vector. This truncated formula yields the same accuracy as that given in Ref. 6.5 but is much simpler to use. It also meets the requirements of the sun-pointing of the huge solar panels of the ISS. Thus, we can stop at this stage for this application and use the following equation:

$$\begin{aligned}\theta &= \phi - 1.8\left[\left(1-0.0285\right)-\cos\left(\phi-15^\circ\right)\right]\\ &= \phi - 1.7487 + 1.8\cos\left(\phi-15^\circ\right)\end{aligned} \tag{6.37}$$

(3) The coefficients A'', B'', and C'' vary from year to year and are related to a_0, a_1, and b_1 in Eq. (6.34) through the constants A', B', and C' (the details being unnecessary). Throughout the nineteen-year period from 1989 to 2007, inclusion of the A'', B'', and C'' terms typically leads to results with errors less than 0.025 deg in the right ascension and declination of the sun vector. This is more than sufficient for the requirements of many applications.

(4) The coefficients A''' and C''' vary from year to year and are related to a_2 and b_2 in Eq. (6.34). Throughout the nineteen-year period from 1989 to 2007, inclusion of the A''' and C''' terms typically leads to results with errors less than 0.0025 deg in the right ascension and declination of the sun vector. This is sufficient for the requirements of practically all applications.

(5) The only inputs into Eq. (6.36) are ϕ, which depends on t_{VE} (the UT time of vernal equinox in the year of interest), and t (the day plus fraction thereof from January $0^d.0$ in the year of interest).

(6) The UT time of vernal equinox for the year of interest was computed using Sunlit Design's The Sun API,[6.8] a solar value calculation freeware program. It is extremely accurate and yields results to within a few seconds of those obtained using the U. S. Naval Observatory's programs for equinox computations. Table 6.3 gives the times of the vernal equinox for the 100 years from 1961 to 2060.

(7) Using the times of vernal equinox from 1989 to 2007 in this table and the right ascension and declination of the sun from the *Astronomical Almanac* during the same period, we obtained values of the coefficients A'', B'', A''', and C''' in Eq. (6.36) as described above and replaced them simply by their average values for years beyond 2007. The values of C'' obtained in this period are replaced by the best linear fit beyond 2007. As a test of goodness of fit, the right ascension and declination of the sun in the year 2008 are computed using this information and then compared to the corresponding values in the 2008 *Astronomical Almanac,*

Table 6.3. Times of the Vernal Equinox, 1961–2060

Year	Time of Vernal Equinox	Year	Time of Vernal Equinox	Year	Time of Vernal Equinox	Year	Time of Vernal Equinox
1961	79.85566875	1986	79.91856905	2011	79.9725679	2036	80.04309918
1962	80.10385685	1987	80.16117959	2012	80.21822807	2037	79.28429502
1963	80.34699542	1988	80.40197355	2013	79.45952563	2038	79.52758648
1964	80.5902155	1989	79.64469547	2014	79.70616165	2039	79.77162354
1965	79.83666607	1990	79.88840101	2015	79.94785142	2040	80.00749046
1966	80.07841733	1991	80.12633595	2016	80.18749867	2041	79.25411512
1967	80.31725039	1992	80.36672793	2017	79.43637726	2042	79.49472051
1968	80.5570038	1993	79.61158129	2018	79.67717171	2043	79.72696347
1969	79.79739333	1994	79.85279223	2019	79.91534084	2044	79.97194242
1970	80.03915012	1995	80.09338649	2020	80.15925408	2045	79.21294405
1971	80.27654286	1996	80.3355203	2021	79.40078184	2046	79.45620617
1972	80.51489312	1997	79.57966111	2022	79.64791807	2047	79.70259208
1973	79.75868516	1998	79.82956377	2023	79.89165286	2048	79.93955301
1974	80.00460592	1999	80.07353258	2024	80.12916385	2049	79.1858519
1975	80.24769905	2000	80.3162208	2025	79.37571068	2050	79.42957527
1976	80.49282098	2001	79.56310966	2026	79.61486418	2051	79.66531313
1977	79.73779198	2002	79.80295326	2027	79.85012506	2052	79.91319707
1978	79.98166192	2003	80.04159547	2028	80.09482747	2053	79.15715465
1979	80.22359315	2004	80.28375843	2029	79.33424953	2054	79.39820862
1980	80.46511692	2005	79.52317216	2030	79.57732744	2055	79.64415138
1981	79.71035227	2006	79.76770518	2031	79.81961629	2056	79.88200562
1982	79.95545088	2007	80.00507046	2032	80.05635999	2057	79.1298023
1983	80.19355562	2008	80.24180157	2033	79.30697852	2058	79.37777207
1984	80.43360632	2009	79.48858214	2034	79.55334562	2059	79.61339886
1985	79.6762363	2010	79.73057556	2035	79.79313935	2060	79.85939588

just published as of this writing. They yield the sun vector accurate to approximately 5×10^{-3} deg.

(8) The right ascension α and declination δ of the sun are computed from the true longitude θ by the following equations:

$$\tan\alpha = \cos\varepsilon \, \tan\theta \tag{6.38}$$

$$\sin\delta = \sin\varepsilon \, \sin\theta \tag{6.39}$$

where ε is the obliquity of the ecliptic (the angle between Earth's equatorial plane and the plane of Earth's orbit around the sun). The value of ε is time-dependent, but a sufficiently accurate formula is

$$\varepsilon = 23^{\circ}.438251 - 0^{\circ}.000130(\text{Year} - 2008) \tag{6.40}$$

6.5 Sample Orbit of the ISS

The orbital elements for the ISS on 18 March 2007 at 19 hr 33 min 51 sec UT were:

semimajor axis $a = 6721.646$ km
eccentricity $e = 0.0020328$
inclination $i = 51.634487$ deg
longitude of ascending node $\Omega = 210.794349$ deg
argument of perigee $\omega = 2.284813$ deg
mean anomaly $M = 359.747937$ deg

From these orbital elements, we obtain:

altitude $h \approx 344$ km
eccentric anomaly $E = 359.7479281$ deg
true anomaly $v = 359.7474151$ deg
argument of latitude $u \equiv \omega + v = 2.032228125$ deg

Those values were obtained with the following equations:

$$E - e\sin E = M \tag{6.41}$$

$$\tan\left(\frac{v}{2}\right) = \sqrt{\frac{1+e}{1-e}}\tan\left(\frac{E}{2}\right) \tag{6.42}$$

The mean motion (or average angular velocity) n is given by:[6.9]

$$n = 3.1252977 \times 10^{9} a^{-3/2} \quad (\text{deg/ day}) \qquad \text{where } a \text{ is in km} \tag{6.43}$$

For the ISS, we obtain $n = 3.938$ deg/min so that the orbital period is 91.409 min and there are 15.753 orbits/day. Because $e \ll 1$, we may regard the ISS orbit as circular for illustrative purposes. Thus, we may write

$$u = n\left(t - t_{\text{eq}}\right) \tag{6.44}$$

where t_{eq} is the time of equatorial crossing on ascension.

The longitude of ascending node Ω precesses because of Earth's oblateness according to the formula[6.9]

$$\left(\frac{d\Omega}{dt}\right)_{J_2} = -2.06474\times10^{14} a^{-7/2}\left(1-e^2\right)^{-2}\cos i \quad (\text{deg}/\,day) \qquad \text{where } a \text{ is in km} \tag{6.45}$$

For the ISS, we obtain $(d\Omega/dt)_{J2} = -5.147$ deg/day. This value compares well with the value of $d\Omega/dt = -5.051125895$ deg/day obtained from flight data. We shall use the latter value for the precession of the longitude of ascending node. Thus, we write

$$\Omega = \Omega_{\text{eq}} + \left(\frac{d\Omega}{dt}\right)\left(t - t_{\text{eq}}\right) \tag{6.46}$$

where Ω_{eq} is the value of the ascending node at t_{eq}. From the preceding information, we find that t_{eq} for this orbit occurred on 18 March 2007 at 19 h 33 min 20.039 sec and $\Omega_{\text{eq}} = 210.796159$ deg.

In Section 6.3, we derived the transformation between the inertial system and the ISS body system. The matrix Q in Eq. (6.32) gives the transformation of a vector from the inertial system to the ISS body system. Because this transformation is orthogonal, the inverse transformation Q^{-1} from the ISS body system to the inertial system is equal to the transpose matrix Q^T. That is, we have

$$Q^{-1} = Q^T = \begin{bmatrix} (-c_\Omega s_u - s_\Omega c_i c_u) & (-s_\Omega s_i) & (-c_\Omega c_u + s_\Omega c_i s_u) \\ (-s_\Omega s_u + c_\Omega c_i c_u) & (c_\Omega s_i) & (-s_\Omega c_u - c_\Omega c_i s_u) \\ (s_i c_u) & (-c_i) & (-s_i s_u) \end{bmatrix} \tag{6.47}$$

In the ISS body system described in Section 6.2, the X-axis is in the direction of the ISS velocity vector (roll axis), the Y-axis is along the starboard trusses (pitch axis), and the Z-axis points toward Earth (yaw axis). We wish to illustrate how the three base vectors $\hat{\mathbf{X}}$, $\hat{\mathbf{Y}}$, and $\hat{\mathbf{Z}}$ change as the ISS goes through an illustrative orbit. Let $\hat{\mathbf{X}}^*$, $\hat{\mathbf{Y}}^*$, and $\hat{\mathbf{Z}}^*$ respectively denote these three vectors transformed to the inertial system. Let $\hat{\mathbf{X}}_I$, $\hat{\mathbf{Y}}_I$, and $\hat{\mathbf{Z}}_I$ denote the three unit base vectors in the inertial system; that is, $\hat{\mathbf{X}}_I$ points in the direction of the vernal equinox, $\hat{\mathbf{Z}}_I$ is perpendicular to Earth's equator, and $\hat{\mathbf{Y}}_I$ completes the right-handed triad. Then, we obtain

$$\begin{aligned} \widehat{\mathbf{X}^*} &= Q^T\,\widehat{\mathbf{X}} = -(c_\Omega s_u + s_\Omega c_i c_u)\widehat{\mathbf{X}_I} + (c_\Omega c_i c_u - s_\Omega s_u)\widehat{\mathbf{Y}_I} + s_i c_u \widehat{\mathbf{Z}_I} \\ \widehat{\mathbf{Y}^*} &= Q^T\,\widehat{\mathbf{Y}} = -s_\Omega s_i \widehat{\mathbf{X}_I} + c_\Omega s_i \widehat{\mathbf{Y}_I} - c_i \widehat{\mathbf{Z}_I} \\ \widehat{\mathbf{Z}^*} &= Q^T\,\widehat{\mathbf{Z}} = (s_\Omega c_i s_u - c_\Omega c_u)\widehat{\mathbf{X}_I} - (s_\Omega c_u + c_\Omega c_i s_u)\widehat{\mathbf{Y}_I} - s_i s_u \widehat{\mathbf{Z}_I} \end{aligned} \tag{6.48}$$

Equations (6.44) and (6.46) and the value of the inclination i are substituted into Eq. (6.48) to obtain the time evolution of these three ISS body system unit vectors in the inertial system. We recall that the argument of latitude u is rapidly varying with time (360 deg/orbit), whereas the longitude of ascending node Ω is slowly varying with time (= –0.327 deg/orbit). Therefore, $\hat{\mathbf{X}}^*$ and $\hat{\mathbf{Z}}^*$ go through 360 deg while $\hat{\mathbf{Y}}^*$ is essentially constant in direction throughout one orbit. ($\hat{\mathbf{Y}}^*$ is in the opposite direction to the angular momentum vector, which precesses slowly as a result of Earth's oblateness.)

Next, we compute the sun vector at the time t_{eq} in the inertial system using Eqs. (A.12) through (A.14) of Appendix A. We obtain the right ascension α = 358.00 deg and declination δ = –0.867 deg. Therefore, the unit sun vector $\hat{\mathbf{S}}$ is given by

$$\hat{\mathbf{S}} = \cos\alpha \, \cos\delta \, \widehat{\mathbf{X}_I} + \sin\alpha \, \cos\delta \, \widehat{\mathbf{Y}_I} + \sin\delta \, \widehat{\mathbf{Z}_I} \tag{6.49}$$

The direction of this vector is also slowly varying throughout one orbit of the ISS. A little consideration reveals that, in the ISS body system, the sun vector $\hat{\mathbf{S}}$ essentially traces out part of a right circular cone whose axis is the $\hat{\mathbf{Y}}^*$ vector during the time the ISS orbit is not in Earth's shadow. The cone angle γ between $\hat{\mathbf{Y}}^*$ and $\hat{\mathbf{S}}$ is given by

$$\cos\gamma = -\sin\Omega \, \sin i \cos\alpha \, \cos\delta + \cos\Omega \, \sin i \sin\alpha \, \cos\delta - \cos i \sin\delta \tag{6.50}$$

If we substitute the values of Ω, i, α, and δ into Eq. (6.50), we obtain γ = 65.464 deg. This cone is illustrated in Fig. 6.7. The direction of the motion of the sun vector in the ISS body system is counterclockwise looking along the port direction.

6.6 Annual Variation of the Sun Vector in the ISS Body System

In the ISS orbit, the inclination is maintained at what is essentially a constant value of approximately 51.634 deg. The other three angles (Ω, α, and δ) vary annually much more than the inclination. We shall investigate how the cone angle γ varies throughout the year because of their variations. The rate of precession of the ascending node Ω varies somewhat, but it may be assumed to be maintained at the approximate value of –5.051 deg/day. Thus, from the orbital elements given in the previous section, we obtain Ω = 243.8485874 deg on January $0^d.0$, 2007. We then compute Ω, α, and δ at five-day intervals. The results are shown in Fig. 6.8.

It is seen that the sun vector cone angle in the ISS body system goes through approximately 6 cycles in a year. This variation is the result of the effects of the eastward drift of the sun vector at an average of 1 deg per day and also the westward drift of the longitude of the ascending node at approximately 5 deg per day in the inertial system. Thus, there is a relative drift of approximately 6 deg per

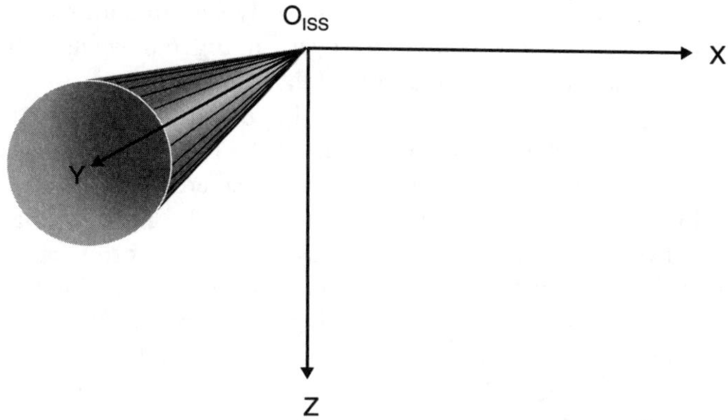

Figure 6.7. Cone traced out by the sun vector in the ISS body system.

day or, equivalently, 360 deg in 60 days. Therefore, these two variables line up every two months, which is the period of each cycle. Hence, there are 6 such cycles in one year, in accordance with Fig. 6.8.

In each of these cycles, the cone angle γ has a variation of approximately 100 deg. Moreover, it goes through 90 deg twice in each cycle. When the cone angle is less than 90 deg, it is on the starboard side. If it starts at the low point in a cycle, it gradually increases and reaches 90 deg, at which instant it lies on the (X, Z)-plane of the ISS body system. Then, it switches to the port side and continues to increase until it reaches the high point of the cycle. Then, it begins to decrease and once

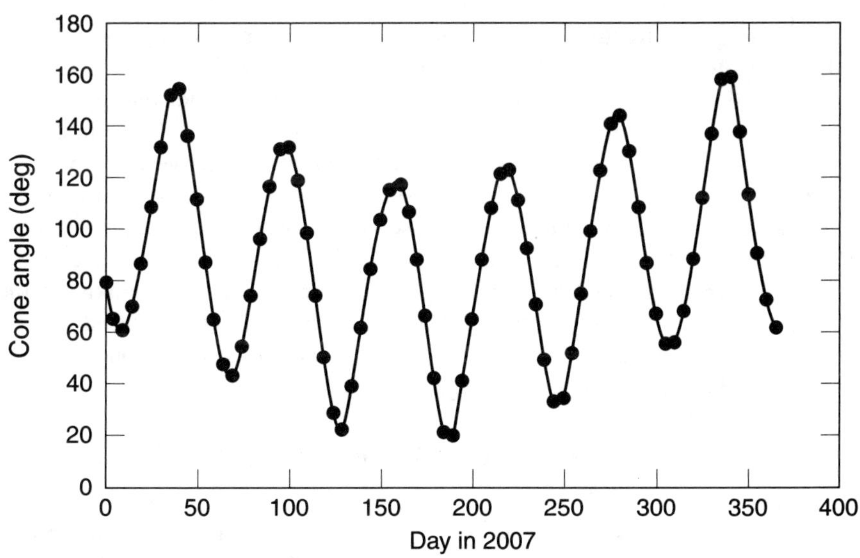

Figure 6.8. Annual variation of sun vector cone angle.

again goes through the (X, Z)-plane of the ISS body system until it is on the starboard side and reaches the low point of the cycle. In Fig. 6.8, we note that the low points and their respective high points are not the same from cycle to cycle. In one year, the cone angle γ goes through a range of 140 deg from 20 to 160 deg.

In Section 6.5, we studied only one orbit of the ISS. Because the sun vector and the longitude of the ascending node were considered frozen, we concluded that, in the ISS body system, the sun vector traced out a right circular cone. In reality, these two quantities are slowly varying over an orbit, and there are approximately 15.753 orbits in a day. Therefore, the sun vector actually traces out a path on a sheet that is tangent along a straight line with an osculating right circular cone. (This phenomenon is very much the same as the orbit of a satellite moving around a nonspherical central body being tangent at every point with an osculating Keplerian orbit.) Only that part of the sheet is applicable when the ISS orbit is not in Earth's shadow.

The direction of the motion of the sun vector in the ISS body system is counterclockwise looking along the port direction. We know that when the cone angle is 90 deg, the sun vector lies in the (X, Z)-plane of the ISS body system. Therefore, in this special case, the solar panels undergo a simple rotation about the Y-axis (instead of two gimbal angles, one about the Y-axis and the other about the axis of the solar panels). To illustrate the computation of the collision probability, we shall consider the simple case for which the solar panels are rotated 45 deg about the Y-axis. Other orientations of the solar panels are also possible depending on the direction of the sun vector, and the ascending node and argument of latitude of the ISS. However, examination of Fig. 6.8 indicates that there cannot be any direction of the normal within a cone of 20 deg on the starboard and also the port directions. Even though Fig. 6.8 is specifically for the year 2007, this statement is generally valid for other years as well.

We shall next study three cases for which the normal to the solar panels lies in the (X, Z)-plane and makes an angle of 30 deg with the X-axis. In the first case, the secondary body approaches the ISS head-on so that the relative velocity $\mathbf{v}_{sp}$ of the secondary with respect to the ISS is along the negative X-axis. That is, $\mathbf{v}_{ps}$ is along the positive X-axis. In the second case, the secondary body approaches the ISS broadside so that the relative velocity $\mathbf{v}_{sp}$ of the secondary with respect to the ISS is along the negative Y-axis. That is, $\mathbf{v}_{ps}$ is along the positive Y-axis. In the third case, the secondary body approaches the ISS from above (overhead) so that the relative velocity $\mathbf{v}_{sp}$ of the secondary with respect to the ISS is along the positive Z-axis. That is, $\mathbf{v}_{ps}$ is along the negative Z-axis.

6.7 Case Study I: Head-On Collision Probability

In this case, the velocity of the secondary object is toward the ISS along the negative $\hat{\mathbf{X}}$ direction so that we have $\hat{\mathbf{y}} \equiv \hat{\mathbf{v}}_{ps} = \hat{\mathbf{X}}$. Suppose at time $t = t_{\text{ISS}}$ the "nominal" closest approach occurs between the center of mass of the ISS and the secondary. At this instant, suppose the secondary is horizontally at a distance x_e on the port side of the ISS so that we have $\hat{\mathbf{x}} = \hat{\mathbf{Y}}$. In this simple case, we can easily conclude that $\hat{\mathbf{z}} = -\hat{\mathbf{Z}}$. However, we wish to illustrate the general procedure for an arbitrary approach direction. Then, we write the right ascension and declination of these two vectors

$$\alpha_x = \pi / 2, \;\; \delta_x = 0, \;\; \alpha_y = 0, \;\; \delta_y = 0 \tag{6.51}$$

Hence, the transformation matrix (6.25) becomes

$$S = \begin{bmatrix} 0 & 1 & 0 \\ 1 & 0 & 0 \\ 0 & 0 & -1 \end{bmatrix} \tag{6.52}$$

In the ISS ($\hat{\mathbf{X}}, \hat{\mathbf{Y}}, \hat{\mathbf{Z}}$) body system, let us consider the ith component. Suppose it is a flat plate of arbitrary shape. We recall that the unit normal and its centroid are denoted by

$$\widehat{\mathbf{N}}_i \equiv (U_i, V_i, W_i) \qquad \widehat{\mathbf{R}}_i \equiv (X_i, Y_i, Z_i) \tag{6.53}$$

By Eqs. (6.11), (6.12), and (6.52), these vectors in the ($\hat{\mathbf{x}}, \hat{\mathbf{y}}, \hat{\mathbf{z}}$) encounter system are given by

$$\widehat{\mathbf{n}}_i \equiv (u_i, v_i, w_i) = (V_i, U_i, -W_i) \tag{6.54}$$

$$\widehat{\mathbf{r}}_i \equiv (x_i, y_i, z_i) = ((x_e + Y_i), X_i, -Z_i) \tag{6.55}$$

At time t_{ISS} the ith component may not necessarily be at its nominal closest point of approach with respect to the secondary object. However, by Eq. (6.16), its closest point of approach occurs at time $t = t_i$, given by

$$t_i = t_{\text{ISS}} - X_i / v_{ps} \tag{6.56}$$

Let A_i denote the area of this plate. By Eq. (6.17), the area A of its projection onto its own encounter plane is

$$A = \left| \widehat{\mathbf{n}} \cdot \widehat{\mathbf{y}} \right| A_i = \left| U_i \right| A_i \tag{6.57}$$

If θ is the rotation angle to transform the combined covariance so that it has only diagonal terms $\sigma_{x'}^2$ and $\sigma_{z'}^2$ in the ISS center of mass encounter plane, then Eq. (6.18) yields the additional rotation angle γ to make the combined covariance diagonal in the ith component encounter plane. The nominal miss distance $x_{e,i}$ for the ith component is given by Eq. (6.19). From Eq. (6.55), it follows that

$$\tan\gamma = \frac{-Z_i}{(x_e + Y_i)} \tag{6.58}$$

$$x_{e,i} = \sqrt{\left[(x_e + Y_i)^2 + Z_i^2\right]} \tag{6.59}$$

Equations (6.58) and (6.59) are then substituted into (6.20) to obtain the coordinates of the centroid of the ith component in its own encounter plane. This result and that given by Eq. (6.57) are substituted into Eqs. (6.6) and (6.7) to obtain u and v. Equation (6.10) is used to compute the probability of collision of the ith component with the secondary object. This procedure is performed for every plate or cuboid. In the case of a cylinder, depending on whether we include its end, we use Eq. (6.3) or (6.4) to obtain the projected area A in its own encounter plane.

Under the assumption of no occultation of one component by another except at common interfaces, the probability of collision of the ISS with the secondary object is obtained by summing all the probabilities associated with the individual components. For this head-on approach we take the normal vector of each flat-plate component as shown in the exploded view, except we rotate the huge solar panels (PVA-US) so that the normal makes an angle of 30 deg with the X-axis.

In this case study, the secondary object (space debris) approaches the front of the ISS head-on but is displaced respectively at 10, 1, and 0.1 km to the port side. For simplicity, we consider the two standard deviations $\sigma_{x'} = \sigma_{z'} \equiv \sigma = 5$ and 1 km. We determine the collision probability for combinations of the input collision parameters.

The probability of a head-on collision of the ISS with the secondary object is shown in Table 6.4.

Table 6.4. Probability of Collision for Head-On Approach

$\sigma_{x'}$ (km)	5	5	5	1	1	1
$\sigma_{z'}$ (km)	5	5	5	1	1	1
Miss distance (km)	10	1	0.1	10	1	0.1
Collision probability	3.71×10^{-6}	2.68×10^{-5}	2.74×10^{-5}	1.32×10^{-25}	4.15×10^{-4}	6.81×10^{-4}

6.8 Case Study II: Broadside Collision Probability

We shall proceed as in Case Study I and change the details where appropriate. Now, the velocity of the secondary object is toward the ISS along the $-\hat{\mathbf{Y}}$ direction so that we have $\hat{\mathbf{y}} \equiv \hat{\mathbf{v}}_{ps} = \hat{\mathbf{Y}}$. At the instant $t = t_{\mathrm{ISS}}$ of "nominal" closest approach between the center of mass of the ISS and the secondary, suppose the secondary is horizontally at a distance x_e in front of the ISS so that we have $\hat{\mathbf{x}} = -\hat{\mathbf{X}}$. In this simple case, we can easily conclude that $\hat{\mathbf{z}} = -\hat{\mathbf{Z}}$. Again, we wish to illustrate the general procedure for an arbitrary approach direction. Then, we write the right ascension and declination of these two vectors

$$\alpha_x = \pi, \quad \delta_x = 0, \quad \alpha_y = \pi / 2, \quad \delta_y = 0 \tag{6.60}$$

Hence, the transformation matrix (6.25) becomes

$$S = \begin{bmatrix} -1 & 0 & 0 \\ 0 & 1 & 0 \\ 0 & 0 & -1 \end{bmatrix} \tag{6.61}$$

In the ISS $(\hat{\mathbf{X}}, \hat{\mathbf{Y}}, \hat{\mathbf{Z}})$ body system, let us consider a flat plate of arbitrary shape as the ith component. Again, we recall that the unit normal and its centroid are denoted by

$$\widehat{\mathbf{N}}_i \equiv (U_i, V_i, W_i) \qquad \widehat{\mathbf{R}}_i \equiv (X_i, Y_i, Z_i) \tag{6.62}$$

By Eqs. (6.11), (6.12), and (6.52), these vectors in the $(\hat{\mathbf{x}}, \hat{\mathbf{y}}, \hat{\mathbf{z}})$ encounter system are given by

$$\widehat{\mathbf{n}}_i \equiv (u_i, v_i, w_i) = (-U_i, V_i, -W_i) \tag{6.63}$$

$$\hat{\mathbf{r}}_i \equiv (x_i, y_i, z_i) = ((x_e - X_i), Y_i, -Z_i) \tag{6.64}$$

By Eq. (6.16), the closest point of approach with respect to the secondary object occurs at time $t = t_i$, given by

$$t_i = t_{ISS} - Y_i / v_{ps} \tag{6.65}$$

Let A_i denote the area of this plate. By Eq. (6.17), the area A of its projection onto its own encounter plane is

$$A = \left|\hat{\mathbf{n}} \cdot \hat{\mathbf{y}}\right| A_i = \left|V_i\right| A_i \tag{6.66}$$

The additional rotation angle γ to make the combined covariance diagonal in the ith component encounter plane, and the nominal miss distance $x_{e,i}$ for the ith component, are given by

$$\tan\gamma = \frac{-Z_i}{(x_e - X_i)} \tag{6.67}$$

$$x_{e,i} = \sqrt{\left[(x_e - X_i)^2 + Z_i^2\right]} \tag{6.68}$$

Equations (6.67) and (6.68) are then substituted into (6.20) to obtain the coordinates of the centroid of the ith component in its own encounter plane. This result and that given by Eq. (6.66) are substituted into Eqs. (6.6) and (6.7) to obtain u and v. Equation (6.10) is used to compute the probability of collision of the ith component with the secondary object. This procedure is performed for every plate or cuboid.

In the case of a cylinder, depending on whether we include its end, we use Eq. (6.3) or (6.4) to obtain the projected area A in its own encounter plane.

For this broadside approach, we take the same configuration as in the case of head-on approach (i.e., the normal vector of each flat-plate component shown in the exploded view), except we rotate the huge solar panels (PVA-US) so that the normal makes an angle of 30 deg with the X-axis.

In this case study, the space debris approaches the starboard of the ISS but is displaced respectively at 10, 1, and 0.1 km to the front. Again, we consider the two standard deviations $\sigma_{x'} = \sigma_{z'} \equiv \sigma = 5$ and 1 km. We determine the collision probability for combinations of the input collision parameters.

The probability of a broadside collision of the ISS with the secondary object is shown in Table 6.5.

Table 6.5. Probability of Collision for Broadside Approach

$\sigma_{x'}$ (km)	5	5	5	1	1	1
$\sigma_{z'}$ (km)	5	5	5	1	1	1
Miss distance (km)	10	1	0.1	10	1	0.1
Collision probability	6.93×10^{-7}	5.02×10^{-6}	5.12×10^{-6}	2.47×10^{-26}	7.76×10^{-5}	1.27×10^{-4}

6.9 Case Study III: Overhead Collision Probability

We shall proceed as in Case Studies I and II and change the details where appropriate. Now, the velocity of the secondary object is toward the ISS along the $\hat{\mathbf{Z}}$ direction so that we have $\hat{\mathbf{y}} \equiv \hat{\mathbf{v}}_{ps} = -\hat{\mathbf{Z}}$. At the instant $t = t_{\text{ISS}}$ of "nominal" closest approach between the center of mass of the ISS and the secondary, suppose the secondary is vertically at a distance x_e in front of the ISS so that we have $\hat{\mathbf{x}} = -\hat{\mathbf{X}}$. In this simple case, we can easily conclude that $\hat{\mathbf{z}} = -\hat{\mathbf{Y}}$. Again, we wish to illustrate the general procedure for an arbitrary approach direction. Then, we write the right ascension and declination of these two vectors

$$\alpha_x = \pi, \quad \delta_x = 0, \quad \alpha_y = \text{undefined (anything)}, \quad \delta_y = -\pi/2 \tag{6.69}$$

Hence, the transformation matrix (6.25) becomes

$$S = \begin{bmatrix} -1 & 0 & 0 \\ 0 & 0 & -1 \\ 0 & -1 & 0 \end{bmatrix} \tag{6.70}$$

In the ISS $(\hat{\mathbf{X}}, \hat{\mathbf{Y}}, \hat{\mathbf{Z}})$ body system, let us consider a flat plate of arbitrary shape as the ith component. Again, we recall that the unit normal and its centroid are denoted by

$$\widehat{\mathbf{N}}_i \equiv (U_i, V_i, W_i) \qquad \widehat{\mathbf{R}}_i \equiv (X_i, Y_i, Z_i) \tag{6.71}$$

By Eqs. (6.11), (6.12), and (6.52), these vectors in the $(\hat{\mathbf{x}}, \hat{\mathbf{y}}, \hat{\mathbf{z}})$ encounter system are given by

$$\widehat{\mathbf{n}}_i \equiv (u_i, v_i, w_i) = (-U_i, -W_i, -V_i) \tag{6.72}$$

$$\hat{\mathbf{r}}_i \equiv (x_i, y_i, z_i) = ((x_e - X_i), -Z_i, -Y_i) \tag{6.73}$$

By Eq. (6.16), the closest point of approach with respect to the secondary object occurs at time $t = t_i$, given by

$$t_i = t_{\text{ISS}} + Z_i / v_{ps} \tag{6.74}$$

Let A_i denote the area of this plate. By Eq. (6.17), the area A of its projection onto its own encounter plane is

$$A = \left|\hat{\mathbf{n}} \cdot \hat{\mathbf{y}}\right| A_i = \left|W_i\right| A_i \tag{6.75}$$

The additional rotation angle γ to make the combined covariance diagonal in the ith component encounter plane, and the nominal miss distance $x_{e,i}$ for the ith component, are given by

$$\tan\gamma = \frac{-Y_i}{(x_e - X_i)} \tag{6.76}$$

$$x_{e,i} = \sqrt{\left[(x_e - X_i)^2 + Y_i^2\right]} \tag{6.77}$$

Equations (6.76) and (6.77) are then substituted into (6.20) to obtain the coordinates of the centroid of the ith component in its own encounter plane. This result and that given by Eq. (6.75) are substituted into Eqs. (6.6) and (6.7) to obtain u and v. Equation (6.10) is used to compute the probability of collision of the ith component with the secondary object. This procedure is performed for every plate or cuboid. In the case of a cylinder, depending on whether we include its end, we use Eq. (6.3) or (6.4) to obtain the projected area A in its own encounter plane.

For this overhead approach, we take the same configuration as in the head-on and broadside approaches (i.e., the normal vector of each flat-plate component, as shown in the exploded view), except we rotate the huge solar panels (PVA-US) so that the normal makes an angle of 30 deg with the X-axis.

In this case study, the space debris approaches the top of the ISS but is displaced respectively at 10, 1, and 0.1 km to the rear. Again, we consider the two standard deviations $\sigma_{x'} = \sigma_{z'} \equiv \sigma = 5$ and 1 km. We determine the collision probability for combinations of the input collision parameters.

The probability of an overhead collision of the ISS with the secondary object is shown in Table 6.6.

6.10 Comparison with the Spherical Model

If we sum appropriately all lengths of the trusses and parts of the protruding P6 and S6 photovoltaic arrays - US (PVA-US) of the ISS given in Section 6.2, we

Table 6.6. Probability of Collision for Overhead Approach

$\sigma_{x'}$ (km)	5	5	5	1	1	1
$\sigma_{z'}$ (km)	5	5	5	1	1	1
Miss distance (km)	10	1	0.1	10	1	0.1
Collision probability	2.44×10^{-6}	1.76×10^{-5}	1.80×10^{-5}	8.68×10^{-26}	2.73×10^{-4}	4.48×10^{-4}

obtain a total of 110.79 m from end to end along the *Y*-axis. This compares well with the value of 110 m reported in *Jane's Space Directory.*[6.10] Similarly, if we sum the lengths of all the components starting from one end of the P4 photovoltaic arrays to the other and include the P4 truss and the approximate spacing of 6 m in between, we obtain 72.19 m, which is the largest linear dimension of the ISS along the *X*-axis. This compares quite well with the value of 73.15 used by NASA.[6.2] Finally, if we sum the lengths of all the components starting from the top of the science power platform photovoltaic arrays (SPP-PVA) to the bottom of the universal docking module (UDM), we obtain 35.76 m, which is the largest linear dimension of the ISS along the *Z*-axis.

Thus, if we contain the ISS in a cuboid with faces perpendicular to the *X*, *Y*, and *Z* axes, the smallest cuboid has dimensions of 110.79 × 72.19 × 35.76 m. Next, if we inscribe this cuboid in a sphere, the diameter of the sphere is $\sqrt{[(110.79)^2 + (72.19)^2 + (35.76)^2]} = 137$ m.

In Sections 6.7, 6.8, and 6.9, we considered three case studies for combinations of the input collision parameters: miss distance $x_e = 10$, 1, and 0.1 km, and standard deviations $\sigma_{x'} = \sigma_{z'} \equiv \sigma = 5$ and 1 km. Thus, if we approximate the ISS by a sphere, it has a cross-sectional radius $r_A = 68.5$ m ≈ 70 m.

For these collision parameters, we used the four algorithms in Chapter 5 to compute the collision probability when the ISS is modeled as a sphere. The results are shown in Table 6.7.

Table 6.7. Collision Probabilities for the Spherical ISS Model

$\sigma_{x'}$ (km)	5	5	5	1	1	1
$\sigma_{z'}$ (km)	5	5	5	1	1	1
Cross-sectional radius (km)	0.07	0.07	0.07	0.07	0.07	0.07
Miss distance (km)	10	1	0.1	10	1	0.1
Chan's collision probability	1.326×10^{-05}	9.605×10^{-05}	9.789×10^{-05}	5.015×10^{-25}	1.485×10^{-03}	2.435×10^{-03}
NASA (Foster's) collision probability	1.326×10^{-05}	9.605×10^{-05}	9.605×10^{-05}	5.015×10^{-25}	1.485×10^{-03}	2.435×10^{-03}
Patera's collision probability	1.326×10^{-05}	9.605×10^{-05}	9.605×10^{-05}	5.015×10^{-25}	1.485×10^{-03}	2.435×10^{-03}
Alfano's collision probability	1.326×10^{-05}	9.605×10^{-05}	9.605×10^{-05}	5.015×10^{-25}	1.485×10^{-03}	2.435×10^{-03}

As demonstrated in Chapter 5, we again find that these four algorithms yield essentially the same values for the probability of collision.

6.11 Discussion

In Sections 6.7, 6.8, and 6.9, we studied respectively the cases of head-on, broadside, and overhead collision of the ISS with an oncoming object. Specifically, we considered the huge solar panels (photovoltaic arrays, PVA-US) to be tilted 30 deg in the (X, Z)-plane. From Tables 6.4, 6.5, and 6.6, we can observe that the probability of collision is between one and two orders of magnitude smaller than the value obtained for the spherical model of the ISS, as shown in Table 6.7.

This result is not totally unexpected for the following reason: If we consider the case of a head-on collision, we note that the ISS presents the smallest collision cross section when the solar panels are in the (X, Y)-plane. For this configuration, the effective area is provided by the ESA lab, Node 2, the Japanese experiment module and its collateral equipment, and the exposed parts of the trusses. Thus, the projected area is approximately $110 \times 5 = 550\ \text{m}^2$. However, if the ISS is considered as a sphere of radius 70 m, the effective cross section is $\pi \times 70^2 = 15{,}393\ \text{m}^2$. Therefore, the ratio of areas is $550/15{,}393 = 3.5 \times 10^{-2}$.

On the other hand, the ISS presents the largest collision cross section when the solar panels are in the (Y, Z)-plane. For this configuration, we have an additional effective area of $4 \times 72.19 \times 11.68 = 3373\ \text{m}^2$. Thus, the total effective cross-sectional area is $550 + 3373 = 3923\ \text{m}^2$. Therefore, the ratio of areas is $3923/15{,}393 = 2.5 \times 10^{-1}$.

If the solar panels are tilted, the effective frontal cross-sectional area lies between these two extremes. Hence, we also expect the same for the collision probability. The same statement, based on similar reasoning, applies to the cases of broadside and overhead collision of the ISS with an oncoming object.

6.12 Conclusion

In general terms, the probability of collision when the ISS is approached by an oncoming object from any direction is expected to be between one and two orders of magnitude smaller than the value obtained from a spherical model. However, the actual value must be obtained by using the detailed model developed in this chapter. The Excel macro used for computing the collision probability of the ISS also provides the collision probability for each component, including the solar panels, the trusses, the U.S. lab, U.S. habitat, ESA lab, Japanese experiment module, Canadarm2, Russian Zarya, and Zvezda.

6.13 Summary

In Section 6.1, we derived expressions for computing the areas of plates and solids projected onto a plane orthogonal to the projecting rays. We also obtained expressions for the centroids of these projections. These equations were then applied to the projection of the components of the ISS onto the encounter plane of an approaching secondary object.

In Section 6.2, we provided geometric specifications of the ISS obtained from the NASA Web site. We also derived the centroids of the ISS's main components and directions of the surface normals.

In Section 6.3, we derived the matrix for transforming from the inertial system to the ISS body system.

In Section 6.4, we outlined a novel algorithm for computing the sun vector in the mean of date inertial frame. This algorithm is based on simple analytical expressions for in-line computation for any time during a hundred-year span from 1961 to 2060 and is accurate to approximately 5×10^{-3} deg.

In Section 6.5, we gave the orbital elements of a sample ISS orbit.

In Section 6.6, we obtained results for the annual variation of the sun vector in the ISS body system. The cone angle between this vector and the ISS angular momentum vector undergoes approximately 6 cycles of oscillations in one year. This cone angle cannot be less than 20 deg.

In Sections 6.7, 6.8, and 6.9, we computed the corresponding probability of head-on, broadside, and overhead collision for several representative close encounters.

In Section 6.10, we modeled the ISS as a sphere and computed the collision probability for the same cases of close encounters.

In Section 6.11, we compared all these cases and observed that the collision probability of a realistic model of the ISS is generally between one and two orders of magnitude less than that obtained from the spherical model. We also provided an explanation for this outcome.

In Section 6.12, we concluded that the collision probability obtained from a realistic model is generally the result to be expected when the ISS encounters another object approaching it from any direction.

6.14 References

[6.1] G. Birkhoff and S. MacLane, *A Survey of Modern Algebra*, 3rd ed. (MacMillan, New York, NY, 1965), pp. 268–273.

[6.2] NASA, "Space Station Structure," <http://www.nasa.gov/mission_pages/station/structure> (31 July 2007).

[6.3] NASA, "HSF-ISS Scale Model Drawing Package," <http://www.spaceflight.nasa.gov/gallery/images/station/models> (31 July 2007).

[6.4] H. Goldstein, *Classical Mechanics* (Addison-Wesley Publishing, Reading, MA, 1959), pp. 107–109.

[6.5] *The Astronomical Almanac for the Year 2007*, prepared jointly by the Nautical Almanac Office, United States Naval Observatory, and Her Majesty's Almanac Office, United Kingdom Hydrographic Office; published by the U.S. Government Printing Office.

[6.6] *Almanac for Computers*, 1986, prepared by the Nautical Almanac Office, United States Naval Observatory; published by the U.S. Government Printing Office.

[6.7] F. K. Chan, "A Novel Algorithm for Computing the Sun Vector," 2007 (unpublished; this appears as Appendix A).

[6.8] Sunlit Design, documentation of sdxFindAnnFeatx function in full online documentation, "The Sun API," 2007, < http://www.sunlit-design.com/products/thesunapi/documentation/sdxFindAnnFeatx.php > (12 July 2007).

[6.9] W. J. Larson and J. R. Wertz, *Space Mission Analysis and Design* (published jointly by Microcosm, Inc., Torrance, CA, and Kluwer Academic Publishers, Dordrecht, Netherlands, 1992), pp. 137, 141.

[6.10] *Jane's Space Directory 2007–2008*, 23rd ed., edited by Bill Sweetman (Cambridge University Press, Great Britain, 2007), p. 292.

Chapter 7: Maneuvers to Mitigate Potential Collision Threats

Closely related to the problem of computing the collision probability between two orbiting objects is that of deciding, planning, and implementing maneuvers so that the two objects will have a reduced chance of colliding.[7.1] One of the orbiting objects (the primary) is assumed to be an active controllable spacecraft. The other object (the secondary) may not be controllable, as in the case of a rogue satellite or space debris. Suppose we are faced with a situation of high imminent collision probability or one that is above a specified acceptable threshold value. We wish to perform an orbital maneuver that is optimal in the sense that it requires the minimum velocity change to mitigate the potential collision threat and reduce the collision probability accordingly.

7.1 Intrack Thrusting

In Eq. (5.26) of Chapter 5, we showed that we may use the following expression for the collision integral to obtain results with three or four significant digits of accuracy under a wide range of input collision parameters:

$$P = e^{-v/2}\left(1 - e^{-u/2}\right) \tag{7.1}$$

The dimensionless variables u and v are defined in terms of the mean standard deviation σ, the companion standard deviation σ^*, the miss distance x_e, and the radius r_A of collision cross-sectional integration by

$$u = \left(\frac{r_A}{\sigma}\right)^2 > 0 \tag{7.2}$$

$$v = \left(\frac{x_e}{\sigma^*}\right)^2 > 0 \tag{7.3}$$

$$\sigma^2 = \sigma_{x'}\sigma_{z'} = \sigma_x\sigma_z(1 - \rho_{xz}{}^2) \tag{7.4}$$

$$\sigma^{*2} = \sigma_{z'}{}^2\left\{1 + \left[\left(\frac{\sigma_{z'}}{\sigma_{x'}}\right)^2 - 1\right]\cos^2\theta\right\}^{-1} \tag{7.5}$$

$$\theta = \frac{1}{2}\tan^{-1}\left[\frac{2\rho_{xz}\sigma_x\sigma_z}{(\sigma_x^{\ 2} - \sigma_z^{\ 2})}\right] \tag{7.6}$$

where θ is the angle of rotation from the encounter plane (x,z)-axes to the principal (x',z')-axes.

We note that we may also invert Eq. (7.1) and express the "nominal" miss distance x_e in terms of the desired collision probability P as

$$x_e = \sigma^* \sqrt{2\left[\ln\left(1 - e^{-r_A^{\ 2}/2\sigma^2}\right) - \ln P\right]} \tag{7.7}$$

This is the crucial relation for use in the determination of optimal orbital maneuvers to reduce the collision probability to a specified threshold value. One of the advantages of possessing such an analytical expression is that we do not need to resort to trial and error iteration. Other reasons are that it offers more insight into the problem and it is not computationally intensive.

In Chapter 2, we discussed details for computing the minimum separation M from initial conditions when the primary P and the secondary S enter the encounter region. We obtained the equation

$$M^2 = H^2 + K^{*2} \tag{7.8}$$

where H is the "height" or minimum distance between the two planes perpendicular to the cross product $\mathbf{n} \equiv \mathbf{v}_p \times \mathbf{v}_s$. One plane contains the velocity $\mathbf{v}_p$ of the primary and the other plane contains the velocity $\mathbf{v}_s$ of the secondary. K^* is defined by Eq. (2.42) in Chapter 2. The reader is urged to refer to Section 2.4 of Chapter 2 for other symbols that follow.

7.1.1 The Direct Problem

If we are given a threshold collision probability P', we may use Eq. (7.7) to obtain the required minimum distance M' between the primary and the secondary so that the collision probability is equal to P'. There are two cases to consider.

Case 1: If M' is much larger than the requisite change $|\Delta a_p|$ in the semimajor axis associated with the maneuver, then the required distance $K^{*\prime}$ is given by

$$M'^2 = H^2 + K^{*\prime 2} \tag{7.9}$$

It follows from Eqs. (7.8) and (7.9) that

$$\frac{K^{*\prime}}{K^*} = \sqrt{\frac{M'^2 - H^2}{M^2 - H^2}} \equiv \rho \tag{7.10}$$

From the important property of similar triangles in the projective plane containing the motion of P and S_{image}, we have

$$\frac{I^{*\prime}}{I^*} = \frac{J^{*\prime}}{J^*} = \frac{K^{*\prime}}{K^*} = \rho \tag{7.11}$$

Prior to the maneuver, we defined P to be at a distance L from Q when S_{image} transits the point Q. After the maneuver is accomplished by an intrack thrusting, let us define P to be at a distance L' from Q when S_{image} transits Q. Thus, the analog of Eq. (2.44) in Chapter 2 is

$$L' = I^{*\prime} \pm \left(\frac{J^{*\prime}}{v_s}\right) v_p = I^{*\prime} \pm \frac{J^{*\prime}}{\lambda} \tag{7.12}$$

It follows from Eqs. (7.11) and (7.12) and the algebraic theory of ratios that

$$\frac{L'}{L} = \rho \tag{7.13}$$

To achieve the threshold minimum distance M', we need to increase the intrack distance by the amount $(L' - L)$. From the equation for the mean motion n_p of the primary spacecraft

$$n_p = \sqrt{\frac{\mu}{a_p^{\,3}}} \tag{7.14}$$

we obtain the change in the mean velocity $\Delta v_{intrack}$:

$$\Delta v_{\text{intrack}} \simeq a_p \Delta n_p = -\frac{3}{2}\sqrt{\frac{\mu}{a_p^{\,3}}}\,\Delta a_p \tag{7.15}$$

where a_p is the semimajor axis of the primary and μ is the gravitational constant GM_E = 398,600.436 km^3/sec^2. Equations (7.13) and (7.15) may be combined to yield the more convenient form for applications:

$$\Delta a_p = \pm T\frac{(L' - L)}{D} = \pm\frac{TL(\rho - 1)}{D} \tag{7.16}$$

where both Δa_p and $(L' - L)$ are measured in the same units of length and T is defined by

$$T \equiv \frac{1}{129{,}600}\sqrt{\frac{a_p^{\;3}}{\mu}} \tag{7.17}$$

if D is expressed in days of the maneuver before the close encounter. In Eq. (7.16), the plus sign applies to the case where S_{image} transits Q ahead of P and the minus sign applies to the case where P transits Q ahead of S_{image}.

Note that the final equation, Eq. (7.16), does not explicitly involve λ, ϕ, I^*, J^*, K^*, $I^{*\prime}$, $J^{*\prime}$, $K^{*\prime}$, and L'. It depends only on L, H, M, and M'. The minimum separation M and the distance L are computed according to the discussion in Chapter 2. The height H between the two planes normal to the cross product $\mathbf{n} \equiv \mathbf{v}_p \times \mathbf{v}_s$ may be determined using equations of three-dimensional analytical geometry. The minimum separation M' corresponding to the specified threshold collision probability P' is computed using Eq. (7.7). Note that we were able to derive Eq. (7.16) without computing $K^{*\prime}$, $I^{*\prime}$, $J^{*\prime}$, and L' as intermediate variables using Eqs. (7.9), (7.11), and (7.12) or performing a tremendous amount of analysis solving for minimum separation distance between the two orbiting objects moving in trajectories in three-dimensional space.

As an example, if a_p = 7151 km, then Eq. (7.17) yields T = 1/135 and Eq. (7.16) becomes $\Delta a_p = \pm(L' - L)/(135D)$. Because of the impending collision with a relatively high probability P, we need to reduce it to a lower value P'. It follows that L' is larger than L. Suppose $(L' - L)$ = 540 m. If S_{image} transits the point Q ahead of P, we may increase a_p by 8 m if we maneuver a half-day before to slow down the primary. If P transits the point Q ahead of S_{image}, we may decrease a_p by 8 m if we maneuver a half-day before to speed up the primary.

Case 2: If M' is of the same order as the requisite change $|\Delta a_p|$ in the semi-major axis associated with the maneuver, then the required distance $K^{*\prime}$ is given by

$$M'^2 = H'^2 + K^{*\prime 2} \tag{7.18}$$

where

$$H' = H - \gamma \Delta a_p \tag{7.19}$$

$$\gamma = \widehat{\mathbf{H}} \cdot \widehat{\mathbf{r}}_p \tag{7.20}$$

This is illustrated in Fig. 7.1.

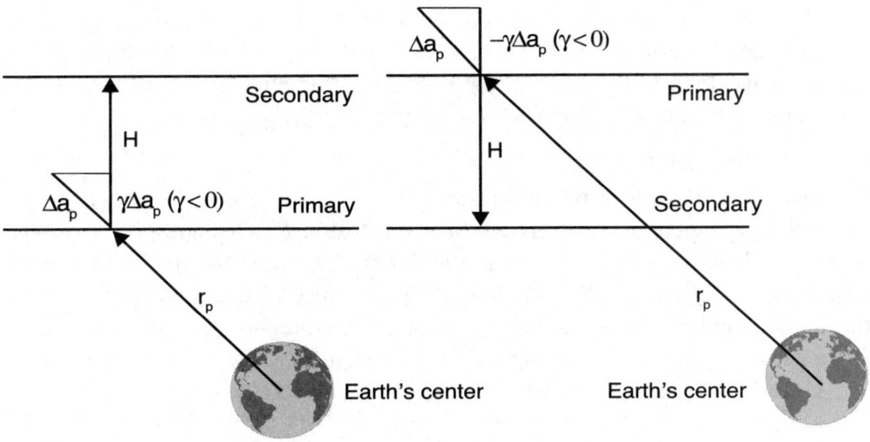

Figure 7.1. Geometric relation for $\Delta a_p > 0$.

By similar analysis, we obtain the following analogs of Eqs. (7.10) and (7.16):

$$\frac{K^{*\prime}}{K^*} = \sqrt{\frac{M'^2 - H'^2}{M^2 - H^2}} \equiv \rho' \tag{7.21}$$

$$\Delta a_p = \frac{TL(\rho' - 1)}{D} \tag{7.22}$$

If we substitute Eqs. (7.19) and (7.21) into (7.22) and then square both sides, we obtain a quadratic equation in Δa. By solving this equation and taking the appropriate root, we obtain

$$\Delta a_p = \frac{-B + \sqrt{\left(B^2 - AC\right)}}{A} \tag{7.23}$$

where

$$A = H^2 - M^2 - \gamma^2\tau^2 \quad B = \tau\left(H^2 - M^2 + H\gamma\tau\right)$$

$$C = \tau^2\left(M'^2 - M^2\right) \quad \tau \equiv \frac{TL}{D} \tag{7.24}$$

The foregoing analysis considers the problem for which we are given the threshold collision probability P' because of the imminent high probability of collision. We use Eq. (7.7) to compute M' and then we obtain the necessary maneuver Δa_p by using Eqs. (7.16) and (7.23) for cases 1 and 2 respectively.

7.1.2 The Inverse Problem

The inverse problem is also of interest. For this, we are given Δa or $\Delta v_{\text{intrack}}$, and we wish to compute the new probability of collision P'. One approach is to perform high-precision orbit propagation and then determine the minimum separation numerically and finally compute the probability of collision. However, we may circumvent this laborious task by inverting the foregoing equations to express M' in terms of Δa_p and then computing P' by using Eq. (7.1).

Case 1: We obtain the following equations:

$$\rho = \frac{D\Delta a_p}{TL} + 1 \tag{7.25}$$

$$M'^2 = \rho^2\left(M^2 - H^2\right) + H^2 \tag{7.26}$$

$$P' = e^{-M'^2/2\sigma^2}\left(1 - e^{-r_A^2/2\sigma^2}\right) \tag{7.27}$$

Case 2: We obtain the following equations:

$$\rho' = \frac{D\Delta a_p}{TL} + 1 \tag{7.28}$$

$$M'^2 = \rho'^2\left(M^2 - H^2\right) + \left(H - \gamma\Delta a_p\right)^2 \tag{7.29}$$

$$P' = e^{-M'^2/2\sigma^2}\left(1 - e^{-r_A^2/2\sigma^2}\right) \tag{7.30}$$

This completes the discussion on preemptive maneuvers to avert potential collisions for the case of applying intrack thrusting only.

7.2 General Thrusting

We now extend our analysis to the case of thrusting to include crosstrack and radial components in addition to the intrack component. There are two parts to this analysis: minimum separation and optimum thrusting. Even though the method described in the previous section is applicable to the determination of minimum separation between two orbiting objects, that formulation turns out to be especially suitable for intrack thrusting. This is because it gives the requisite intrack thrusting to yield the increase in the intrack separation so as to achieve the necessary threshold probability of collision. For the present general case, we may perform numerous computer simulations involving high-precision orbit propagation to determine the optimum thrusting that would yield the desired threshold collision probability. However, it turns out that this problem is also amenable to analytical solution as follows:

Let $\mathbf{r}_p(t)$ and $\mathbf{r}_s(t)$ respectively denote the position of the primary and the secondary at any time t. Let $f(t, \boldsymbol{\alpha}, \boldsymbol{\beta})$ denote the separation between them; that is,

$$f(t,\alpha,\beta) = \left|\mathbf{r}_p(t) - \mathbf{r}_s(t)\right| \tag{7.31}$$

where $\boldsymbol{\alpha}$ denotes all modeling parameters such as geopotential coefficients for a nonspherical Earth, atmospheric drag, solar radiation pressure, etc., and $\boldsymbol{\beta}$ denotes perturbations on epoch orbital elements of the primary at time $t = 0$. There are many components in $\boldsymbol{\alpha}$ but only 6 elements in $\boldsymbol{\beta}$ ($\Delta\mathbf{r}_o$ and $\Delta\mathbf{v}_o$). For thrusting, $\Delta\mathbf{r}_o = 0$ and $\Delta\mathbf{v}_o \neq 0$. Figure 7.2 illustrates this separation as a function of t and $\boldsymbol{\beta}$ in an eight-dimensional space.

For a specified $\boldsymbol{\beta}$ corresponding to a given epoch set of elements, this separation is a function of t only as illustrated in Fig. 7.3.

Let t_m denote the time of minimum separation between the unperturbed primary and the secondary. The value t_m may be determined using the analytical method discussed in Section 2.4 of Chapter 2 instead of using high-precision orbit propagation and search by trial and error. Let t_m' denote the minimum separation when the primary has undergone a general thrusting. For convenience, we let $g(t, \boldsymbol{\alpha}, \boldsymbol{\beta})$ denote the rate of separation; that is,

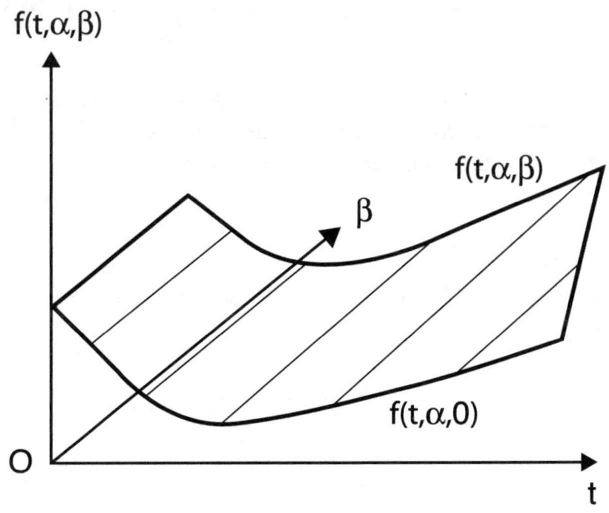

Figure 7.2. Separation distance as a function of time and thrusting.

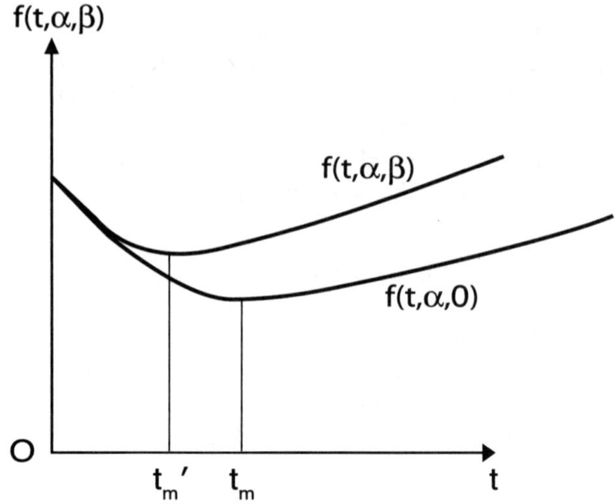

Figure 7.3. Separation distance as a function of time for a specified thrusting.

$$g(t,\alpha,\beta) \equiv \frac{\partial f(t,\alpha,\beta)}{\partial t} \tag{7.32}$$

If the thrusting is small so that the perturbations in the epoch elements are small, then we may use a first-order expansion about the point (t_m, $\boldsymbol{\alpha}$, $\mathbf{0}$):

$$g(t_m{}', \boldsymbol{\alpha}, \boldsymbol{\beta}) = g(t_m, \boldsymbol{\alpha}, \mathbf{0}) + g_t(t_m, \boldsymbol{\alpha}, \mathbf{0})(t_m{}' - t_m) + \sum_i g_{\beta_i}(t_m, \boldsymbol{\alpha}, \mathbf{0})\beta_i + \cdots \tag{7.33}$$

where, without any undue confusion, the subscript of $g(t, \boldsymbol{\alpha}, \boldsymbol{\beta})$ denotes differentiation with respect to the particular variable and then evaluation at the value of that variable as indicated in the argument. But we have by definition

$$g(t_m{}', \alpha, \beta) \equiv 0 \quad \text{and} \quad g(t_m, \alpha, 0) \equiv 0 \tag{7.34}$$

Thus, if we retain the first-order terms in Eq. (7.33), we may solve for $t_m{}'$ in terms of t_m and $\boldsymbol{\beta}$:

$$t_m{}' = t_m - \frac{\sum_i g_{\beta_i}(t_m, \boldsymbol{\alpha}, \mathbf{0})\beta_i}{g_t(t_m, \boldsymbol{\alpha}, \mathbf{0})} \tag{7.35}$$

If we desire more accuracy, we may go to a second-order expansion, but must be careful to choose the correct sign to be associated with the appropriate solution of the quadratic equation. These details are omitted in the present discussion as they distract from the main ideas.

Our next task is to obtain the new minimum separation $f(t_m', \boldsymbol{\alpha}, \boldsymbol{\beta})$. To accomplish this, we proceed as follows: Let $F(t, \boldsymbol{\alpha}, \boldsymbol{\beta})$ denote any continuous function of its arguments. Then, we may symbolically write ad infinitum the following series expansion about the point $(t,\mathbf{0},\mathbf{0})$.

$$F(t,\boldsymbol{\alpha},\boldsymbol{\beta}) = F(t,\mathbf{0},\mathbf{0}) + \sum_i F_{\alpha_i}(t,\mathbf{0},\mathbf{0})\alpha_i + \frac{1}{2}\sum_i\sum_j F_{\alpha_i\alpha_j}(t,\mathbf{0},\mathbf{0})\alpha_i\alpha_j + \cdots$$
$$+\sum_i F_{\beta_i}(t,\mathbf{0},\mathbf{0})\beta_i + \frac{1}{2}\sum_i\sum_j F_{\beta_i\beta_j}(t,\mathbf{0},\mathbf{0})\beta_i\beta_j + \cdots$$
$$+\sum_i\sum_j F_{\alpha_i\beta_j}(t,\mathbf{0},\mathbf{0})\alpha_i\beta_j + \cdots \tag{7.36}$$

A little consideration reveals that we may subtract and add the term $F(t,\mathbf{0},\mathbf{0})$, re-collect terms into three infinite series, and write Eq. (7.36) in the form

$$F(t,\alpha,\beta) = F(t,\alpha,\mathbf{0}) - F(t,\mathbf{0},\mathbf{0}) + F(t,\mathbf{0},\beta) + \text{Cross Terms Series} \tag{7.37}$$

If we apply Eq. (7.37) to $f(t_m', \boldsymbol{\alpha}, \boldsymbol{\beta})$, we obtain

$$f(t_m',\alpha,\beta) = f(t_m',\alpha,\mathbf{0}) - f(t_m',\mathbf{0},\mathbf{0}) + f(t_m',\mathbf{0},\beta) + \text{Cross Terms Series} \tag{7.38}$$

The first term on the right-hand side (RHS) can be obtained by high-precision orbit propagation while the second and third terms can be obtained from Keplerian motion because α is zero. The fourth term may be neglected, as its contribution is usually small compared to those of the other terms because maneuvers are performed in a relatively short time (within a day or two) before the spacecraft conjunction.

It is interesting to note that Eq. (7.37) may also be applied to any component of the position or velocity of an orbiting object. That is, we may use it to obtain a whole slew of trajectories of the primary with different thrustings by performing only one high-precision orbit propagation represented by the first term on the RHS. This results in achieving substantial computational efficiency.

With a slight twist in interpretation of the second term on the RHS of Eq. (7.37) as a Keplerian backward propagation, Patera and Peterson[7.2] devised an algorithm for an efficient orbit propagation when many orbit propagations have to be performed to study the effects of different impulses $\Delta\mathbf{v}$ applied at a specific point in a spacecraft trajectory. This procedure involves (1) high-precision orbit propagation with no impulse, (2) backward Keplerian propagation with no impulse, and (3) forward Keplerian propagation with impulse $\Delta\mathbf{v}$. This procedure is especially efficient for simulations that normally involve numerous time-consuming high-precision orbit propagations. Peterson has shown by numerical studies that this methodology yields extremely accurate results throughout two weeks for the case of geosynchronous orbits where the effects of atmospheric drag and higher gravitational harmonics are comparatively negligible. Moreover, even for the case of low Earth orbits above 600 km altitude where these effects are not negligible, it is still applicable for at least four days. Below 400 km altitude, it is valid for one day.

Equation (7.38) gives the expression of the new minimum separation $f(t_m', \boldsymbol{\alpha}, \boldsymbol{\beta})$ corresponding to an applied orbital perturbation $\boldsymbol{\beta}$. Thus, by using Eq. (7.1), we may compute P' in terms of $\boldsymbol{\beta}$. However, what we want is to determine the optimum thrusting $\boldsymbol{\beta}$ in terms of the specified threshold collision probability P'. To proceed, we need to conceptually construct surfaces of constant P as a function of the three thrusting components. This is illustrated in Fig. 7.4.

Let the intrack, radial, and crosstrack directions be labeled by the vectors $\mathbf{x}_1$, $\mathbf{x}_2$, and $\mathbf{x}_3$. Let the corresponding components of $\boldsymbol{\beta}$ be labeled as β_1, β_2, and β_3. That is, we have

$$\boldsymbol{\beta} = \beta_1 \widehat{\mathbf{x}_1} + \beta_2 \widehat{\mathbf{x}_2} + \beta_3 \widehat{\mathbf{x}_3} \tag{7.39}$$

Therefore, ∇P (gradient of P, a vector) in the $\boldsymbol{\beta}$-space may be written as

$$\nabla P = \frac{\partial P_c}{\partial \beta_1} \widehat{\mathbf{x}_1} + \frac{\partial P_c}{\partial \beta_2} \widehat{\mathbf{x}_2} + \frac{\partial P_c}{\partial \beta_3} \widehat{\mathbf{x}_3} \tag{7.40}$$

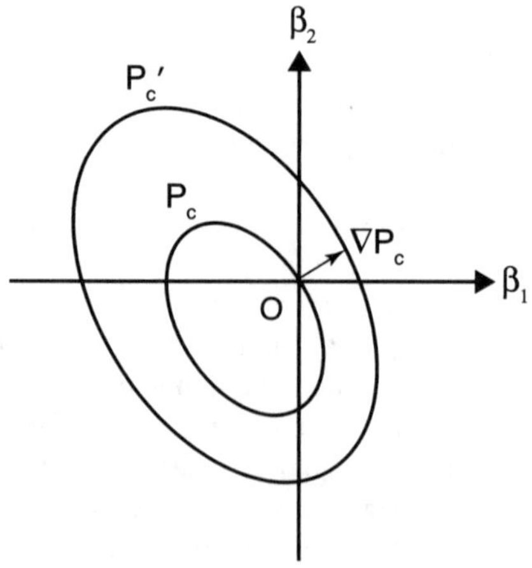

Figure 7.4. Surfaces of constant *P*.

Because the applied thrust $\boldsymbol{\beta}$ is usually small, therefore the optimum thrust is in the same direction as $-\nabla P$ evaluated at the origin of the $\boldsymbol{\beta}$-space (not the physical three-dimensional $[x,y,z]$-space). Moreover, because the logarithm of P is a monotonic function, it follows that the optimum thrust is in the same direction as the $-\nabla(\ln P)$. However, from Eq. (7.1), we have

$$P = e^{-f^2/2\sigma^{*2}}\left(1 - e^{-r_A^2/2\sigma^2}\right) \tag{7.41}$$

so that

$$\ln P = -\frac{f^2}{2\sigma^{*2}} + \ln(1 - e^{-r_A^2/2\sigma^2}) \tag{7.42}$$

$$\nabla \ln P = -\frac{f}{\sigma^{*2}}\nabla f \tag{7.43}$$

where ∇f is evaluated at the origin of the $\boldsymbol{\beta}$-space, and the minimum separation ϕ is a function of the applied thrust $\boldsymbol{\beta}$ and the conjunction time t_m'; that is,

$$f = f(t_m', \alpha, \beta) \tag{7.44}$$

If we next expand $f(tm', \boldsymbol{\alpha}, \boldsymbol{\beta})$ about the point $(tm, \boldsymbol{\alpha}, \boldsymbol{\beta})$, we have

$$f(t_m', \boldsymbol{\alpha}, \boldsymbol{\beta}) = f(t_m, \boldsymbol{\alpha}, \mathbf{0}) + f_t(t_m, \boldsymbol{\alpha}, \mathbf{0})(t_m' - t_m) + \sum_i f_{\beta_i}(t_m, \boldsymbol{\alpha}, \mathbf{0})\beta_i + \cdots \tag{7.45}$$

But from Eqs. (7.32) and (7.34), we note that

$$f_t(t_m, \alpha, \mathbf{0}) \equiv \left[\frac{\partial f(t, \alpha, \mathbf{0})}{\partial t}\right]_{t=t_m} \equiv g(t_m, \alpha, \mathbf{0}) \equiv 0 \tag{7.46}$$

Hence, if we retain only the first-order terms in Eq. (7.45), we obtain

$$f(t_m', \boldsymbol{\alpha}, \boldsymbol{\beta}) = f(t_m, \boldsymbol{\alpha}, \mathbf{0}) + \sum_i f_{\beta_i}(t_m, \boldsymbol{\alpha}, \mathbf{0})\beta_i \tag{7.47}$$

If we take the gradient in the $\boldsymbol{\beta}$-space of both sides of Eq. (7.47) and evaluate at the origin, it follows that the first term on the RHS drops out and we have a first-order approximation

$$\left[\nabla f(t_m{}',\boldsymbol{\alpha},\boldsymbol{\beta})\right]_{\boldsymbol{\beta}=\mathbf{0}} = \sum_i f_{\beta_i}(t_m,\boldsymbol{\alpha},\mathbf{0})\widehat{\mathbf{x}_i} \equiv \left[\nabla f(t_m,\boldsymbol{\alpha},\boldsymbol{\beta})\right]_{\boldsymbol{\beta}=\mathbf{0}} \equiv \nabla f(t_m,\boldsymbol{\alpha},\mathbf{0}) \tag{7.48}$$

Because the thrust $\boldsymbol{\beta}$ is in the direction of ∇f, let us introduce a scalar χ and write

$$\boldsymbol{\beta} = \chi\left[\nabla f(t_m,\boldsymbol{\alpha},\boldsymbol{\beta})\right]_{\boldsymbol{\beta}=\mathbf{0}} \tag{7.49}$$

In view of Eq. (7.49), it follows that (7.47) takes the form

$$f(t_m{}',\boldsymbol{\alpha},\boldsymbol{\beta}) = f(t_m,\boldsymbol{\alpha},\mathbf{0}) + \chi\left|\nabla f(t_m,\boldsymbol{\alpha},\mathbf{0})\right|^2 \tag{7.50}$$

By solving for the scalar χ in Eq. (7.50) and then substituting the resulting value into (7.49), we obtain the requisite thrust $\boldsymbol{\beta}$ for optimum maneuver to achieve the threshold collision probability P':

$$\boldsymbol{\beta} = \frac{f(t_m{}',\boldsymbol{\alpha},\boldsymbol{\beta}) - f(t_m,\boldsymbol{\alpha},\mathbf{0})}{\left|\nabla f(t_m,\boldsymbol{\alpha},\mathbf{0})\right|^2}\nabla f(t_m,\boldsymbol{\alpha},\mathbf{0}) \tag{7.51}$$

In this equation, $f(t_m{}', \boldsymbol{\alpha}, \boldsymbol{\beta})$ is computed from P'. The term $f(t_m, \boldsymbol{\alpha}, \mathbf{0})$ may be obtained from high-precision orbit propagations of the primary and the secondary according to Eq. (7.31). Its gradient is obtained by taking the three numerical partial derivatives $[\nabla f(t_m, \boldsymbol{\alpha}, \boldsymbol{\beta})]_{\boldsymbol{\beta}=0}$ evaluated at the origin of the $\boldsymbol{\beta}$-space.

This completes the discussion on preemptive maneuvers to avert potential collisions for the general case of thrusting.

7.3 Discussion

Compared to general thrusting, intrack thrusting is much simpler to implement for analysis and simulations on a computer and also much simpler to execute operationally for spacecraft maneuvers. In fuel expenditure, it is only slightly more costly than the more general approach in the case of only one collision-avoidance maneuver. However, its most salient feature is that it is perhaps even more effective in the long run when there is a complementary adjustment to bring the spacecraft back to the original orbit. This is because it involves orbit phasing to either slow down or speed up the spacecraft so as to achieve the requisite minimum separation to ensure meeting the collision probability threshold requirements. After the close encounter, it could be used again to regain the proper phasing of the spacecraft in its nominal trajectory. This is especially important if the primary spacecraft is one member of a large constellation moving in some prescribed configuration.

On the other hand, by executing a general thrusting in the crosstrack and radial directions in addition to an intrack component, the primary spacecraft can be made to change its orbital characteristics quite drastically. Then, to restore its proper position in the constellation, it would have to undergo another maneuver involving three-component thrusting. In general, this operation requires more intricate analysis and is more complicated to execute.

7.4 Conclusion

In view of this discussion, it is recommended that intrack thrusting be applied to spacecraft maneuvers to mitigate potential collision threats.

7.5 Summary

In Section 7.1, we derived the equations for performing intrack thrusting so as to decrease the collision probability to a specified acceptable threshold value. The analysis is simple and the maneuver is also simple to perform.

In Section 7.2, we derived the equations for general thrusting with crosstrack and radial components. The analysis is complicated and the maneuver is difficult to perform.

In Section 7.3, we discussed that, except for cases of immediate exigency, we should not base a maneuver on myopic considerations of near-term reduction of collision probability but must also take into consideration subsequent scenarios.

In Section 7.4, we recommended performing a simple intrack thrusting.

7.6 References

[7.1.] F. K. Chan, "Spacecraft Maneuvers to Mitigate Potential Collision Threats," *AIAA/AAS Astrodynamics Specialist Conference* (Monterey, CA, 5–8 August 2002).

[7.2.] R. P. Patera and G. E. Peterson, "Space Vehicle Maneuver Method to Lower Collision Risk to an Acceptable Level," *J. Guidance, Control and Navigation* **26** (2), 233–237 (2003).

Chapter 8: Analytical Expressions for Long-Term Encounters

Around the year 2000, Chan predicted in an analysis (and Peterson subsequently confirmed by examining the resident space objects catalog) that certain pairs of geosynchronous satellites have low relative velocity (low enough to be measured in meters per second), so that the time they spend in the encounter region is appreciable. (This analysis now appears as Chapters 2 and 3.) During this period, which can extend to well beyond a day, the relative velocity is no longer constant in direction nor can the combined covariance error ellipsoid be treated as constant. In contrast to the existing short-term encounter models discussed in Chapter 5 for which the assumption of constant relative velocity is valid, the long-term encounter model requires a different approach to computing the collision probability.[8.1]

To analyze the general case of long-term encounter, we must account for the covariance error ellipsoid changing in shape, size, and orientation. Thus, we can no longer consider the three Cartesian coordinates representing the relative position uncertainty as random variables in the physical space. Instead, we must choose three different random variables as a common basis so that we can meaningfully compute collision probability. This probability is determined by evaluating a three-dimensional integral over the appropriate region corresponding to the values of the random variables.

8.1 Choice of Random Variables

Consider Fig. 8.1, which illustrates a reference set of coordinate axes (x, y, z) in the physical space. As in Chapter 3, we consider a sphere with radius $\rho \equiv r_A$ equal to the combined radius of two spherical satellites. In this space, there is a volume V swept out by the passage of the sphere.

Suppose we have a 1-σ covariance ellipsoid at time $t = 0$ with principal semiaxes (a, b, c) in (x', y', z'). Let P denote the transformation matrix between corresponding vectors in these two systems; that is,

$$\vec{r}' = P\vec{r} \quad \text{where} \quad P^T = P^{-1} \tag{8.1}$$

Suppose at time t, this 1-σ covariance ellipsoid has undergone a rotation R with principal directions (x'', y'', z''). Let this 1-σ ellipsoid also have undergone a "stretching" D (a general term used here for denoting expansion or compression) of the principal semiaxes (α, β, γ) so that it appears as shown in the coordinate system (x''', y''', z'''). Then, we have the following transformations:

$$\vec{r}'' = R\vec{r}' \quad \text{where} \quad R^T = R^{-1} \tag{8.2}$$

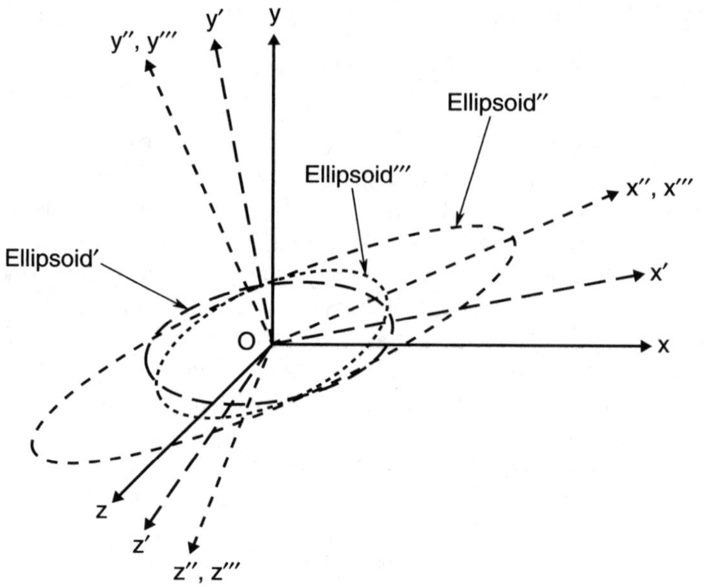

Figure 8.1. Transformation of coordinate systems.

$$\vec{r}''' = D\vec{r}'' \quad \text{where} \quad D^T \equiv D \tag{8.3}$$

To have a standard basis for comparison, it is convenient (but not necessary) to choose a coordinate system in which the 1-σ ellipsoid is mapped into the sphere with radius σ. Let this be accomplished by the scale transformation S:

$$\vec{r}^* = S\vec{r}''' \quad \text{where} \quad S^T = S \tag{8.4}$$

Thus, we have an isotropic probability density function (pdf) $f^*(x^*, y^*, z^*)$ in this coordinate system (x^*, y^*, z^*). In this space, there is a volume V^* corresponding to V swept out by the sphere of radius ρ.

Because the covariance matrix is time-dependent, it is meaningless to perform integration over the physical space as was done simply and harmlessly in the case of short-term encounters in Chapters 4 and 5. The covariance there was treated as constant, and (x, y, z) were chosen as the random variables. Thus, we have to devise a common frame of reference for which the pdf is constant and random variables (x^*, y^*, z^*) can be defined meaningfully. Once this is accomplished, we then transform the volume V to the corresponding volume V^* in this new coordinate system. Finally, we evaluate the probability by integrating $f^*(x^*, y^*, z^*)$ over the volume V^*.

It follows that, by combining all the transformations, we have

$$\vec{r}^* = S\,D\,R\,P\,\vec{r} \tag{8.5}$$

For convenience, let us define the transformation T by

$$T \equiv S\,D \Rightarrow T^T = T \tag{8.6}$$

so that Eq. (8.5) becomes

$$\vec{r}^* = M\,\vec{r} \quad \text{where} \quad M \equiv T\,R\,P \tag{8.7}$$

Hence, we have

$$\vec{r} = M^{-1}\vec{r}^*; \quad \vec{r}^{*T} = \vec{r}\,M^T; \quad \vec{r}^T = \vec{r}^{*T}\,(M^{-1})^T \tag{8.8}$$

8.2 Transformation of a Sphere

We shall next transform a sphere of radius ρ with center at (x_C, y_C, z_C) at time t in the physical space:

$$(x - x_c)^2 + (y - y_c)^2 + (z - z_c)^2 = \rho^2 \tag{8.9}$$

$$(\vec{r} - \vec{r}_c)^T(\vec{r} - \vec{r}_c) = (\vec{r}^T - \vec{r}_c^{\,T})(\vec{r} - \vec{r}_c) = \rho^2 \tag{8.10}$$

Because we can substitute Eq. (8.8) into (8.10), therefore

$$(\vec{r}^{*T} - \vec{r}_c^{\,*T})(M^{-1})^T(M^{-1})(\vec{r}^* - \vec{r}_c^{\,*}) = \rho^2 \tag{8.11}$$

From the second equation of each pair in (8.1), (8.2), and (8.7), it follows that

$$M^{-1} = (TRP)^{-1} = P^{-1}R^{-1}T^{-1} = P^T R^T T^{-1} \tag{8.12}$$

$$(M^{-1})^T = (P^T R^T T^{-1})^T = (T^{-1})^T RP \tag{8.13}$$

Consequently, from the second equation in (8.6), as well as Eqs. (8.12) and (8.13), we obtain

$$(M^{-1})^T(M^{-1}) = (T^{-1})^T RPP^{-1}R^{-1}T^{-1} = (T^{-1})^T T^{-1} = (T^T)^{-1}T^{-1} = T^{-1}T^{-1} = (TT)^{-1} = (T^2)^{-1} \tag{8.14}$$

Therefore, Eq. (8.11) takes the unexpectedly simple form

$$(\vec{r}^{\,*T} - \vec{r}_c^{\,*T})(T^2)^{-1}(\vec{r}^{\,*} - \vec{r}_c^{\,*}) = \rho^2 \tag{8.15}$$

Equation (8.15) describes an ellipsoid with principal axes along (x^*, y^*, z^*) with center at the point (x_c^*, y_c^*, z_c^*). This "derived ellipsoid" has been transformed from the original sphere with radius ρ, and its shape depends on the time-dependent diagonal matrix $(T^2)^{-1}$. We note that the transformation matrix T involves only expansion and contraction but not rotation of the covariance ellipsoid. The effects of the covariance ellipsoid rotation matrix R show up in the transformation of the center (x_c, y_c, z_c) to (x_c^*, y_c^*, z_c^*) at time t through the equation

$$\vec{r}_c^{\,*} = M\vec{r}_c \quad \text{where} \quad M \equiv T\,R\,P \tag{8.16}$$

Thus, we may state the following important theorem, which reiterates what has already been proved:

THEOREM 8.1. *Suppose the covariance matrix C is time-dependent (involving changes in shape, size, and orientation) and is transformed to the (x^*, y^*, z^*)-space of random variables by Eq. (8.5). Then, the sphere of radius ρ in the physical space (x, y, z)-space is transformed to an ellipsoid in the (x^*, y^*, z^*)-space. The principal axes of this ellipsoid are always along the (x^*, y^*, z^*) coordinate axes. Its shape and size depend only on the time-dependent diagonal matrix $(T^2)^{-1}$ where T, defined by Eq. (8.6), involves only expansion and contraction but not rotation.*

In particular, even if the hard-body sphere does not move in the (x, y, z) coordinate system but the covariance ellipsoid rotates, the center (x_c, y_c, z_c) will move along a circular arc in the (x^*, y^*, z^*) coordinate system. In general, the trajectory of the center depends on both the motion of the sphere and the rotation of the covariance ellipsoid as dictated by Eq. (8.16). Thus, the tangent to the trajectory is in the direction of the following vector derivative of the center position in the (x^*, y^*, z^*) coordinate system:

$$\frac{d\vec{r}_c^{\,*}}{dt} = M\frac{d\vec{r}_c}{dt} + \frac{dM}{dt}\vec{r}_c \tag{8.17}$$

It is important to note that this tangent vector is not the same as the "physical" velocity $(d\vec{r}_c / dt)$ of the center transformed to the (x^*, y^*, z^*) coordinate system. This "physical" velocity, like the position vector $\vec{r}_c$ of the center, transforms from the (x, y, z) coordinate system to the (x^*, y^*, z^*) system according to Eq. (8.16), which comprises only the first term of Eq. (8.17). It is not tangent to the trajectory of the center in the (x^*, y^*, z^*) coordinate system. Equation (8.17) contains another term resulting from the time-varying nature of the covariance. This is a very important point.

8.3 Motion of a Sphere in Physical Space

We next obtain the equations describing the motion of the center of the hard-body sphere according to the laws of dynamics. This is given by the relative motion of one satellite with respect to the other. Because we are concerned with a long-term encounter between two geosynchronous satellites, we may safely use the Clohessy-Wiltshire equations as a first approximation. The reason is that their orbits are essentially circular and are far enough away to justify the validity of the assumption of Keplerian motion. The equations of motion in a rotating rectangular coordinate system are given in terms of the initial relative position (x_o, y_o, z_o) and relative velocity $(\dot{x}_o, \dot{y}_o, \dot{z}_o)$:[8.2]

$$x_c = x_o + \left(6\omega y_o - 3\dot{x}_o\right)t + 2\frac{\dot{y}_o}{\omega}\left(1 - \cos\omega t\right) + \left(4\frac{\dot{x}_o}{\omega} - 6y_o\right)\sin\omega t \tag{8.18}$$

$$y_c = 4y_o - 2\frac{\dot{x}_o}{\omega} + \left(2\frac{\dot{x}_o}{\omega} - 3y_o\right)\cos\omega t + \frac{\dot{y}_o}{\omega}\sin\omega t \tag{8.19}$$

$$z_c = \frac{\dot{z}_o}{\omega}\sin\omega t + z_o\cos\omega t \tag{8.20}$$

The expressions on the right-hand side (RHS) are used for the motion of the center (x_c, y_c, z_c) of the sphere in the (x, y, z)-space. By using the transformation in Eq. (8.16), we obtain the trajectory of (x_c^*, y_c^*, z_c^*) in the (x^*, y^*, z^*)-space. Even though we subsequently use Eqs. (8.18) through (8.20), they are not easily amenable to simple physical interpretation.

We shall rewrite these equations in the "phase-amplitude" form frequently used for expressing signals in electrical engineering:

$$x_c = C + Dt + A\sin(\omega t + \phi) \tag{8.21}$$

$$y_c = \frac{2D}{3\omega} + \frac{1}{2}A\cos(\omega t + \phi) \tag{8.22}$$

$$z_c = B\cos(\omega t - \psi) \tag{8.23}$$

The six parameters corresponding to the initial relative position and relative velocity are now replaced by the constant C, the drift D, the amplitude A for the x and y motion, the amplitude B for the z motion, the phase ϕ for the x and y motion, and the phase $-\psi$ for the z motion. Note that the amplitude of the y motion in Eq.

(8.22) is one-half of that of the x motion in Eq. (8.21). It may be shown that these parameters are related by the following equations:

$$A^2 = \left(2\frac{\dot{y}_o}{\omega}\right)^2 + \left(4\frac{\dot{x}_o}{\omega} - 6y_o\right)^2 \tag{8.24}$$

$$B^2 = z_o^{\,2} + \left(\frac{\dot{z}_o}{\omega}\right)^2 \tag{8.25}$$

$$C = x_o + 2\frac{\dot{y}_o}{\omega} \tag{8.26}$$

$$D = 6\omega y_o - 3\dot{x}_o \tag{8.27}$$

$$\phi = \tan^{-1}\left(\frac{-2\dfrac{\dot{y}_o}{\omega}}{4\dfrac{\dot{x}_o}{\omega} - 6y_o}\right) \tag{8.28}$$

$$\psi = \tan^{-1}\left(\frac{-z_o\omega}{\dot{z}_o}\right) \tag{8.29}$$

Figure 8.2 illustrates an instantaneous (x, y)-profile of the relative orbit without any drift motion. Note that it is an ellipse with a 2:1 aspect ratio. Under no circumstances can it be a circle. If there is drift ($D > 0$) along the positive x-direction, then the center of the osculating ellipse moves in the radial-intrack plane, as shown in Fig. 8.3. Similarly, the center of the osculating ellipse moves in the intrack-crosstrack plane, as shown in Fig. 8.4.

8.4 Volume of Integration

Finally, it remains to discuss how we obtain the volume of integration V^* for computing the probability of collision between the two satellites. If we substitute Eqs. (8.18) through (8.20) into (8.16), then we obtain (x_c^*, y_c^*, z_c^*) as functions of time t. Next, we substitute these into Eq. (8.15) and obtain an equation written symbolically as

$$F(x^*, y^*, z^*, t) = 0 \tag{8.30}$$

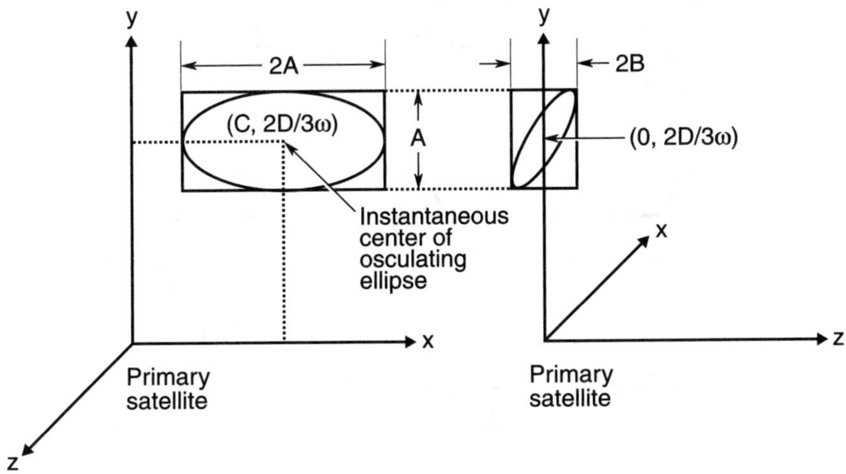

Figure 8.2. Two orthogonal profiles of the relative motion.

We had noted that this "derived ellipsoid" has been transformed from the original hard-body sphere, and its shape depends on the time-dependent diagonal matrix $(T^2)^{-1}$. The trajectory of the center (x_c*, y_c*, z_c*) moves according to Eqs. (8.16) and (8.18) through (8.20). We may consider time t as a parameter characterizing a family of such ellipsoids. During an interval of time, let a surface E*

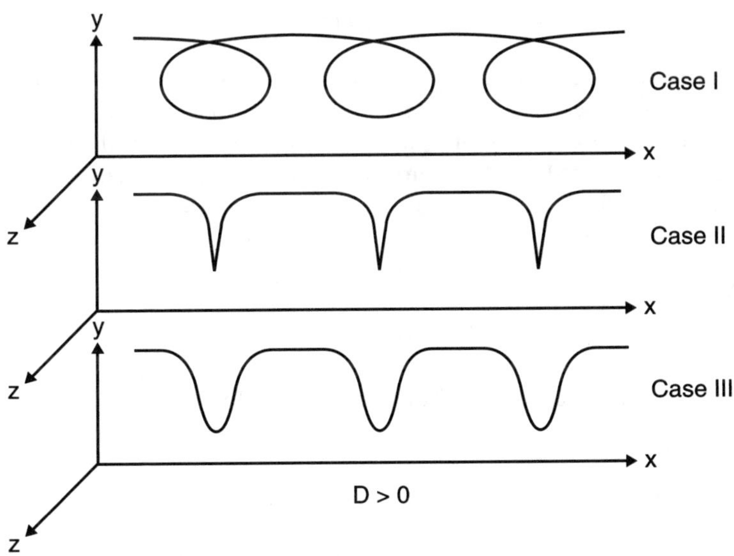

Figure 8.3. Radial and intrack profile of relative orbit.

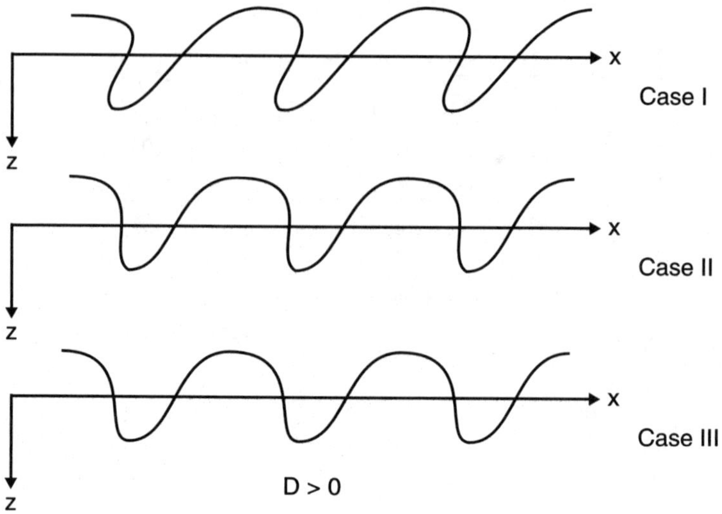

Figure 8.4. Intrack and crosstrack profile of relative orbit.

denote an envelope to this family of ellipsoids such that each of them is tangent to E^* along a locus of points. We now have a problem that is the generalization of the classic case of an envelope tangent to a family of curves.[8.3] For the general case, we shall use a different approach, as follows: If we are given a family of surfaces

$$F(x_1,x_2,...x_n,t)=0 \tag{8.31}$$

with t as a parameter characterizing each surface, then we may consider Eq. (8.31) as describing a "hypersurface" in the $(n + 1)$-dimensional space of the variables so that if we take cuts of constant t, we recover each member of the family. Next, we consider an extended family of surfaces $F(x_1, x_2, ...x_n, t) = c$, of which $c = 0$ is a member. Thus, for a surface E^* to be tangent to the family indicated in Eq. (8.31), we must have

$$\frac{\partial}{\partial t}F(x_1,x_2,...x_n,t)=0 \tag{8.32}$$

It follows that the envelope E^* of the family of ellipsoids (8.30) has to satisfy

$$\frac{\partial}{\partial t}F(x^*,y^*,z^*,t)=0 \tag{8.33}$$

By eliminating t between Eqs. (8.33) and (8.30), we obtain the equation of the envelope E^*:

$$\Phi(x^*, y^*, z^*) = 0 \tag{8.34}$$

Equation (8.34) describes a surface which bounds a volume V^* in the (x^*, y^*, z^*)-space. The general nature of this surface is very complicated. It depends on both the motion of the sphere and the time variation of the covariance ellipsoid. Even if the covariance ellipsoid does not change much in time in both its dilation and rotation, the envelope E^* still depends on the motion of the center and the radius of the sphere. If the radius of curvature of the motion of the center is smaller than the radius of the sphere, this surface can cut back on itself, and we have to be extremely cautious in determining the volume bounded by it. On the other hand, if the radius of curvature is large compared to the radius of the sphere, this surface resembles a gently bending tube with an undulating cross section, as depicted in Fig. 8.5.

8.5 Examples of Volumes V and V^*

8.5.1 Torus in Volume V

We may represent the torus as symmetric about the z-axis with r the radius of the circular cross section and R the radius of the circular locus of the center of the cross section. The equation for this surface may be obtained simply, as described in books on mensuration, by rotating a circle of radius r with center at a distance R from the z-axis. However, to illustrate the foregoing method, we wish to obtain this equation as the envelope of a family of spheres of radius r whose center moves in a circle of radius R.

Thus, the family of moving spheres parameterized by time t takes the form

$$(x - R\sin t)^2 + (y - R\cos t)^2 + z^2 = r^2 \tag{8.35}$$

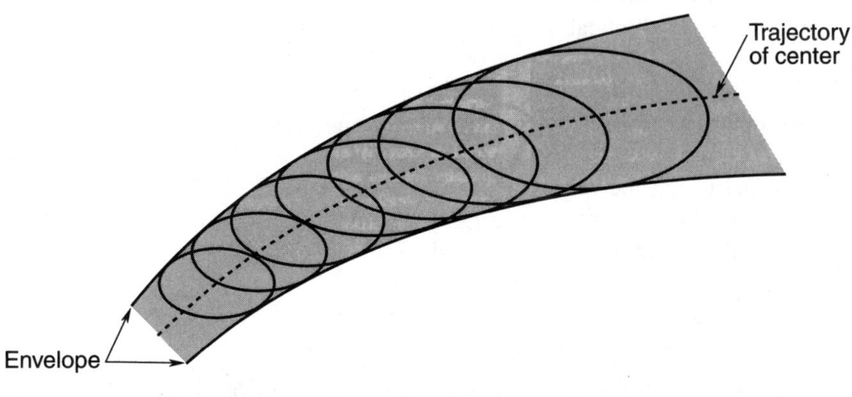

Figure 8.5. Envelope of a family of ellipsoids.

which is equivalently

$$(x^2 + y^2) - 2R(x\sin t + y\cos t) + R^2 + z^2 = r^2 \tag{8.36}$$

By differentiating with respect to t and setting to zero, we obtain the following envelope condition:

$$x\cos t - y\sin t = 0 \tag{8.37}$$

which yields

$$\sin t = x\Big/\sqrt{x^2 + y^2} \quad \text{and} \quad \cos t = y\Big/\sqrt{x^2 + y^2} \tag{8.38}$$

By substituting Eq. (8.38) into (8.36) and then regrouping terms, we obtain the envelope

$$\left(\sqrt{x^2 + y^2} - R\right)^2 + z^2 = r^2 \tag{8.39}$$

8.5.2 Elliptical Doughnut in Volume V*

We shall next consider the case of elliptical relative motion about the origin. With $C = D = 0$ in the Clohessy-Wiltshire equations (8.21) through (8.23), the motion of the center becomes

$$x_c = A\sin\tau, \quad y_c = \frac{1}{2}A\cos\tau \quad \text{and} \quad z_c = 0 \quad \text{where} \quad \tau \equiv \omega t + \phi \tag{8.40}$$

In this special case, the trajectory of the center is a closed curve, and this surface resembles an elliptical doughnut with a somewhat (but not exactly) elliptical cross section.

For simplicity, we consider the case of covariance that is time-independent and isotropic so that we now have a sphere of constant radius with center moving along the ellipse described by Eq. (8.40). Hence, the volume V in the (x, y, z)-space is the same as the volume V^* in the (x^*, y^*, z^*)-space. Moreover, because of this simplification, we note that in Eq. (8.7) the matrix M is equal to the identity matrix I so that we may omit the asterisk in this special case.

Equation (8.30) now takes the form

$$(x - A\sin\tau)^2 + \left(y - \frac{1}{2}A\cos\tau\right)^2 + z^2 = \rho^2 \tag{8.41}$$

which is equivalent to

$$(x^2+y^2)-2A(x\sin\tau+\frac{1}{2}y\cos\tau)+\frac{1}{4}A^2+\frac{3}{4}A^2\sin^2\tau+z^2=\rho^2 \tag{8.42}$$

By differentiating with respect to t, we obtain from Eq. (8.33)

$$2Ax\cos\tau-A\sin\tau\left(y+\frac{3}{2}A\cos\tau\right)=0 \tag{8.43}$$

By multiplying Eq. (8.42) by $\cos\tau$ and (8.43) by $\sin\tau$, using the identity $\sin^2\tau+\cos^2\tau=1$, and then eliminating terms, we obtain the following cubic equation in $\cos\tau$:

$$\frac{3}{4}A^2\cos^3\tau+\left(x^2+y^2+z^2-\frac{1}{2}A^2-\rho^2\right)\cos\tau-Ay=0 \tag{8.44}$$

This equation is already in the "reduced" form, because the second-degree term is absent. It may be readily solved for cost by Cardan's method.[8.4] Thus, we define

$$p=4\left(x^2+y^2+z^2-\frac{1}{2}A^2-\rho^2\right)\Big/3A^2,\quad q=-4y/3A=0\quad\text{and}\quad Q=\left(\frac{p}{3}\right)^3+\left(\frac{q}{2}\right)^2 \tag{8.45}$$

The solution is then given by

$$\cos\tau=\sqrt[3]{-\frac{q}{2}+\sqrt{Q}}+\sqrt[3]{-\frac{q}{2}-\sqrt{Q}} \tag{8.46}$$

The resultant expression may then be substituted into either Eq. (8.41) or (8.43) to obtain the equation for the envelope, Eq. (8.34). Caution must be exercised to determine if the surface cuts back on itself. If the radius ρ of the circular cross section is smaller than $A/2$, then the elliptical doughnut will not cut back on itself and there will only be one hole. This surface of genus 1 is called a "torus" (Fig. 8.6).

A little consideration will reveal that if $\rho \geq A/2$, then there will be no hole. This surface of genus 0 may be called a "sphere" (Fig. 8.7). Thus, for a sphere of constant radius $\rho \geq A/2$ with center moving along an ellipse, there cannot be a surface generated of genus 2 called a "pretzel."

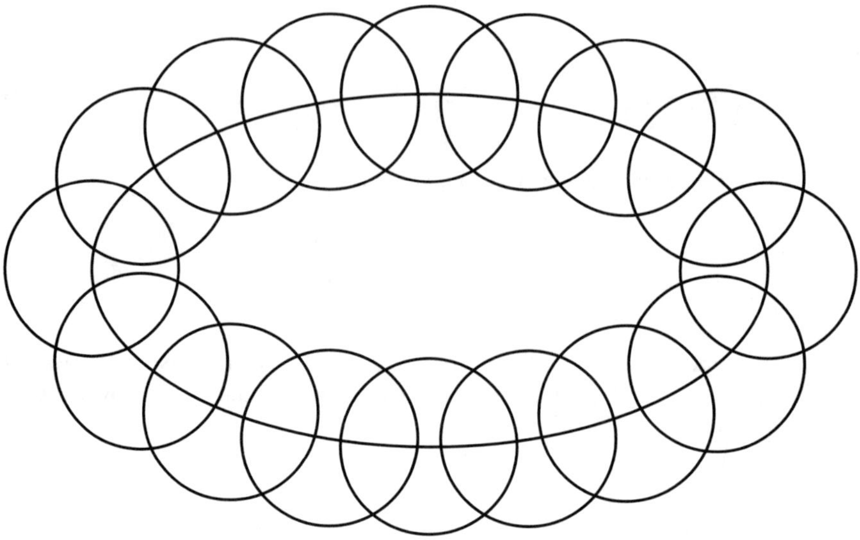

Figure 8.6. "Torus" (surface of genus 1) for $\rho < A/2$.

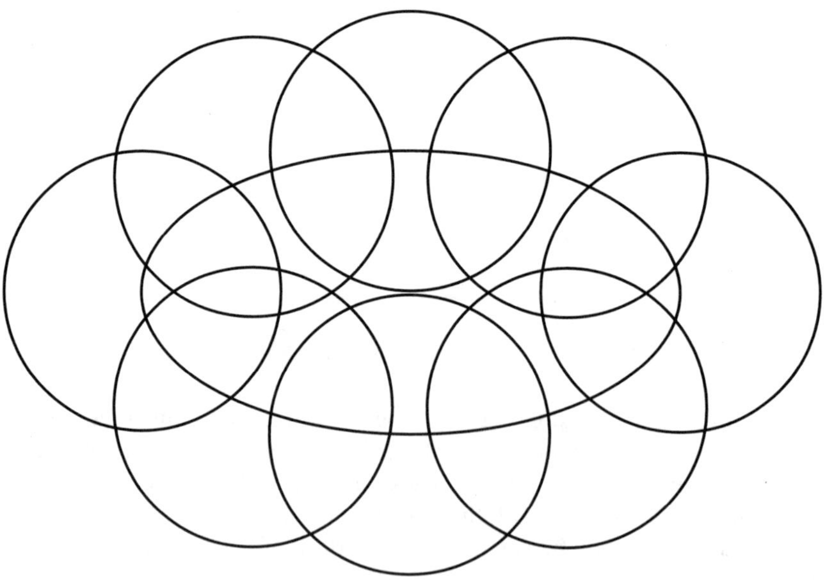

Figure 8.7. "Sphere" (surface of genus 0) for $\rho \geq A/2$.

The foregoing classifications take after those of differential geometry except for issues pertaining to differentiability.[8.5] Whatever the nature of this surface, it determines the volume of integration V for the isotropic three-dimensional Gaussian pdf to compute the probability of collision for the case of long-term encounters. Because of the possibility of the surface intersecting itself, we cannot simply determine the probability of collision by considering cylindrical disks (with normal in the direction of the instantaneous tangent) that are covered by the motion of the center during infinitesimal periods of time. Moreover, because of the curvature of the trajectory of the center, these cylindrical slices have the additional problem of overlapping on the concave side and introducing gaps on the convex side of the curved trajectory. Thus, the principles of calculus cannot be applied even in the limit of infinitesimal slices.

8.6 Probability of Collision

From the foregoing discussion, we compute the probability of collision P by integrating the three-dimensional isotropic Gaussian pdf over the volume V^* in the (x^*, y^*, z^*)-space:

$$P = \frac{1}{(2\pi)^{3/2}\sigma^3} \iiint_{V^*} e^{-(x^{*2}+y^{*2}+z^{*2})/2\sigma^2} dx^* \, dy^* \, dz^* \tag{8.47}$$

The volume V^* is bounded by the enveloping surface E^* given by $\Phi(x^*, y^*, z^*) = 0$ as in Eq. (8.34). In general, this surface E^* and hence the volume V^* are very complicated. Moreover, we do not usually have the explicit matrices needed in Eq. (8.7) to transform from V to V^*. Hence, we resort to simplifying assumptions as in the example discussed previously with the elliptical doughnut. Unless we specify how the covariance changes with time, all we have at our disposal are the comparatively simple cases of closed relative trajectories as shown in Figs. 8.2 and 8.6. Even this meager information is sufficient to illustrate vital differences between short-term and long-term encounters. Thus, we work with Eqs. (8.21) through (8.23), which yield

$$x_c = C + A\sin\tau, \quad y_c = \frac{1}{2}A\cos\tau \quad \text{and} \quad z_c = 0 \quad \text{where} \quad \tau \equiv \omega t + \phi \tag{8.48}$$

Hence, we have an elliptical doughnut described by Eqs. (8.41) through (8.44), but displaced by a constant C on the x-axis. The integral P may be evaluated numerically, and this can be very time-consuming. Moreover, this approach yields little insight and has to be repeated whenever the input collision parameters, such as the standard deviation σ, the spherical radius ρ, the trajectory semimajor axis A, and the displacement C, are changed.

An alternative approach is to exploit the method of equivalent cross-section areas (MECSA), discussed in Section 5.6 of Chapter 5, which has been found to be numerically accurate to approximately three significant figures in computing the collision probability for most spacecraft encounters. We need now to make a slight change of viewpoint, because we no longer apply it to collision cross-sectional areas but to general integration areas. For convenience, we shall refer to this as the method of equivalent areas (MEA). We proceed as follows.

First, we revisit Fig. 8.6, but here show only the outlines of the envelope, in Fig. 8.8.

Even though these two outlines are not true ellipses, we shall approximate them by ellipses: the outer, with semimajor axis $(A + \rho)$ and semiminor axis $(A/2 + \rho)$; the inner, with semimajor axis $(A - \rho)$ and semiminor axis $(A/2 - \rho)$. Thus, their respective areas are given by

$$A_{\text{outer}} = \pi(A+\rho)(A/2+\rho) \quad \text{and} \quad A_{\text{inner}} = \pi(A-\rho)(A/2-\rho) \tag{8.49}$$

We approximate each ellipse by a circle of equal area. Thus, we have

$$R_{\text{outer}} = \sqrt{(A+\rho)(A/2+\rho)} \quad \text{and} \quad R_{\text{inner}} = \sqrt{(A-\rho)(A/2-\rho)} \tag{8.50}$$

We now essentially have the situation of a circular torus with radius R from the symmetry axis (parallel to the z-axis and displaced along the x-axis by a distance C) and radius r of cross section given by

$$R = (R_{\text{outer}} + R_{\text{inner}})/2 \quad \text{and} \quad r = (R_{\text{outer}} - R_{\text{inner}})/2 \tag{8.51}$$

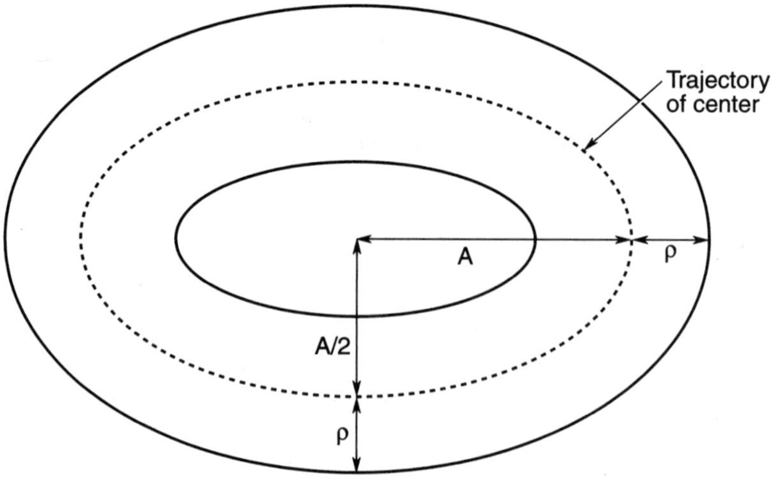

Figure 8.8. Outlines of envelope from Fig. 8.6 in (x, y)-plane.

This circular torus is shown in Fig. 8.9.

Let us next consider a two-dimensional integral I over the area of the plane $z = \beta$ within the circular torus. This (x, y)-integration area is an annulus A' bounded by two concentric circles of radii $(R + \alpha)$ and $(R - \alpha)$ centered at the point $(C, 0)$. It is easily shown that we have

$$\alpha = \sqrt{r^2 - z^2} \tag{8.52}$$

The integral I is given by

$$I = \frac{1}{2\pi\sigma^2} \iint_{\text{Annulus } A'} e^{-(x^2+y^2)/2\sigma^2} \, dxdy \tag{8.53}$$

Let the integrals $I_{R+\alpha}$ and $I_{R-\alpha}$ be defined by

$$I_{R+\alpha} = \frac{1}{2\pi\sigma^2} \iint_{\substack{\text{Circle} \\ \text{Radius} \\ (R+\alpha)}} e^{-(x^2+y^2)/2\sigma^2} \, dxdy \quad \text{and} \quad I_{R-\alpha} = \frac{1}{2\pi\sigma^2} \iint_{\substack{\text{Circle} \\ \text{Radius} \\ (R-\alpha)}} e^{-(x^2+y^2)/2\sigma^2} \, dxdy \tag{8.54}$$

We can transform the two-dimensional integral $I_{R+\alpha}$ into a one-dimensional integral involving the Rician pdf, and we obtain the following result accurate to approximately three significant figures:

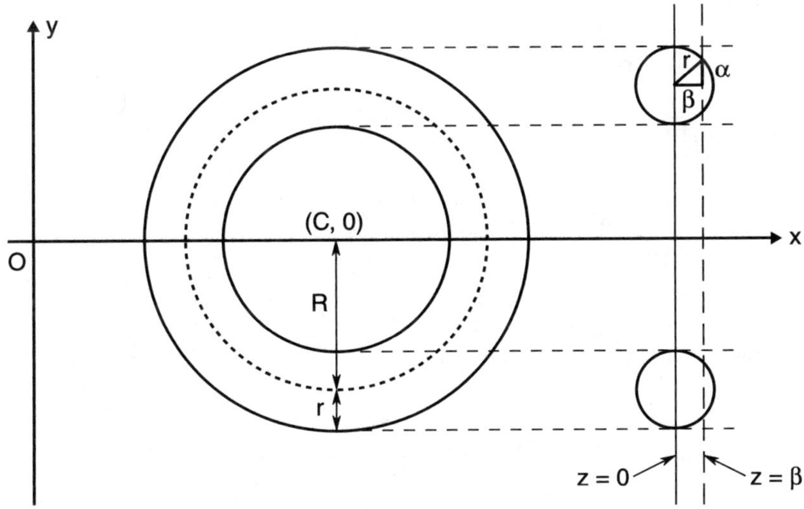

Figure 8.9. Outline of circular torus.

$$I_{R+\alpha} = e^{-v/2}(1 - e^{-u_{R+\alpha}/2}) \quad \text{where} \quad u_{R+\alpha} \equiv \left(\frac{R+\alpha}{\sigma}\right)^2 \quad \text{and} \quad v \equiv \left(\frac{C}{\sigma}\right)^2 \tag{8.55}$$

Similarly, the two-dimensional integral $I_{R-\alpha}$ can be transformed into the following one-dimensional integral:

$$I_{R-\alpha} = e^{-v/2}(1 - e^{-u_{R-\alpha}/2}) \quad \text{where} \quad u_{R-\alpha} \equiv \left(\frac{R-\alpha}{\sigma}\right)^2 \quad \text{and} \quad v \equiv \left(\frac{C}{\sigma}\right)^2 \tag{8.56}$$

Therefore, the integral I over the annulus A' is given by

$$\begin{aligned} I &= I_{R+\alpha} - I_{R-\alpha} \\ &= e^{-v/2}(e^{-u_{R-\alpha}/2} - e^{-u_{R+\alpha}/2}) \\ &= e^{-v/2}(e^{-(R^2-2R\alpha+\alpha^2)/2\sigma^2} - e^{-(R^2+2R\alpha+\alpha^2)/2\sigma^2}) \\ &= e^{-v/2}e^{-(R^2+\alpha^2)/2\sigma^2}(e^{R\alpha/\sigma^2} - e^{-R\alpha/\sigma^2}) \\ &= e^{-v/2}e^{-(R^2+r^2-z^2)/2\sigma^2}(e^{R\sqrt{r^2-z^2}/\sigma^2} - e^{-R\sqrt{r^2-z^2}/\sigma^2}) \end{aligned} \tag{8.57}$$

Hence, the collision probability P in Eq. (8.47) takes the form

$$\begin{aligned} P &= \frac{1}{\sqrt{2\pi}\sigma}\int_{-r}^{r} Ie^{-z^2/2\sigma^2}\,dz \\ &= \frac{2}{\sqrt{2\pi}\sigma}e^{-v/2}e^{-(R^2+r^2)/2\sigma^2}\int_{0}^{r}(e^{R\sqrt{r^2-z^2}/\sigma^2} - e^{-R\sqrt{r^2-z^2}/\sigma^2})\,dz \\ &= \frac{4}{\sqrt{2\pi}\sigma}e^{-(C^2+R^2+r^2)/2\sigma^2}\int_{0}^{r}\sinh\left(\frac{R\sqrt{r^2-z^2}}{\sigma^2}\right)dz \end{aligned} \tag{8.58}$$

It appears at first sight that the RHS of Eq. (8.58) has to be evaluated numerically. However, a little consideration reveals that we may express the integrand as

$$\sinh\xi = \sum_{n=0}^{\infty}\frac{\xi^{2n+1}}{(2n+1)!} \tag{8.59}$$

Thus, we obtain the following expression

$$P = \frac{4}{\sqrt{2\pi}\sigma} e^{-(C^2+R^2+r^2)/2\sigma^2} \int_0^r \sum_{n=0}^{\infty} \frac{\xi^{2n+1}}{(2n+1)!} dz \quad \text{where} \quad \xi \equiv \frac{R\sqrt{r^2 - z^2}}{\sigma^2} \tag{8.60}$$

Let us introduce a new variable θ defined by

$$z = r\sin\theta \quad \text{so that} \quad dz = r\cos\theta\, d\theta \tag{8.61}$$

Then, it is easily shown that

$$\xi = \frac{Rr}{\sigma^2}\cos\theta, \quad \xi dz = \frac{Rr^2}{\sigma^2}\cos^2\theta\, d\theta \quad \text{and} \quad \xi^{2n+1} dz = \frac{Rr^2}{\sigma^2}\left(\frac{Rr}{\sigma^2}\right)^{2n} \cos^{2n+2}\theta\, d\theta \tag{8.62}$$

By substituting Eq. (8.62) into (8.60) and interchanging the order of integration and summation, we obtain

$$P = \frac{4}{\sqrt{2\pi}} e^{-(C^2+R^2+r^2)/2\sigma^2} \frac{Rr^2}{\sigma^3} \sum_{n=0}^{\infty} \frac{1}{(2n+1)!}\left(\frac{Rr}{\sigma^2}\right)^{2n} \int_0^{\pi/2} \cos^{2n+2}\theta\, d\theta \tag{8.63}$$

The integral on the RHS can be obtained in closed form:[8.5]

$$\int_0^{\pi/2} \cos^{2n+2}\theta\, d\theta = \frac{\pi}{2}\, \frac{1\cdot 3\cdot 5\cdot 7\cdots(2n+1)}{2\cdot 4\cdot 6\cdot 8\cdots(2n+2)} = \frac{\pi}{2}\, \frac{(2n+1)!}{2^{2n+1} n!(n+1)!} \tag{8.64}$$

Consequently, Eq. (8.63) becomes

$$P = \sqrt{2\pi}\, e^{-(C^2+R^2+r^2)/2\sigma^2} \frac{Rr^2}{\sigma^3} \sum_{n=0}^{\infty} \left(\frac{Rr}{\sigma^2}\right)^{2n} \frac{1}{2^{2n+1} n!(n+1)!} \tag{8.65}$$

It is easily seen that the infinite series on the RHS is rapidly convergent for all values of the parameters C, R, r, and σ, because it is termwise dominated by the exponential series. The combined hard-body radius r is approximately 10 m. For most long-term geosynchronous spacecraft encounters, we are probably dealing with R on the order of 10 km or less. We may assume that the effective combined standard deviation σ is on the order of 1 km. Hence, the ratio $(Rr/\sigma^2)^2$ of successive terms in the infinite series is approximately 0.01. It probably suffices to take only the first two terms in Eq. (8.65) to obtain the probability of collision for most long-term spacecraft encounters. However, if we are dealing with a value of R on the order of 100 km, then we may need about 4 or 5 terms. Instead of evaluating the terms individually and then summing them, it is more efficient and more accurate to use the following recursion relation:

$$T_o = \frac{1}{2}, \quad T_n = T_{n-1}\left(\frac{Rr}{\sigma^2}\right)^2 \frac{1}{4n(n+1)} \quad \text{for} \quad n = 1,2,3\cdots \tag{8.66}$$

8.7 Discussion

In this analysis, we used the MEA to obtain an analytical expression for the collision probability for the comparatively simple case of an elliptical torus. We can apply this procedure to analyze more complex volumes of integration by effectively using equivalent areas as shown in Chapter 5. However, we may have to resort to numerical evaluation of areas of integration before we can convert these to circles of the same area. Once we do this, we have essentially converted the problem to one described by the Rician pdf and we can then exploit results previously obtained in Chapter 4, which gives Eqs. (8.55) and (8.56) in this chapter.

Finally, we proceed to integrate along the remaining direction. There are no rigid rules that govern which two integration variables to use first and which to use last. In the example given here, we used the (x, y)-plane first because of the simplicity of performing that conversion to existing available results. Any other choice would have made the analysis more complicated. However, for other more complex volumes of integration, it is possible that a different choice may prove more advantageous. For enveloping surfaces that cut back on themselves, it is also possible that we may simplify the integration by breaking the volume into a number of components that are easier to handle and then applying MEA.

8.8 Conclusion

An analytical expression has been obtained for computing the probability of collision between two spacecraft that spend a substantial period of time in the same vicinity. The main results are given by Eq. (8.65). The advantages of using this expression are:

- It eliminates the numerical evaluation of the collision integral by a computer program that may be difficult to develop logically.
- It circumvents time-consuming Monte Carlo simulations of potential collisions that can take as much as several days to complete.
- It rapidly yields results if the collision parameters such as the standard deviation σ, the radius ρ, the trajectory semimajor axis A, and the displacement C are changed, without having to repeat the computer runs.

8.9 Summary

In this chapter, we considered the case of long-term encounters for which the assumption of rectilinear motion for evaluating the collision integral is not valid.

In Section 8.1, we discussed the need to define an appropriate set of random variables (x^*, y^*, z^*) consistent with the formulation of the probability integral. If the covariance error ellipsoid changes in shape, size, and orientation or the relative motion within the encounter region is curved, we can no longer consider the Cartesian coordinates (x, y, z) representing the relative position uncertainty in the physical space as random variables.

In Section 8.2, we derived equations for the transformation of a sphere in the (x, y, z)-space to the (x^*, y^*, z^*)-space. We also obtained the tangent to the trajectory in the (x^*, y^*, z^*)-space. This tangent is not in the same direction as the "physical" velocity transformed to the (x^*, y^*, z^*)-space.

In Section 8.3, we discussed the relative motion in the physical space consistent with the laws of dynamics. These are the well-known Clohessy-Wiltshire equations as a first approximation.

In Section 8.4, we derived the equation of an envelope generated by an object moving in a three-dimensional space. This is a generalization of the classical case of an envelope in a two-dimensional plane. The volume within this envelope is required for integration to obtain the collision probability.

In Section 8.5, we worked out details of obtaining an envelope for a torus and an elliptical doughnut.

In Section 8.6, we derived an expression for the collision probability for relative in-plane motion for which we have an ellipse with aspect ratio of 2. This solution is in the form of an infinite series convergent for all values of the input collision parameters.

In Section 8.7, we briefly advocated the use of a combination of numerical evaluation of areas and the method of equivalent areas before we can apply the Rician distribution to compute the collision probability for the case of long-term encounters.

In Section 8.8, we stated the advantages of having an analytical expression for the collision probability for a simple case of long-term encounters.

8.10 References

[8.1] F. K. Chan, "Spacecraft Collision Probability for Long-Term Encounters," *AIAA/AAS Astrodynamics Specialist Conference* (Big Sky, MT, 3–7 August 2003).

[8.2] V. A. Chobotov, *Orbital Mechanics, 2nd ed.* (AIAA Education Series, 1996), pp. 157–158.

[8.3] P. Franklin, *Methods of Advanced Calculus* (McGraw-Hill, 1944) pp. 343–344.

[8.4] G. A. Korn and T. M. Korn, *Mathematical Handbook for Scientists and Engineers* (McGraw-Hill, 1968), pp. 23 and 974.

[8.5] W. Gellert, S. Gottwald, M. Hellwich, H. Kastner, and H. Kustner, eds., *Concise Encyclopedia of Mathematics, 2nd ed.* (Van Nostrand Reinhold, 1989), p. 570.

Chapter 9: Short-Term vs. Long-Term Spacecraft Encounters

In this chapter, we use the equations for computing the collision probabilities obtained in Chapters 5 and 7 to compare the differences between short-term and long-term encounters.[9.1] First, we derive the equation for the minimum distance between any point on an ellipse and any point on the major axis of the same ellipse.

9.1 Distance of Closest Approach

Consider Fig. 9.1, which illustrates an ellipse with semimajor axis A and semiminor axis A/m (i.e., the ellipse has an aspect ratio m). The equation of this ellipse is

$$x^2 + m^2 y^2 = A^2 \tag{9.1}$$

At the point $P(x_o, y_o)$ on this ellipse, the normal **n** is given by

$$\mathbf{n} = x_o \hat{\mathbf{i}} + m^2 y_o \hat{\mathbf{j}} \tag{9.2}$$

Therefore, the equation of this normal is

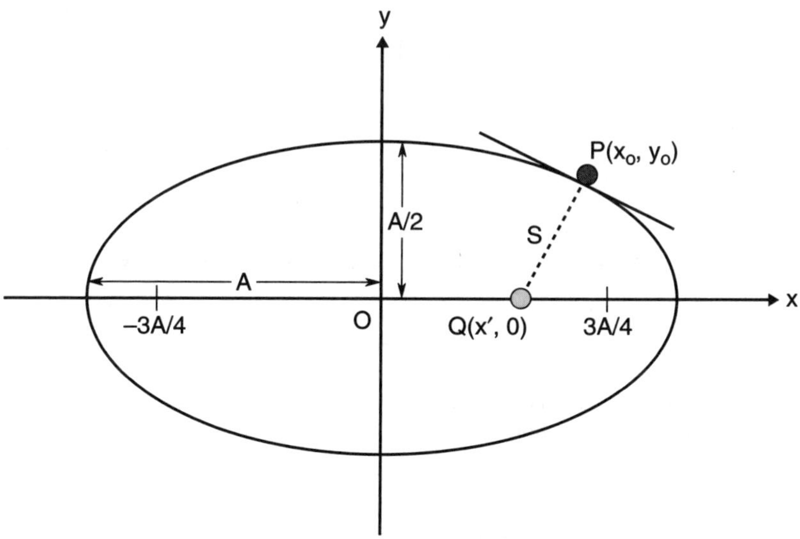

Figure 9.1. Distance of closest approach.

$$y = y_o + \frac{m^2 y_o}{x_o}\left(x - x_o\right) \tag{9.3}$$

If $y_o \neq 0$, then this line intersects the x-axis at some point we denote by $Q(x', 0)$. Hence, we have

$$y_o + \frac{m^2 y_o}{x_o}\left(x' - x_o\right) = 0 \tag{9.4}$$

Because $y_o \neq 0$, therefore we may cancel the common factor y_o to obtain

$$1 + \frac{m^2}{x_o}\left(x' - x_o\right) = 0 \tag{9.5}$$

which yields

$$x' = \left(\frac{m^2 - 1}{m^2}\right) x_o \tag{9.6}$$

The distance S from P to Q is given by

$$S^2 = \left(x' - x_o\right)^2 + y_o^{\,2} \tag{9.7}$$

Substitution of Eq. (9.5) into (9.7) yields

$$m^4 S^2 = x_o^{\,2} + m^4 y_o^{\,2} \tag{9.8}$$

Because the point $P(x_o, y_o)$ lies on the ellipse, therefore we have

$$x_o^{\,2} + m^2 y_o^{\,2} = A^2 \tag{9.9}$$

By eliminating y_o between Eqs. (9.8) and (9.9) and dividing by m^2 (noting that m cannot be zero), we obtain

$$m^2 S^2 = A^2 - \left(\frac{m^2 - 1}{m^2}\right) x_o^{\,2} \tag{9.10}$$

We recall that Eq. (9.10) was derived under the assumption that the normal **n** intersects the x-axis. If the point $P(x_o, y_o)$ is on the x-axis, then the intersection point $Q(x', 0)$ is not defined. However, we can consider the limit as $x_o \to A$ in Eq. (9.10). We note that

$$\lim_{x_o \to A} S = \frac{A}{m^2} \equiv S^* \tag{9.11}$$

By using Eq. (9.6), we can also write (9.10) in terms of x' instead of x_o. Thus, we have

$$m^2 S^2 = A^2 - \left(\frac{m^2}{m^2 - 1} \right) x'^2 \tag{9.12}$$

Let C denote the distance of any point on the x-axis displaced from the center of the ellipse. In accordance with the usage of x_e as the distance of closest approach (or miss distance in spacecraft encounters), it follows from the present discussion that

$$\text{If } |C| \leq (A - S^*), \text{ then } x_e = S = \frac{1}{m} \sqrt{\left[A^2 - \frac{m^2 C^2}{(m^2 - 1)} \right]} \tag{9.13}$$

$$\text{If } |C| > (A - S^*), \text{ then } x_e = |A - C| \tag{9.14}$$

For our application to relative orbits with semimajor axis A and semiminor axis $A/2$, we see that $m = 2$. Thus, Eqs. (9.13) and (9.14) become specifically

$$\text{If } |C| \leq (3A/4), \text{ then } x_e = S = \frac{1}{2} \sqrt{\left[A^2 - \frac{4C^2}{3} \right]} \tag{9.15}$$

$$\text{If } |C| > (3A/4), \text{ then } x_e = |A - C| \tag{9.16}$$

For illustration, Fig. 9.2 depicts the distance of closest approach for the case of $A = 4$ km. Note that this distance is a nonlinear function of C from the origin up to 3 km. After that, it decreases linearly until it reaches zero. Thereafter, it increases linearly as C increases.

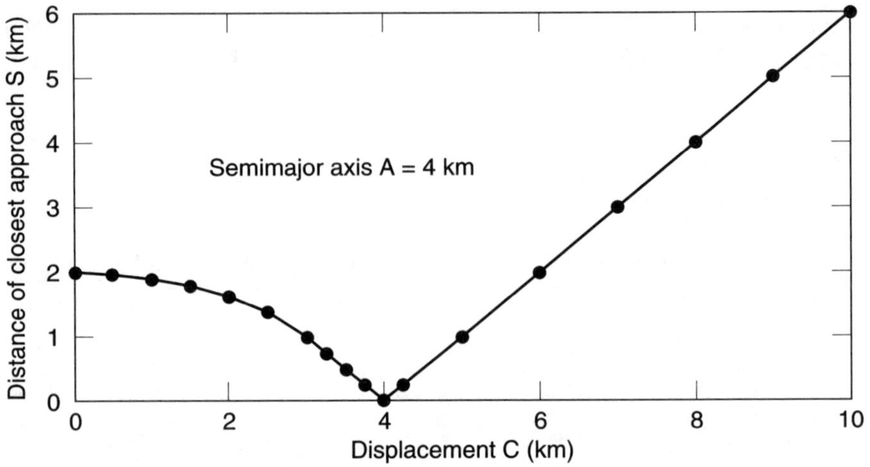

Figure 9.2. Distance of closest approach for the case of A = 4 km.

9.2 Short-Term Encounters

In Chapter 5, an analytical solution was obtained for the collision probability in the form of an infinite series convergent for all values of the relevant parameters. It turns out that, for spacecraft encounters of interest, truncation after the first term yields an error that appears in the third or fourth significant digit. Thus probability of collision for most short-term spacecraft encounters is expressed with sufficient accuracy as

$$P = e^{-v/2}(1 - e^{-u/2}) \tag{9.17}$$

where the dimensionless variables u and v are defined in terms of the mean standard deviation σ, the companion standard deviation σ^*, the miss distance x_e, and the radius r_A of collision cross-sectional integration by

$$u \equiv \left(\frac{r_A}{\sigma}\right)^2 > 0 \tag{9.18}$$

$$v \equiv \left(\frac{x_e}{\sigma^*}\right)^2 > 0 \tag{9.19}$$

$$\sigma^2 \equiv \sigma_{x'}\sigma_{z'} \quad \text{and} \quad \sigma^{*2} \equiv \sigma_{z'}^{\,2}\left\{1 + \left[\left(\frac{\sigma_{z'}}{\sigma_{x'}}\right)^2 - 1\right]\left(\frac{x_p'^2}{x_p'^2 + z_p'^2}\right)\right\}^{-1} \tag{9.20}$$

A simple alternative form of Eq. (9.19) devoid of the nonessential singularity at $x'_p = 0$ and $z'_p = 0$ is simply

$$v = \frac{x_p'^2}{\sigma_{x'}^2} + \frac{z_p'^2}{\sigma_{z'}^2} \tag{9.21}$$

9.3 Long-Term Encounters

In Chapter 8, we considered the special case of relative motion for in-plane motion and no drift:

$$x_c = C + A\sin\tau, \quad y_c = \frac{1}{2}A\cos\tau \quad \text{and} \quad z_c = 0 \quad \text{where} \quad \tau \equiv \omega t + \phi \tag{9.22}$$

Thus, the secondary spacecraft moves in an ellipse relative to the primary in the orbital plane of the primary with semimajor axis A and semiminor axis $A/2$. The volume of integration for determining the collision probability is an elliptical doughnut, which is approximated by a circular torus using the method of equivalent areas.

Let R be the radius of the center of the cross section from the axis of symmetry of the torus and let r be the radius of the cross section. (See Chapter 8, Fig. 8.9.)

For simplicity, we considered the case of an isotropic and time-independent covariance. Hence, we have a sphere of radius ρ (or r_A) moving along an ellipse described by Eq. (9.22). The parameters R and r are defined in terms of A and ρ by the following equations:

$$R_{\text{outer}} = \sqrt{(A+\rho)(A/2+\rho)} \quad \text{and} \quad R_{\text{inner}} = \sqrt{(A-\rho)(A/2-\rho)} \tag{9.23}$$

$$R = (R_{\text{outer}} + R_{\text{inner}})/2 \quad \text{and} \quad r = (R_{\text{outer}} - R_{\text{inner}})/2 \tag{9.24}$$

From Eqs. (9.23) and (9.24), we can easily show that the following identities hold for all values of A, ρ, R, and r:

$$Rr \equiv \frac{3}{4}A\rho \tag{9.25}$$

$$R^2 + r^2 \equiv \frac{1}{2}A^2 + \rho^2 \tag{9.26}$$

For $\rho < A/2$, by using Eqs. (9.23) and (9.24), we obtain the series expansions

$$R = \frac{A}{\sqrt{2}}\left[1 - \frac{\rho^2}{8A^2} - \frac{37\rho^4}{128A^4} + O\left(\frac{\rho^6}{A^6}\right)\right] \tag{9.27}$$

$$r = \frac{3\rho}{2\sqrt{2}}\left[1 + \frac{\rho^2}{8A^2} + \frac{39\rho^4}{128A^4} + O\left(\frac{\rho^6}{A^6}\right)\right] \tag{9.28}$$

When the probability density function (pdf) does not vary much over a region whose dimensions are of the magnitude of A (for example, the case of $A < \sigma$), an analytical solution is obtained for the collision probability in the form of an infinite series that is convergent for all values of the relevant parameters. It turns out that, for the spacecraft encounters of interest, truncation after the first term yields an error that appears in the third or fourth significant digit. Thus, the probability of collision for most long-term spacecraft encounters may be expressed with sufficient accuracy as

$$P = \sqrt{2\pi}\, e^{-(C^2+R^2+r^2)/2\sigma^2} \frac{Rr^2}{2\sigma^3} \tag{9.29}$$

In this equation, we need to invoke Eqs. (9.23) and (9.24) to compute R and r from A and ρ. However, by substituting Eqs. (9.25) and (9.28) into (9.29), we further obtain the following extremely simple approximate form directly involving A and ρ.

$$P \cong \frac{9\sqrt{\pi}A\rho^2}{16\sigma^3} e^{-(A^2+2\rho^2+2C^2)/4\sigma^2} \tag{9.30}$$

In view of Eq. (9.28), Eq. (9.30) is accurate to one or two significant digits for $(\rho/A) < 0.1$ and is accurate to 15% for $(\rho/A) = 0.5$. As with Eq. (9.29), we know that this equation is valid for $A < \sigma$, and we may also verify that it is accurate even for values of A slightly greater than σ (say approximately up to 1.5σ). Equation (9.29), rather than (9.30), is preferred for computations because it is accurate to four significant digits up to $(\rho/A) = 0.5$. However, it is not as useful for trend analysis; in that area, the latter equation gives a more insightful relation.

Beyond the range $0 \le A \le 1.5\sigma$ (approximate), the approach using these equations for computing the collision probability is replaced by the methodology discussed in Appendix A. The formulation described there is valid for all values of A and C, provided that $(\rho/\sigma) < 0.05$ (approximate), as is the case for most applications. In most spacecraft encounters, the value of ρ is usually between 0.5 m and 50 m, and σ is of the order of 100 m and 1 to 3 km. Only A and C will change, and they are determined by the initial conditions of the relative motion.

9.4 Case Study I: Concentric Ellipses, Primary at Center

For this case, we have the following family of concentric ellipses, each of which describes the relative motion of a secondary spacecraft around the primary spacecraft according to

$$x^2 + 4y^2 = A^2 \tag{9.31}$$

This is illustrated in Fig. 9.3. Thus, the displacement of the center of the ellipses from the primary spacecraft $C = 0$ in Eq. (9.22). (The displacement C is positive if the ellipses are to the right of the primary, negative if to the left.) For simplicity, we let the standard deviation $\sigma = 1$ km, thc collision cross-sectional radius $\rho = 0.005$ km, and the amplitude A range from 0.1 to 1.5 km. It is obvious that the distance of closest approach S for each of these ellipses is equal to the semiminor axis $A/2$ as shown in Fig. 9.4. Because (A/σ) is at most 1.5, Eq. (9.29) may be used to compute the probability of collision P.

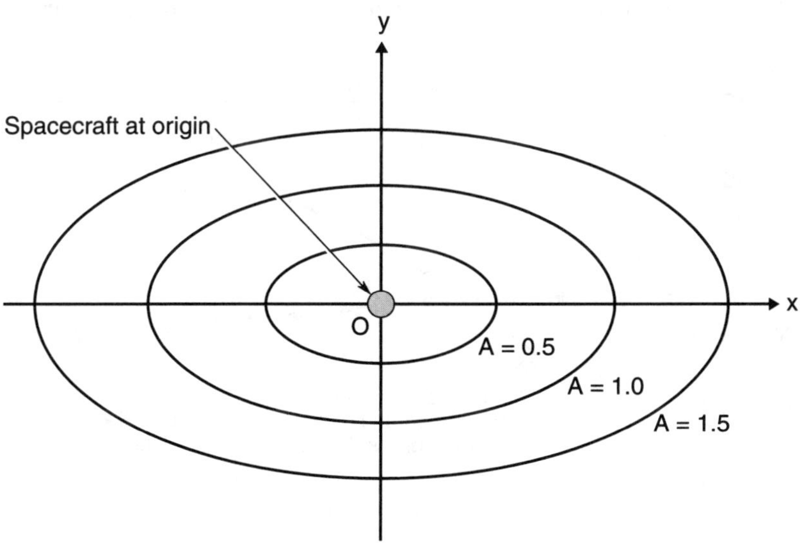

Figure 9.3. Concentric ellipses, primary at center.

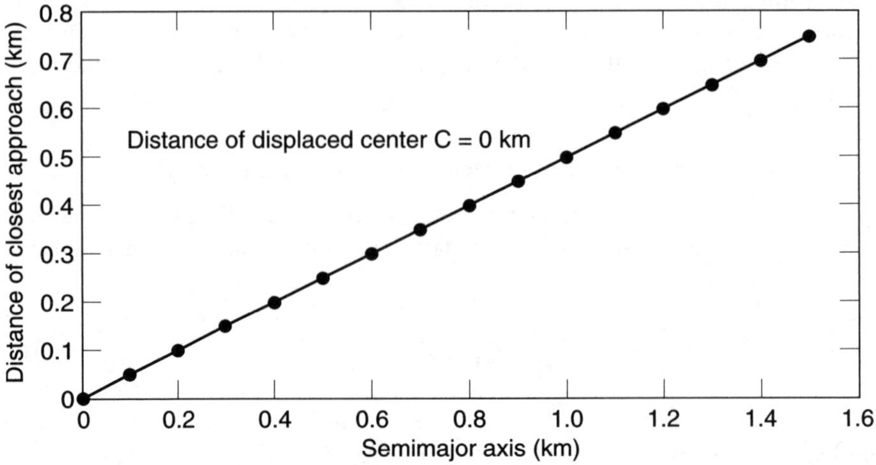

Figure 9.4. Distance of closest approach for concentric ellipses.

Figure 9.5 shows P as a function of A. Note that P increases to a maximum value of approximately 2×10^{-5} when $A \cong 1.4$ km, and then it decreases. This is expected because the volume of integration is small when A is small, thus yielding a small value of P. As A increases, the volume of integration increases, thus resulting in a higher value of P. However, as A further increases, the pdf decreases and even though the volume of integration increases, the net effect is that P decreases.

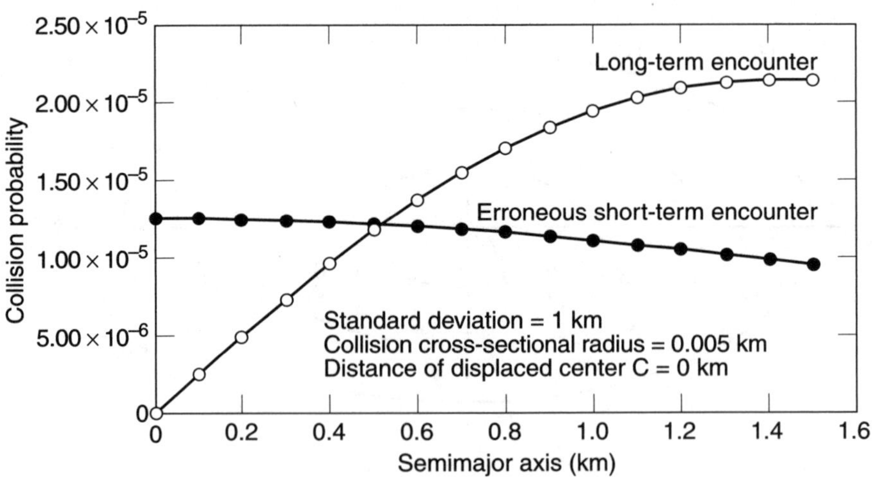

Figure 9.5. Collision probability for concentric ellipses.

In Fig. 9.5 is also plotted the erroneous collision probability that would have been unwarily computed if we had considered the spacecraft encounter to be of the short-term nature. Observe that the erroneous value obtained for the short-term encounter is larger than the correct value obtained for the long-term encounter when $(A/\sigma) < 0.5$ and smaller when $(A/\sigma) > 0.5$. The reason is that there is respectively excessive and insufficient integration volume allowed for by the improper short-term modeling in these ranges.

Of specific interest is the following: If we write Eq. (9.30) as

$$P = MAe^{-A^2/4\sigma^2} \quad \text{where} \quad M \equiv \frac{9\sqrt{\pi}\rho^2}{16\sigma^3} e^{-(\rho^2+C^2)/2\sigma^2} \tag{9.32}$$

then differentiation yields

$$\frac{\partial P}{\partial A} = Me^{-A^2/4\sigma^2}\left(1 - \frac{A^2}{2\sigma^2}\right) \tag{9.33}$$

The function $P(A)$ is maximum when $(\partial P/\partial A) = 0$, and we obtain

$$A = \sqrt{2}\sigma \tag{9.34}$$

Equation (9.34) holds for all families of concentric ellipses for which C is constant, not just zero. This is manifested in Fig. 9.5. Equation (9.34) also holds for all values of the cross-sectional radius ρ provided that Eq. (9.30) is valid. For these, only the value of the maximum value (dependent on C and ρ) of the collision probability P changes. The most important conclusion is that we need to ensure we avoid the situation in which the amplitude A is approximately 1.4σ.

9.5 Case Study II: Fixed-Size Ellipses, Variable Apsidal Distances

For this case, we have a family of fixed-size ellipses, each of which describes the relative motion of a secondary spacecraft with reference to the primary spacecraft according to

$$(x - C)^2 + 4y^2 = A^2 \tag{9.35}$$

These ellipses are illustrated in Fig. 9.6. In this family, the center of each ellipse is displaced a distance C along the x-axis from the primary. For simplicity, we let the standard deviation $\sigma = 1$ km, the collision cross-sectional radius $\rho = 0.005$ km, the amplitude $A = 0.4$ km, and the displacement C range from 0 to 1.2 km.

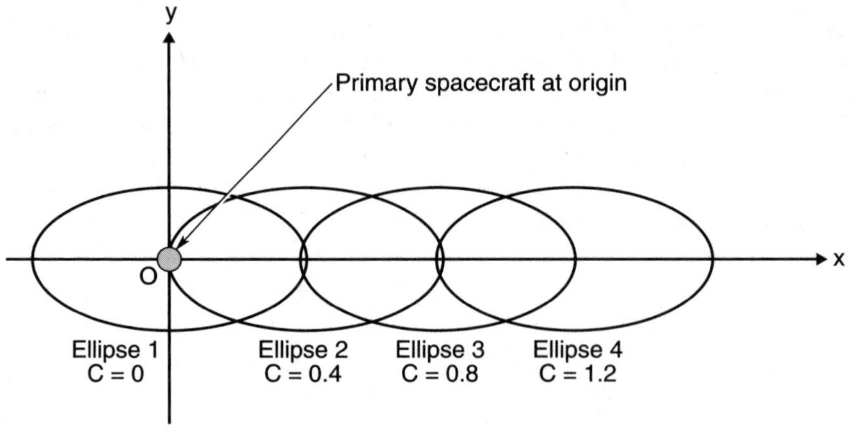

Figure 9.6. Fixed-size ellipses, variable apsidal distances.

The distance of closest approach S is determined according to the analysis given in Section 9.1. It is shown as a function of C in Fig. 9.7. When $C = 0$, the primary is at the center of the ellipse and $S = A/2$ as illustrated by Ellipse 1. As C increases, S decreases to the value zero when $C = A$ as illustrated by Ellipse 2. This is the transition point for the primary being inside or outside the ellipse traced out by the secondary. Thereafter, S increases linearly as a function of C as illustrated by Ellipses 3 and 4. Because $(A/\sigma) = 0.4$, Eq. (9.29) may again be used to compute the probability of collision P.

Figure 9.8 shows P as a function of C. Note that P decreases monotonically from a maximum of approximately 9.6×10^{-6} when $C = 0$. In Fig. 9.8 is also

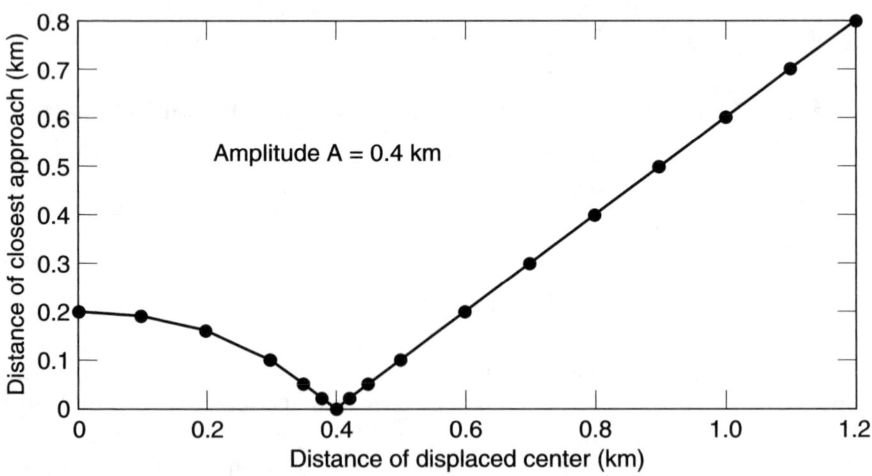

Figure 9.7. Distance of closest approach for fixed-size ellipses.

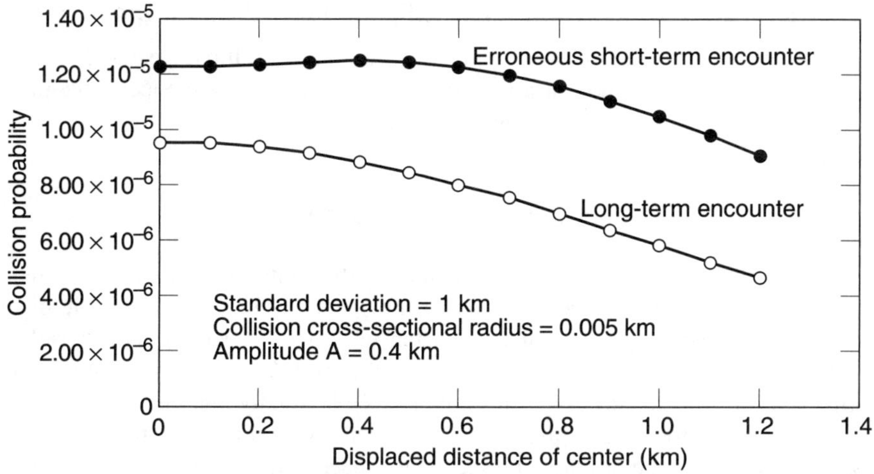

Figure 9.8. Collision probability for fixed-size ellipses.

plotted the erroneous higher collision probability that would have been computed if we had considered the spacecraft encounter to be of the short-term nature. It is noted that the erroneous value obtained for the short-term encounter is always larger than the correct value obtained for the long-term encounter. The reason is that there is excessive integration volume allowed for by the improper short-term modeling in these ranges.

Just as before, if we write Eq. (9.30) as

$$P = Ne^{-C^2/2\sigma^2} \quad \text{where} \quad N \equiv \frac{9\sqrt{\pi}A\rho^2}{16\sigma^3} e^{-(A^2+2\rho^2)/4\sigma^2} \tag{9.36}$$

then differentiation yields

$$\frac{\partial P}{\partial C} = -Ne^{-C^2/2\sigma^2}\frac{C^2}{\sigma^2} \tag{9.37}$$

The function $P(C)$ is maximum when $(\partial P/\partial C) = 0$, and we obtain

$$C = 0 \tag{9.38}$$

Equation (9.38) holds for all families of fixed-size ellipses for which A is constant. This is manifested in Fig. 9.8. It also holds for all values of the cross-sectional radius ρ provided that Eq. (9.30) is valid. For these, only the value of the maximum value (dependent on A and ρ) of the collision probability P changes.

The most important conclusion is that we need to ensure we avoid the situation in which the primary spacecraft is at the center of the ellipse (i.e., $C = 0$).

9.6 Case Study III: Variable-Size Ellipses, Fixed Apsidal Distances

For this case, we have the following family of variable-size ellipses, each of which describes the relative motion of a secondary spacecraft with reference to the primary spacecraft according to the equation

$$(x-C)^2 + 4y^2 = A^2 \quad \text{where} \quad A - C = \sigma \tag{9.39}$$

This is illustrated in Fig. 9.9. In this family, the center of each ellipse is displaced a distance C along the x-axis from the primary. For any ellipse, the displacement C is such that the "apsidal distance" D to a specified apse (apsidal point) on the relative orbit is fixed and set equal to σ. (*Note*: Strictly speaking, in normal celestial mechanics usage, apsidal distance is usually measured with reference to one of the foci of the ellipse. For Keplerian orbits, this distinction does not arise. But here, both the primary and secondary spacecraft move under the gravitational attraction of Earth, so the motion of the secondary relative to the primary is not Keplerian. Consequently, the primary is not always at one of the foci of the ellipse of relative motion.) For simplicity, we let the standard deviation $\sigma = 1$ km, the collision cross-sectional radius $\rho = 0.05$ km, and the amplitude A range from 0 to 1.2 km.

Again, the distance of closest approach S is determined according to the analysis given in Section 9.1. It is shown as a function of A in Fig. 9.10. Note that the distance of closest approach $S = 0$ when $A = 0$. Then, it decreases linearly to zero when $A = 0.5$ km. After that, it increases nonlinearly until $A = 4$ km. Beyond that, it stays constant at 1 km for all values of A.

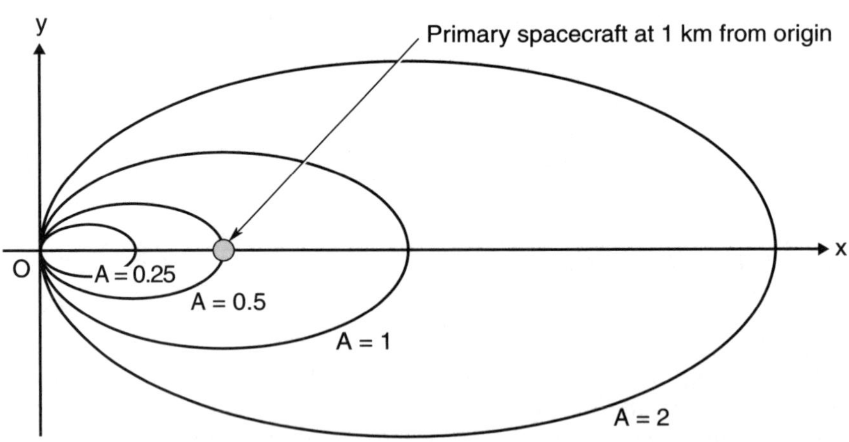

Figure 9.9. Variable-size ellipses, fixed apsidal distances.

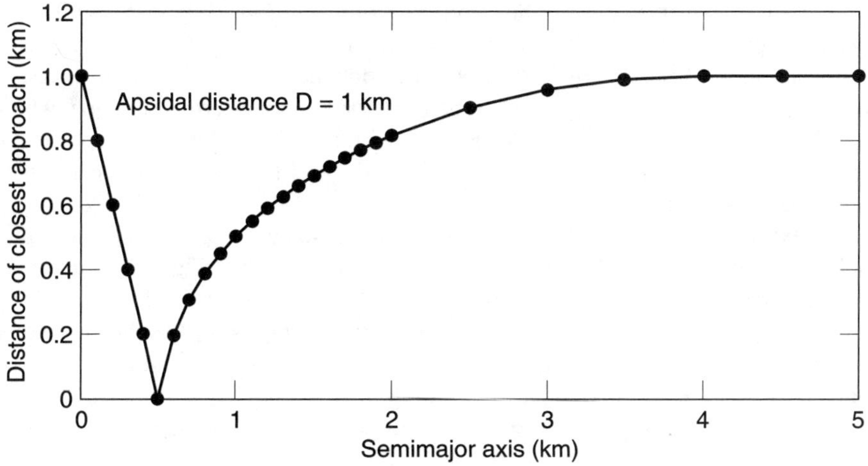

Figure 9.10. Distance of closest approach for variable-size ellipses.

Because (A/σ) is less than 1.5, Eq. (9.29) may again be used to compute the probability of collision *P*. Figure 9.11 shows *P* as a function of *A*. Note that *P* increases to a maximum value of approximately 2×10^{-3} when $A \cong 1.2$ km, and then it decreases. This is expected because the volume of integration is small when *A* is small, thus yielding a small value of *P*. As *A* increases, the volume of integration increases, thus resulting in a higher value of *P*. However, as *A* further increases, the pdf decreases, and even though the volume of integration increases, the net effect is that *P* decreases.

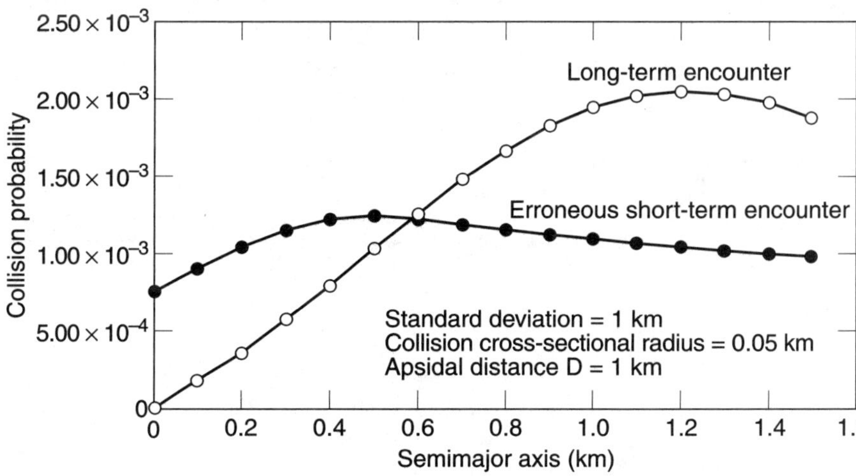

Figure 9.11. Collision probability for variable-size ellipses.

In Fig. 9.11 is also plotted the erroneous collision probability that would have been computed if we had considered the spacecraft encounter to be of the short-term nature. It is seen that the erroneous value obtained for the short-term encounter is larger than the correct value obtained for the long-term encounter when $(A/\sigma) < 0.6$ and smaller when $(A/\sigma) > 0.6$. The reason is that there is respectively excessive and insufficient integration volume allowed for by the improper short-term modeling in these ranges.

Next, if we use the formulation in Appendix B to compute the collision probability, we obtain Fig. 9.12, which covers a larger range than Fig. 9.11. Note that the same features appear in the subrange $0 \le A \le 1.5$ km obtained using Eq. (9.29). However, when A increases, both the correct (long-term) as well as the erroneous (short-term) collision probabilities decrease monotonically after the maximum value of $P \cong 1.9 \times 10^{-3}$ is reached at $A \cong 1.3$ km.

By using the relation $A - C = \sigma$ from Eq. (9.39), we can write Eq. (9.30) as

$$P = QAe^{-(3A^2+4A\sigma)/4\sigma^2} \quad \text{where} \quad Q \equiv \frac{9\sqrt{\pi}\rho^2}{16\sigma^3} e^{-(2\rho^2+\sigma^2)/4\sigma^2} \tag{9.40}$$

Then differentiation yields

$$\frac{\partial P}{\partial A} = Qe^{-(3A^2+4A\sigma)/4\sigma^2}\left[1 + A\frac{(-3A+2\sigma)}{2\sigma^2}\right] \tag{9.41}$$

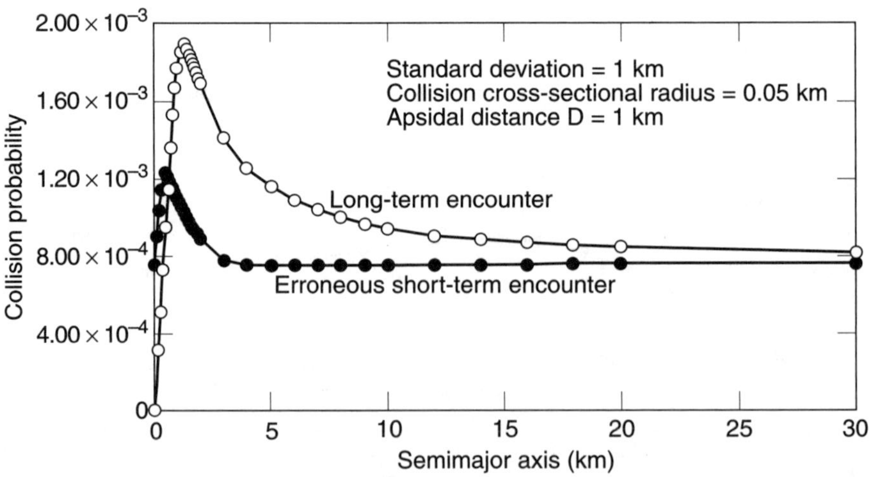

Figure 9.12. Collision probability for variable-size ellipses for larger range of parameters.

The function $P(A)$ is maximum when $(\partial P/\partial A) = 0$, and we obtain

$$A = \frac{1+\sqrt{7}}{3}\sigma \simeq 1.2\sigma \tag{9.42}$$

Equation (9.42) holds for all families of variable-size ellipses for which $A - C = \sigma$. This manifested in Fig. 9.11. It also holds for all values of the cross-sectional radius ρ, provided that Eq. (9.30) is valid. For these, only the value of the maximum value (dependent on ρ) of the collision probability P changes. The most important conclusion is that we need to ensure we avoid the situation in which the amplitude A is approximately 1.3σ.

Finally, if we have the following family of variable-size ellipses, each of which describes the relative motion of a secondary spacecraft with reference to the primary spacecraft according to the equation

$$\left(x - C\right)^2 + 4y^2 = A^2 \quad \text{where} \quad A - C = k\sigma \tag{9.43}$$

then the maximum occurs at the value

$$A = \frac{k + \sqrt{(k^2+6)}}{3}\sigma \tag{9.44}$$

It must be noted that this analysis is valid for $0 \le A \le 1.5\sigma$ (approximate).

9.7 Discussion

The three cases studied in the previous sections elucidate the difference between the results of collision probabilities obtained through long-term encounter modeling under prevailing circumstances and those obtained through short-term encounter simplification used inappropriately under the same circumstances. More important is the application of the long-term analytical formulation to some problems of interest. Specifically, the case of concentric ellipses can be used in the study of secondary objects orbiting around a primary spacecraft. An example of this is the parking of collateral equipment around the International Space Station.

Equation (9.34) shows that the probability of collision is maximum when the amplitude A is approximately 1.4 times the combined standard deviation. Equation (9.33) gives the sensitivity of the collision probability to changing the amplitude. The case of fixed-size ellipses can be applied to a slew of objects orbiting synchronously with small (essentially the same) amplitudes at various distances from a primary. If the orbits were all perfectly circular, then there could be no collision whatsoever from now to eternity. However, such is not the case, because

Earth is not perfectly spherical and perturbations can result from third bodies, solar radiation, and atmospheric drag.

Equation (9.38) states the fact that nearby objects are most likely to collide with the primary (perhaps an intuitively obvious assertion), while Eq. (9.37) gives the rate of decrease of the collision probability with increasing separation.

Finally, the case of variable-size ellipses may be used for analysis of maneuvers in formation flying. If thrusting is applied to a nearby member, then according to Eq. (9.42) we should avoid any amplitude of approximately 1.2 times the combined standard deviations. Equation (9.40) may be used to compute the thrusting, to meet the safety standards set for collision probability. Equation (9.41) gives the sensitivity as a function of amplitude of the resultant relative motion and can be used in trade-off studies when the fuel consumption and the safety margin are to be weighed.

9.8 Conclusion

We observe from Table 3.1 of Chapter 3 that, for low Earth orbits with moderate to large approach angles, it is permissible to invoke the assumption of rectilinear relative motion because the path is essentially straight over a distance that is approximately 1000 times the deflection from linearity.

If the relative velocities are of the order of several kilometers per second, the time spent in the encounter region is only a fraction of a second or at most a few seconds. This condition is satisfied in encounters that are short-term in nature. In contrast, for long-term encounters the time spent in the encounter region is of the order of one orbital period. For some infrequent geosynchronous spacecraft encounters with low relative velocity (so low it is measured in meters per second or even smaller units), this period can extend to considerably more than a day. Relatively simple analytical expressions for computing the collision probability have been given for these two types of encounter.

Three illustrative cases of long-term encounters were studied in detail to compare the results of the correct long-term formulation versus those obtained by inappropriately using the erroneous short-term formulation. For these cases, one collision probability can be greater than the other or vice versa, depending on the range of collision parameters under consideration. Until the requisite computations are performed, it is difficult to make any a priori conclusions from an intuitive point of view. Most encounters between spacecraft are short-term in duration, and it would be misleading to treat all of them the same.

9.9 Summary

In Section 9.1, we derived the expression giving the minimum value of the distance between a point on the ellipse and a point displaced from the center on either the major or minor axis of the ellipse. This minimum distance is not a smooth function of the displacement. For small displacements, it is given by a complicated function, whereas for large displacements it is given by the absolute coordinate difference along the principal axis.

In Section 9.2, we recalled the collision probability results derived earlier for short-term encounters.

In Section 9.3, we recalled the collision probability results derived earlier for long-term encounters.

In Section 9.4, we studied the case of a family of in-plane concentric ellipses, each of which describes the relative motion of a secondary spacecraft around the primary spacecraft. We found that the erroneous short-term encounter collision probability is larger than the correct value obtained for the long-term encounter when $(A/\sigma) < 0.5$ and smaller when $(A/\sigma) > 0.5$, where A is the semimajor axis of the ellipse and σ is the standard deviation of an isotropic Gaussian pdf.

In Section 9.5, we studied the case of a family of fixed-size in-plane ellipses, each of which describes the relative motion of a secondary spacecraft with reference to the primary spacecraft. We found that the erroneous short-term encounter collision probability is always larger than the correct value obtained for the long-term encounter.

In Section 9.6, we studied the case of a family of variable-size in-plane ellipses (with a common apsidal point), each of which describes the relative motion of a secondary spacecraft with reference to the primary spacecraft. We found that the erroneous short-term encounter collision probability is larger than the correct value obtained for the long-term encounter when $(A/\sigma) < 0.6$ and smaller when $(A/\sigma) > 0.6$.

In Section 9.7, we described three applications for these three study cases.

In Section 9.8, we concluded the fallacy of using the short-term encounter formulation to compute the collision probability when the relative motion does not meet the criteria of rectilinear motion.

9.10 Reference

9.1. F. K. Chan, "Short-Term vs. Long-Term Spacecraft Encounters," *AIAA/AAS Astrodynamics Specialist Conference* (Providence, RI, 16–19 August 2004).

Chapter 10: Formation Flying

This chapter outlines onboard procedures to assess probable collisions between spacecraft in formation flight and also between them and other orbiting objects, to minimize collision risk by performing evasive maneuvers, and to design contingency plans for safe haven parking and subsequent system recovery. It draws on analytical expressions derived in previous chapters for computing collision probability. In describing evasive maneuvers, it uses intrack thrusting or general thrusting to mitigate potential collision threat. For safe haven parking in times of emergencies, it takes advantage of information provided by the estimation, guidance, and control systems. This analysis concentrates on the more difficult highly elliptical Earth-orbiting (HEO) satellite formations. Of special emphasis is the proposed algorithm for efficiently generating accurate relative orbits referenced to a highly elliptical orbit around a nonspherical Earth.

10.1 Prologue

The equations for relative motion of an elliptical orbit referenced to a circular orbit were first derived by Hill[10.1] in 1878 for lunar theory. These equations were subsequently rederived by Clohessy and Wiltshire[10.2] in 1960 for analysis and control of one spacecraft with reference to another. These equations are linearized from the two-body equations of motion and are not valid for long periods of time because their first-order solution contains a secular term. Thus, their general applicability is rather restricted for long-term orbital analysis. However, for formation flying the secular term is suppressed by appropriate choice of initial conditions and the Clohessy-Wiltshire equations are then used for preliminary design studies of formations with near-circular orbits. An example of this is the low Earth orbit (LEO) benchmark formation, which is sun-synchronous at 400 km altitude. This comprises two 3-satellite formations inclined at ±26.6 deg. Each formation has circular paths 500 m in diameter about the reference center when projected onto the local horizontal plane. This means that the intersatellite separation is 433 m. The relative positions are to be controlled to within 5 m throughout the entire orbit.

For analyzing the general relative motion in formation flying, it is desirable to have reference orbits that are elliptical. Fortunately, sufficient research has been done for the design architecture and control of satellite formations. This was made possible through the work of Lawden[10.3] in 1963, Tschauner and Hempel[10.4] from 1964 to 1967, and Broucke[10.5] in 2002, among many others within the last few years; however, these analyses are still restricted to a spherical Earth model. On the other hand, Wiesel[10.6] in 2001 studied the case of a near-circular reference orbit in a gravitational field with rotational symmetry (i.e., with only zonal harmonics) and all other harmonics and drag treated as perturbations to the first-order solution. Thus, these approaches are valid for elliptical Keplerian reference orbits or circular non-Keplerian reference orbits.

By extending these analyses to include general elliptical orbits about a nonspherical Earth, we find it is conceivable that their results could be used in satellite formation dynamics estimation and control (although that application would not be easy to accomplish). The algorithms based on these formulations can be very complex whether they are employed on the ground or on board. A case in point is the HEO benchmark constellation of four spacecraft with orbit 1.2 by 18 Earth radii to be spaced 10 km apart on the vertices of a tetrahedron. It is to be constrained to within 1 km deviation throughout the entire orbit. For this orbit, a little consideration reveals that an uncontrolled along-track satellite separation of 10 km at apogee grows to 150 km at perigee! On the other hand, an uncontrolled crosstrack satellite separation of 10 km at apogee diminishes to 0.667 km = 667 m at perigee! This observation presents a somewhat Herculean effort for formation control in order to meet the specifications. It also creates a daunting task for very accurate orbit determination at perigee. Above all, because of tightness of the error budget, it behooves us to take proper measures to anticipate and avert possible disasters or even catastrophes. To prepare for such a predicament, we need to be able to rapidly assess collision risk, mitigate collision threats, and formulate contingency plans for system recovery.

10.2 Collision Assessment

When two spherical orbiting objects are in close proximity, the usual method of computing the probability of collision is that used by NASA. In this formulation, the probability density function (pdf) of the relative position error is given by a three-dimensional Gaussian form having in general three unequal standard deviations. For short-term encounters, one considers an encounter plane that is perpendicular to the relative position at the point of closest approach; and this pdf is then bivariate Gaussian. The collision probability is computed by a two-dimensional numerical integration.[10.7] This approach is not adaptable to onboard collision assessment because it is cumbersome and time-consuming; however, the formulation in Chapter 5 involves only the evaluation of a simple analytical expression as advocated by Carpenter.[10.8] It is especially suited to onboard collision assessment because it is simple to code and is 10,000 times faster than the numerical integration. Moreover, this approach, based on the method of equivalent cross-section areas (MECSA), is also applicable to nonspherical spacecraft. Both formulations give numerical results that agree to three significant digits over an extremely wide range of collision parameters.

During normal times of operations, the satellite positions can be obtained by using Global Positioning System (GPS) and intersatellite range measurements. Their orbits will be determined as independently and simultaneously estimated solutions. The details are not the subject of this collision assessment effort but of the design architects' effort for control and navigation of the system. This task takes advantage of the orbit determination results that are constantly acquired. An activity of this task stores and uses both the relative state vectors and covariances to continuously compute the collision probability between pairs of satellites. This assessment could be performed on board or on the ground using the algorithm based on Eq. (7.36) of Chapter 7.

$$
\begin{aligned}
F(t,\boldsymbol{\alpha},\boldsymbol{\beta}) = F(t,\mathbf{0},\mathbf{0}) &+ \sum_i F_{\alpha_i}(t,\mathbf{0},\mathbf{0})\alpha_i + \frac{1}{2}\sum_i\sum_j F_{\alpha_i\alpha_j}(t,\mathbf{0},\mathbf{0})\alpha_i\alpha_j + \cdots \\
&+ \sum_i F_{\beta_i}(t,\mathbf{0},\mathbf{0})\beta_i + \frac{1}{2}\sum_i\sum_j F_{\beta_i\beta_j}(t,\mathbf{0},\mathbf{0})\beta_i\beta_j + \cdots \\
&+ \sum_i\sum_j F_{\alpha_i\beta_j}(t,\mathbf{0},\mathbf{0})\alpha_i\beta_j + \cdots
\end{aligned}
\tag{10.1}
$$

However, if we do not have a flyby of short duration, then we avail ourselves of the algorithm developed in Chapter 8 for situations where the encounter is of a long-term nature. Such a tool can also be used for computing the probability of collision between a pair of geosynchronous satellites that spend well in excess of a day in the same proximity. The second activity of this task is to maintain on board a running archive of the navigation maneuvers (magnitude and time of impulses for stationkeeping during an orbit) to bring the formation within performance specifications. The third activity is to use the absolute state vectors and covariances to compute the collision probability with orbiting objects that come within threatening close distances. This effort will have to be performed on the ground as it is too demanding for the satellite constellation to keep track of the more than 10,000 objects in the resident space objects catalog.

During times of system failure resulting from malfunction of any spacecraft sensor, it is desirable to have other backup means of orbit determination for that particular space vehicle. Fortunately, the use of intersatellite ranging by the other functioning members of the constellation will provide this information. This is probably more accurate than the information that impromptu ground ranging can provide. This is also why it is advantageous to have independently and simultaneously estimated solutions with decentralized control even though it has been found by simulation[10.9] that there is no noticeable difference between the two of them. On the other hand, during times when every member of the formation suffers from malfunctioning of its sensor system, the strategy described here is not applicable. The probability of this happening is very small unless it is caused by a catastrophic temporary common blackout. In this case, the formation will summon its archived data to pull it through. It will search for (or even use interpolation to identify) the state vector and covariance for each member that most closely match the last known state vector and covariance with approximately the same atmospheric drag (dependent on the solar flux and geomagnetic indices) that has a dominant effect on the intrack motion. Each member satellite will then follow its historical procedure for control and navigation (magnitude and time of impulses during an orbit). All these operations will be performed on board without any commands from the ground as there will be no terrestrial contact possible under these extreme circumstances. If there happens to be a potential collision threat from another orbiting object, there can be no communication for evasive maneuvers.

For each LEO benchmark formation of three 3-axis-stabilized satellites at the vertices of an equilateral triangle with sides of 433 m, the effects of atmospheric drag and solar radiation are approximately the same. However, we know that projected circular formations are unstable because of the disruption of the circular formation by slight differences in nodal and perigee precessions from the J_2 effects. For an 800 km altitude orbit with 1 km separation between member satellites,[10.10] the separation grows by 25% during 4 days. However, for the LEO benchmark constellation, the altitude of 400 km means a higher drag, thus producing more along-track differences. In contrast, the smaller intersatellite separation of 433 m means less inclination difference, thus producing fewer nodal and perigee precession differences.

For the HEO benchmark formation with four satellites at the vertices of a tetrahedron with sides of 10 km, we noted that an uncontrolled along-track satellite separation of 10 km at apogee grows to 150 km at perigee whereas an uncontrolled crosstrack satellite separation of 10 km at apogee diminishes to 667 m at perigee. This means that, if permitted, we can judiciously choose the orientation of the tetrahedron (not the specified orientation of the spin-stabilized spacecraft) so as to minimize the changes of the intersatellite distances. This will greatly minimize the control and navigation of the formation as it orbits Earth.

10.3 Preemptive Maneuvers

When a potential close encounter between members of a formation leading to a collision probability exceeds a threshold value set by safety standards, we need to perform an evasive maneuver to mitigate that collision threat. The principle of a preemptive maneuver is to increase the expected closest distance of approach, thus decreasing the collision probability. Ideally, we would like to perform just the right amount of thrusting so as to achieve the correct miss distance corresponding to the threshold probability. Even then, there is still an infinite number of ways to thrust in the three-dimensional space to achieve this minimum miss distance. Thus, we would want the direction of thrust application yielding the minimum magnitude of thrust. This is called optimal thrusting. The simplest way to determine optimal thrusting is to perform numerical simulations with thrusts in different directions and magnitudes; however, this would require an inordinate number of high-precision orbit propagations that are very time-consuming and also cannot be performed on board a spacecraft.

In contrast, for the HEO constellation with highly elliptical orbits, we need to extend our analysis of thrusting to include crosstrack and radial components in addition to the intrack component. There are two parts to this analysis: minimum separation and optimum thrusting. For the present general case, we may perform numerous computer simulations involving high-precision orbit propagation to determine the optimum thrusting that would yield the desired threshold collision probability.

Our next task is to obtain an accurate relative orbit referenced to a highly elliptical orbit around a nonspherical Earth. To accomplish this, we proceed as follows: Let $F(t, \boldsymbol{\alpha}, \boldsymbol{\beta})$ be a scalar denoting any analytic function of its arguments; then, we may symbolically write ad infinitum the following series expansion about the point $(t,\mathbf{0},\mathbf{0})$. Recall Eq. (10.1):

$$F(t,\boldsymbol{\alpha},\boldsymbol{\beta}) = F(t,\mathbf{0},\mathbf{0}) + \sum_i F_{\alpha_i}(t,\mathbf{0},\mathbf{0})\alpha_i + \frac{1}{2}\sum_i\sum_j F_{\alpha_i\alpha_j}(t,\mathbf{0},\mathbf{0})\alpha_i\alpha_j + \cdots$$

$$+\sum_i F_{\beta_i}(t,\mathbf{0},\mathbf{0})\beta_i + \frac{1}{2}\sum_i\sum_j F_{\beta_i\beta_j}(t,\mathbf{0},\mathbf{0})\beta_i\beta_j + \cdots$$

$$+\sum_i\sum_j F_{\alpha_i\beta_j}(t,\mathbf{0},\mathbf{0})\alpha_i\beta_j + \cdots$$

A little consideration reveals that we may subtract and add the term $F(t,\mathbf{0},\mathbf{0})$, recollect terms into three infinite series, and write Eq. (10.1) in the form

$$F(t,\boldsymbol{\alpha},\boldsymbol{\beta}) = F(t,\boldsymbol{\alpha},\mathbf{0}) - F(t,\mathbf{0},\mathbf{0}) + F(t,\mathbf{0},\boldsymbol{\beta}) + \text{Cross Terms Series} \tag{10.2}$$

In Eq. (10.2), let F denote any element in any set of orbital elements. For example, we can have Cartesian elements (x, y, z, u, v, w), Keplerian elements $(a, e, i, \Omega, \omega, M)$, Delauney elements (L, G, H, l, g, h), equinoctial elements (a, h, k, p, q, λ), etc. Let $\boldsymbol{\alpha}$ denote all modeling parameters such as geopotential coefficients for a nonspherical Earth beyond J_2, atmospheric drag, solar radiation pressure, etc. That is, when $\boldsymbol{\alpha} = \mathbf{0}$ we have a J_2 orbit. Let $\boldsymbol{\beta}$ denote perturbations on epoch orbital elements of the primary at time $t = 0$. There are many components in $\boldsymbol{\alpha}$ but only six elements in $\boldsymbol{\beta}$ ($\Delta\mathbf{r}_o$ and $\Delta\mathbf{v}_o$). For thrusting, $\Delta\mathbf{r}_o = 0$ and $\Delta\mathbf{v}_o \neq 0$.

The first term on the right-hand side can be obtained from high-precision orbit propagation while the second and third terms can be obtained from motion around an oblate Earth because $\boldsymbol{\alpha}$ is zero. The fourth term may be neglected as the contribution is usually small compared to the others because maneuvers are performed in a relatively short time (within a day or two) before spacecraft conjunction.

The reason for the formulation described here is that we do have at our disposal the analytical theories of Kozai[10.11] and Brouwer[10.12] for the main problem of artificial satellite theory. In view of this, we now have an algorithm for determining a whole slew of high-precision orbits with perturbations in terms of only one high-precision orbit (with no perturbations) and the difference between two J_2 orbits (one with perturbations and the other with no perturbations). The first-order solution in J_2 is given in closed form as a finite number of terms if the true anomaly is the independent variable. (See Fitzpatrick.[10.13]) The only inconvenience is that we have to invert Kepler's equation if we are to use time as the independent variable, but this is not difficult computationally. This formulation yields results accurate to the third order in small parameters (the product of first-order terms in thrust and second-order terms in gravitational harmonic coefficients). Typically, the velocity impulses are approximately 5×10^{-4} m/s to change the semimajor axis of a 400 km orbit by 1 m, and the second-order gravitational coefficients are of the order of 10^{-6}. Thus, the relative motion obtained using this method of differencing between two J_2 orbits is very accurate. In addition, it is also very efficient and easy to implement. Using this approach, we can circumvent the difficulties encountered by the other formulations discussed in the introduction for obtaining relative motion of a spacecraft referenced to a general elliptical orbit in a general gravitational field with drag and solar radiation effects. Thus, it would appear that it is possible to perform computations on board for optimal evasive maneuvers involving any two members for both the near-circular LEO and the highly elliptical HEO benchmark satellite formations during an extended period of time. This approach should be given serious consideration for implementation.

Usually, stationkeeping maneuvers are performed to maintain each satellite of the formation within its own box. Hence, there is very little possibility that such a maneuver will result in unwarranted threats of collision with the other remaining satellites. However, if there is imminent threat of colliding with an orbiting object, then we must be cautious that an optimal preemptive maneuver by a member will not lead to subsequent close approaches with the other members. Strategies have to be formulated and algorithms have to be developed to ensure that we achieve an overall optimal maneuver in a longer-term span and not just a one-time event. Again, as with continuous collision assessment discussed in Section 10.2, Collision Assessment, any evasive maneuver with external objects will have to be commanded from the ground.

The discussion so far applies to the formation operating in its normal mode; however, during times of system failure because of malfunction of any spacecraft sensor system, we would have to proceed as discussed in Section 10.2. Suppose we have a close approach involving a pair of satellites in the formation. Then, the other functioning member will perform intersatellite ranging and optimal preemptive maneuver computations in a decentralized mode. If there is still a communications link, it can command that malfunctioning member to thrust accordingly or it can perform the evasive action itself, depending on which one has more fuel to spare. If there is no communications link, then all the remaining satellites of the formation will perform maneuvers as a whole so that they will continue to function as a somewhat smaller constellation. It is better to have this choice than the disruption of service resulting from a collision in which numerous fragments explode in all directions and disable the whole system. Moreover, this course of action averts contamination of the space environment with debris. In fact, this is the most worrisome situation with the HEO benchmark formation near perigee where the crosstrack separations can diminish to hundreds or even tens of meters if a particular satellite should become uncontrollable.

10.4 Safe Haven Parking

In the normal operating mode, everything works nominally. However, in emergencies when a component or the whole system fails to function, then we have to be prepared with strategies to control further damage, allow time for diagnostics and repair, and, it is hoped, bring the system back to nominal operations. The object of collision assessment is to continuously monitor the health and safety of the formation from the standpoint of collision. The object of preemptive maneuvers is to prevent potential collisions from happening. In executing such evasive actions, we take the system out of its normal operating mode. Thus, for every conceivable scenario, it is desirable to have contingency plans and to devise a safe haven configuration whereby we can set the system up for eventual recovery operations. Safe haven parking in times of emergencies will take advantage of the information provided by the estimation, guidance, and control systems from the running archives available on board. If such data is not available, each member of the formation will have the capability to receive commands from the ground to execute corrective actions.

The primary products of this effort should be designs of safe mode configurations, derivation of algorithms, and numerical studies of recovery operations as the constellation goes through an indeterminable period of extenuating circumstances with unexpected large errors in maneuvers, degradations of sensor performance, and failures of communications systems and other onboard components that render nominal operations impossible. Finally, strategies should be devised, algorithms should be developed, and simulation studies should be performed for recovery after the exigencies are over to bring the satellite constellation back to normal operation. It is recommended that this work be performed in close coordination with the NASA/GSFC (Goddard Space Flight Center) Distributed Space Systems personnel using their Formation Flying Testbed for demonstration. It is hoped that the software tools developed will be integrated into their technologies as part of a joint effort with NASA/GSFC.

10.5 Discussion

The investigations described here use as case studies the two benchmark constellations: the near-circular LEO satellite formation and the highly elliptical HEO satellite formation. Even though the first has 400 km altitude and the second has 1.2 by 18 Earth radii, these orbital parameters may be changed and the results can be applied to other similar constellations. Thus, for the first formation, by changing the altitude to 800 km and inclination to 90 deg, we have the constellation presently studied.[10.10] By changing the second formation to have orbits 1.1 by 2.7 Earth radii in the equatorial plane, we have the apogee-at-constant-time-of-day equatorial (ACE) orbits[10.14] for the proposed satellite constellation to off-load daily peaks in geostationary traffic. In addition, the algorithms for computing collision probability for long-term encounters are directly applicable for geosynchronous satellites in the congested geostationary belt where they spend considerable time in proximity to one another.

The case of intrack thrusting is much simpler to implement for analysis and simulations on a computer and also much simpler to execute operationally for spacecraft maneuvers. In fuel expenditure, it is only slightly more costly than the more general approach in the case of only one collision avoidance maneuver. However, the most salient feature is that intrack thrusting is perhaps even more effective in the long run when there is a complementary adjustment to bring the spacecraft back to the original orbit. This is because it involves orbit phasing to either slow down or speed up the spacecraft so as to achieve the requisite minimum separation to ensure meeting the collision probability threshold requirements. After the close encounter, it could be used again to regain the proper phasing of the spacecraft in its nominal trajectory. This is especially important if the primary spacecraft is one member of a large constellation moving in some prescribed configuration. On the other hand, by executing a general thrusting in the crosstrack and radial directions in addition to an intrack component, the primary spacecraft can be made to change its orbital characteristics quite drastically. Then, to restore its proper position in the constellation, it would have to undergo another maneuver involving three-component thrusting. In general, this operation requires more intricate analysis and is more complicated to execute.

The analytical formulations for computing collision probability have several desirable features. First, the exceeding speed and comparative accuracy are crucial when dealing with possibly hundreds of thousands or even millions of conjunctions in launch window and on-orbit studies. This timeliness is especially important because of the increasing number of orbiting objects and also the need to consider more objects of smaller dimensions in the future. Second, the ease of implementation makes it feasible to perform onboard collision probability analyses as part of autonomous navigation. Finally, the applicability to spacecraft of general shape means that we can model the International Space Station more realistically as it is rather than as a sphere.

10.6 Conclusion

Onboard methods have been presented to assess probable collisions between spacecraft in formation flight and also between them and other orbiting objects, to minimize collision risk by performing evasive maneuvers, and to design contingency plans for safe haven parking and subsequent system recovery.

For the continuous collision assessment, the onboard system will take advantage of the information provided by the relative trajectory estimations of the satellites' state vectors during times of nominal operational conditions; however, during times of system failure, it will have to augment the normal estimation procedures by other means. For potential close encounters with other orbiting objects, information has to be provided externally. Each member in the formation can then either thrust autonomously or be commanded from the ground to perform the requisite collision avoidance maneuver.

For preemptive maneuvers, algorithms were derived to mitigate potential collision threats. This orbit maneuver is optimized in fuel consumption when reducing the collision probability to a specified acceptable threshold value. Consideration should be given to the idea that the process of reducing collision probability between two satellites should not cause subsequent problems with the other members in the formation. The same preemptive maneuver strategies should also apply to the case of potential threats from other orbiting objects.

For safe haven parking in times of emergencies, the onboard system will take advantage of the information provided by the estimation, guidance, and control systems. If such data is not available, each member of the formation will have the capability to receive commands from the ground to execute the corrective actions. Algorithms should be developed for recovery after the exigencies are over so as to bring the satellite constellation back to nominal operation.

10.7 Summary

In Section 10.1, we gave a brief historical account covering both relative motion referenced to a circular orbit around a spherical Earth as well as relative motion referenced to a slightly elliptical orbit around an oblate Earth.

In Section 10.2, we discussed the need for collision assessment for a constellation in formation flight. During normal times of operation, the satellites are tracked using GPS and intersatellite range measurements. Their orbits are determined as independently and/or simultaneously estimated solutions. During times of a space vehicle's system failure resulting from malfunction of any spacecraft sensor, it is desirable to have other backup means of orbit determination for that particular vehicle. The use of intersatellite ranging by the other functioning members of the constellation will provide this information.

In Section 10.3, we formulated the outline of a semianalytic algorithm for obtaining very accurate relative motion referenced to a general elliptical orbit around an Earth with unrestricted geopotential. This algorithm can be used for determining a whole slew of high-precision orbits with perturbations in terms of only one high-precision orbit (with no perturbations) and the difference between two J_2 orbits (one with perturbations and the other with no perturbations).

In Section 10.4, we stated the desirability of having contingency plans and of devising a safe haven configuration whereby we can set the system up for eventual recovery operations. Safe haven parking in times of emergencies will take advantage of the information provided by the estimation, guidance, and control systems from the running archives available on board.

In Section 10.5, we advocated using intrack thrusting for mitigating potential collision threats because that technique is much simpler to implement and execute operationally for spacecraft maneuvers than other techniques. After a close encounter, the same technique could be used again to regain the proper phasing of the spacecraft in its nominal trajectory. This is especially important if the primary spacecraft is one member of a large constellation moving in a prescribed configuration.

In Section 10.6, we recommended that the onboard system take advantage of the information provided by the relative trajectory estimations of the satellites' state vectors during times of nominal operational conditions. During emergencies, the onboard system will take advantage of the information provided by the estimation, guidance, and control systems.

10.8 References

[10.1.] G. W. Hill, "Researches in the Lunar Theory," *Am. J. Math.* **1** (1), 5–26 (1878).

[10.2.] W. H. Clohessy and P. S. Wiltshire, "Terminal Guidance System for Satellite Rendezvous," *J. Aerospace Sci.* **27** (9), 653–658 (1960).

[10.3.] D. F. Lawden, *Optimal Trajectories for Space Navigation* (Butterworths, London, 1963) pp. 79–86.

[10.4.] J. Tschauner and P. Hempel, "Rendezvous with a Target in an Elliptical Orbit," *Astronautica Acta* **11** (2), 104–109 (1965).

[10.5.] R. Broucke, "A Solution of the Elliptic Rendezvous Problem with the Time as Independent Variable," *AAS/AIAA Space Flight Mechanics Meeting* (San Antonio, TX, January 2002).

[10.6.] W. E. Wiesel, "Relative Satellite Motion about an Oblate Planet," *J. Guidance, Control, and Dynamics* **25** (4), 776–785 (2002).

[10.7.] J. L. Foster and H. S. Estes, "A Parametric Analysis of Orbital Debris Collision Probability and Maneuver Rate for Space Vehicles," NASA/JSC-25898 (August 1992).

[10.8.] J. R. Carpenter, "Conservative Analytical Collision Probability for Design of Orbital Formations," *Second International Symposium on Formation Flying Missions and Technologies* (Arlington, VA, September 2004).

[10.9.] D. Kelbel et al., "Evaluation of Relative Navigation Algorithms for Formation-Flying Satellites," *NASA/GSFC Flight Mechanics Symposium* (Greenbelt, MD, June 2001).

[10.10.] C. Sabol, R. Burns, and C. McLaughlin, "Satellite Formation Flying Design and Evolution," *AAS/AIAA Space Flight Mechanics Meeting* (Breckenridge, CO, February 1999).

[10.11.] Y. Kozai, "The Motion of a Close Earth Satellite," *Astron. J.* **64** (1274), 367–377 (November 1959).

[10.12.] D. Brouwer, "Solution of the Problem of Artificial Satellite Theory Without Drag," *Astron. J.* **64** (1274), 378–395 (November 1959).

[10.13.] P. M. Fitzpatrick, *Principles of Celestial Mechanics* (Academic Press, New York, 1970) pp. 311–318.

[10.14.] A. E. Turner, "New Non-Geosynchronous Orbits for Communications Satellites to Off-Load Daily Peaks in Geostationary Traffic" *AAS/AIAA Astrodynamics Specialist Conference* (Kalispell, MT, August 1987).

Chapter 11: Maximum Probability of Collision

In this chapter, we consider the following problem: Suppose we are given the Gaussian probability density function (pdf) in the two-dimensional encounter plane. However, we are not given the standard deviations σ_x and σ_z and the cross-correlation coefficient ρ_{xz} or, equivalently, the two standard deviations $\sigma_{x'}$ and $\sigma_{z'}$ in the principal directions. All we know are the distance of closest approach x_e on the x-axis and the combined circular collision cross-sectional area of radius r_A with center $(x_e, 0)$. We would like to determine the maximum probability that can be obtained by assigning different values of $\sigma_{x'}$ and $\sigma_{z'}$ in the $(\sigma_{x'}, \sigma_{z'})$-plane. There are two approaches: the maximum likelihood method and the maximum probability method. The first is an approximation and is valid if the pdf does not vary much over the collision cross-sectional area. The second approach is an exact analysis of the problem as stated and depends only on the accuracy of the analytical expression for the collision probability previously derived in Chapter 5.

11.1 Maximum Likelihood Approach

Let us first illustrate this with the simple example of a one-dimensional Gaussian pdf:

$$f(x) = \frac{1}{\sqrt{2\pi}\sigma} e^{-x^2/2\sigma^2} \tag{11.1}$$

At the point $x = x_e$, we want to determine the value of σ that maximizes the pdf $f(x)$. Hence, we take the derivative of f with respect to σ:

$$\frac{\partial f}{\partial \sigma} = \frac{1}{\sqrt{2\pi}\sigma^2} e^{-x^2/2\sigma^2} \left(\frac{x^2}{\sigma^2} - 1 \right) \tag{11.2}$$

Next, we evaluate this derivative at the value x_e, set it equal to zero, and obtain

$$\sigma = x_e \tag{11.3}$$

Thus, we have the rather simple but also very interesting result for the maximum likelihood method: For a one-dimensional Gaussian pdf, the value of the standard deviation that maximizes the pdf is equal to the value of the random variable x at the particular point. Moreover, if $x_e \neq 0$, the maximum value that can be attained by the pdf is

$$f_{\max}(x_e) = \frac{1}{\sqrt{2\pi}x_e} e^{-1/2} \tag{11.4}$$

Suppose the pdf does not vary much over the interval $[(x_e - r_A), (x_e + r_A)]$. This is particularly true if $r_A << \sigma$. Then, the maximum probability that can be attained is approximately given by

$$P_{\max}(r_A, x_e) \simeq 2r_A f_{\max}(x_e) = \sqrt{\frac{2}{\pi e}}\beta \quad \text{where} \quad \beta \equiv \left(\frac{r_A}{x_e}\right) \tag{11.5}$$

Figure 11.1 illustrates a set of Gaussian curves $f(x, \sigma)$ as a function of the random variable x with the standard deviation σ as a parameter. It is often stated that "as the standard deviation increases the associated probability density decreases." To illustrate that this statement is erroneous, let us consider two Gaussian curves with different standard deviations $\sigma_1 < \sigma_2$. It is obvious that one pdf can be greater or smaller than the other depending on the particular range under consideration. Let $x = x_0$ be the point at which these two curves cross each another. It can easily be shown that

$$x_0 = \sqrt{\frac{2\sigma_1^2\sigma_2^2 \ln(\sigma_2/\sigma_1)}{(\sigma_2^2 - \sigma_1^2)}} \tag{11.6}$$

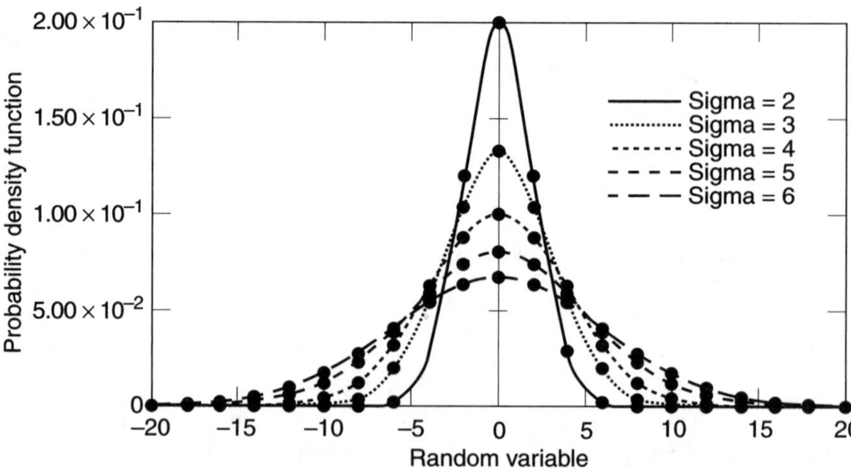

Figure 11.1. Set of Gaussian curves for various standard deviations.

We note that

$$f_1(x) > f_2(x) \quad \text{when} \quad x < x_0$$
$$f_1(x) < f_2(x) \quad \text{when} \quad x > x_0 \tag{11.7}$$

In Fig. 11.1, we depict a set of Gaussian curves as functions of x with σ as a parameter. Alternatively, we may also consider the surface $f(x, \sigma)$ in the three-dimensional (x, σ, f)-space. From Eq. (11.3), we know that, for a given $x = x_e$, the value of σ that maximizes $f(x, \sigma)$ is $\sigma = x_e$. In the (x, σ)-plane, the line $\sigma = x$ gives the graphical relationship for maximum likelihood. This is a line making 45 deg with the x-axis and passing through the origin (0, 0). Note that when $x_e = 0$ so that $\sigma = 0$, we have the delta function at the origin defined by

$$\delta(x) = 0 \quad \text{for} \quad x \neq 0$$
$$\int_{-\infty}^{+\infty} \delta(x)dx = 1 \tag{11.8}$$

Next, we consider the two-dimensional Gaussian pdf expressed in the principal axes (x', z') system derived in Chapter 5:

$$f(x',z') = \frac{1}{2\pi\sigma_{x'}\sigma_{z'}} e^{-\frac{1}{2}\left[\left(\frac{x'}{\sigma_{x'}}\right)^2 + \left(\frac{z'}{\sigma_{z'}}\right)^2\right]} = \frac{1}{\sqrt{2\pi}\sigma_{x'}} e^{-\frac{1}{2}\left(\frac{x'}{\sigma_{x'}}\right)^2} \frac{1}{\sqrt{2\pi}\sigma_{z'}} e^{-\frac{1}{2}\left(\frac{z'}{\sigma_{z'}}\right)^2} \tag{11.9}$$

We wish to determine the standard deviations $\sigma_{x'}$ and $\sigma_{z'}$ that maximize the pdf $f(x', z')$ at the point of closest approach $(x_e \cos\theta, x_e \sin\theta)$ where θ is the angle that the point of closest approach makes with the x'-axis in the encounter (x', z')-plane. Proceeding as in the one-dimensional case above, we take the partial derivatives of f with respect to $\sigma_{x'}$ and $\sigma_{z'}$ respectively:

$$\frac{\partial f(x',z')}{\partial \sigma_{x'}} = \frac{1}{2\pi\sigma_{x'}^2\sigma_{z'}} e^{-\frac{1}{2}\left[\left(\frac{x'}{\sigma_{x'}}\right)^2 + \left(\frac{z'}{\sigma_{z'}}\right)^2\right]} \left(\frac{x'^2}{\sigma_{x'}^2} - 1\right)$$
$$\frac{\partial f(x',z')}{\partial \sigma_{z'}} = \frac{1}{2\pi\sigma_{x'}\sigma_{z'}^2} e^{-\frac{1}{2}\left[\left(\frac{x'}{\sigma_{x'}}\right)^2 + \left(\frac{z'}{\sigma_{z'}}\right)^2\right]} \left(\frac{z'^2}{\sigma_{z'}^2} - 1\right) \tag{11.10}$$

By setting these partial derivatives to zero, we obtain

$$\begin{aligned}\sigma_{x'} &= x_e|\cos\theta| \\ \sigma_{z'} &= x_e|\sin\theta|\end{aligned} \tag{11.11}$$

Thus, for the two-dimensional Gaussian pdf, the values of the standard deviations $\sigma_{x'}$ and $\sigma_{z'}$ that maximize the pdf are respectively equal to the coordinates ($x_e \cos\theta$, $x_e \sin\theta$) of the particular point. Moreover, if $x_e \neq 0$ and $\theta \neq 0$ or $\pi/2$, the maximum value that can be attained by the pdf is

$$f_{\max}(x_e\cos\theta, x_e\sin\theta) = \frac{1}{\pi x_e^{\,2}\sin 2\theta}e^{-1} \tag{11.12}$$

Suppose the pdf does not vary much over the combined circular collision cross-sectional area of radius r_A. This is particularly true if $r_A << \sigma_{x'}$ and $r_A << \sigma_{z'}$. Then, the maximum probability that can be attained is approximately given by

$$P_{\max}(r_A, x_e, \theta) \simeq \pi r_A^{\,2} f_{\max}(x_e\cos\theta, x_e\sin\theta) = \frac{\beta^2}{e\sin 2\theta} \quad \text{where} \quad \beta \equiv \left(\frac{r_A}{x_e}\right) \tag{11.13}$$

We note that the right-hand side of Eq. (11.13) is undefined when $\theta = 0$. Hence, we need to return to Eq. (11.9) as a starting point. We know that when $\sigma \to 0$, the Gaussian pdf tends to become the delta function. The delta function is a special case of what is known as "generalized functions" introduced by mathematicians[11.1] after Dirac introduced it without giving a rigorous foundation. Thus, when $\theta = 0$, Eq. (11.9) is logically replaced by

$$f(x', z') = \frac{1}{\sqrt{2\pi}\sigma_{x'}} e^{-\frac{1}{2}\left(\frac{x'}{\sigma_{x'}}\right)^2} \delta(z') \tag{11.14}$$

Consequently, Eq. (11.13) is replaced by

$$P_{\max}(r_A, x_e, 0) \simeq 2r_A f_{\max}(x_e, 0) = \sqrt{\frac{2}{\pi e}}\left(\frac{r_A}{x_e}\right) \simeq 0.4839\,\beta \quad \text{where} \quad \beta \equiv \left(\frac{r_A}{x_e}\right) \tag{11.15}$$

With either Eq. (11.13) or (11.15), it is easy to compute approximate values of maximum collision probability obtained from the principle of maximum likelihood. Note that Eq. (11.13) involves only the ratio β^2 and the angle θ whereas Eq. (11.15) involves only the ratio β.

11.2 Maximum Probability Approach

Let us next use the following results already derived in Chapter 5 for the probability of collision. Recall that numerical testing verified that the following analytical expression for collision probability is accurate to two or three significant figures (when compared to three other collision probability computation models) for a wide range of the collision parameters r_A, x_e, $\sigma_{x'}$, $\sigma_{z'}$, and θ:

$$P = e^{-v/2}(1 - e^{-u/2}) \tag{11.16}$$

$$u \equiv \left(\frac{r_A^{\,2}}{\sigma_{x'}\sigma_{z'}} \right) > 0 \tag{11.17}$$

$$v \equiv x_c^{\,2} \left\{ 1 + \left[\left(\frac{\sigma_{z'}}{\sigma_{x'}} \right)^2 - 1 \right] \cos^2\theta \right\} \Big/ \sigma_{z'}^{\,2} > 0 \tag{11.18}$$

Here θ is the angle that the point of closest approach makes with the x'-axis in the encounter (x', z')-plane. The model based on Eq. (11.16) is valid for $\beta \equiv r_A/x_e \lesssim 0.3$ and also the aspect ratio $\lambda \equiv \sigma_{x'}/\sigma_{z'} \lesssim 10$. We wish to determine the standard deviations $\sigma_{x'}$ and $\sigma_{z'}$ that maximize the probability $P(x', z')$ at the point of closest approach ($x_e \cos\theta$, $x_e \sin\theta$). Thus, we take the partial derivatives of P with respect to $\sigma_{x'}$ and $\sigma_{z'}$ respectively and set them equal to zero:

$$e^{-u/2} \frac{\partial u}{\partial \sigma_{x'}} - \left(1 - e^{-u/2}\right) \frac{\partial v}{\partial \sigma_{x'}} = 0 \tag{11.19}$$

$$e^{-u/2} \frac{\partial u}{\partial \sigma_{x'}} - \left(1 - e^{-u/2}\right) \frac{\partial v}{\partial \sigma_{x'}} = 0 \tag{11.20}$$

From Eqs. (11.17) and (11.18), we obtain the following partial derivatives:

$$\frac{\partial u}{\partial \sigma_{x'}} = -\frac{r_A^{\,2}}{\sigma_{x'}^{\,2}\sigma_{z'}} \tag{11.21}$$

$$\frac{\partial u}{\partial \sigma_{z'}} = -\frac{r_A^{\,2}}{\sigma_{x'}\sigma_{z'}^{\,2}} \tag{11.22}$$

$$\frac{\partial v}{\partial \sigma_{x'}} = -\frac{2kx_e^2}{\sigma_{x'}^3} \qquad (11.23)$$

$$\frac{\partial v}{\partial \sigma_{z'}} = \frac{2kx_e^2}{\sigma_{x'}^2 \sigma_{z'}} - \frac{2Qx_e^2}{\sigma_{z'}^3} \qquad (11.24)$$

$$k \equiv \cos^2 \theta \qquad (11.25)$$

$$Q \equiv \left\{ 1 + \left[\left(\frac{\sigma_{z'}}{\sigma_{x'}} \right)^2 - 1 \right] k \right\} \qquad (11.26)$$

By substituting Eqs. (11.21) and (11.23) into (11.19) and then multiplying by $\sigma_{x'}^3 \sigma_{z'}^2$, we obtain

$$2\left(1 - e^{-u/2}\right) kx_e^2 \sigma_{z'}^2 - e^{-u/2} r_A^2 \sigma_{x'} \sigma_{z'} = 0 \qquad (11.27)$$

Similarly, by substituting Eqs. (11.22) and (11.24) into (11.20) and then multiplying by $\sigma_{x'}^2 \sigma_{z'}^3$, we obtain

$$-2\left(1 - e^{-u/2}\right) kx_e^2 \sigma_{z'}^2 + 2\left(1 - e^{-u/2}\right) Qx_e^2 \sigma_{x'}^2 - e^{-u/2} r_A^2 \sigma_{x'} \sigma_{z'} = 0 \qquad (11.28)$$

To obtain the values of $\sigma_{x'}$ and $\sigma_{z'}$ that maximize the collision probability P, we have to solve the two extremely nonlinear equations involving these two variables, Eqs. (11.27) and (11.28). This task seems rather daunting at first; however, by subtracting Eq. (11.28) from (11.27) and then judiciously simplifying, it turns out, fortuitously, that we obtain the amazingly simple result

$$\frac{\sigma_{z'}}{\sigma_{x'}} = |\tan \theta| \qquad (11.29)$$

Equation (11.29) states that the values of $\sigma_{x'}$ and $\sigma_{z'}$ that maximize the collision probability P lie on the line that makes an angle θ with the $\sigma_{x'}$-axis in the ($\sigma_{x'}$, $\sigma_{z'}$)-plane. Note that this result is general to the extent that the analytical expression Eq. (11.16) is valid.

Substitution of Eq. (11.29) into (11.27) yields

$$e^{-u/2} = \frac{x_e^2 \sin 2\theta}{r_A^2 + x_e^2 \sin 2\theta} \qquad (11.30)$$

$$u = 2\ln\left(1+\frac{r_A^2}{x_e^2\sin 2\theta}\right) \tag{11.31}$$

By substituting Eqs. (11.29) and (11.31) into (11.17), we solve for $\sigma_{x'}^2$ to obtain

$$\sigma_{x'}^2 = \frac{r_A^2}{2\tan\theta\ln\left(1+\frac{r_A^2}{x_e^2\sin 2\theta}\right)} \tag{11.32}$$

In view of Eq. (11.29), it follows that

$$\sigma_{z'}^2 = \frac{r_A^2\tan\theta}{2\ln\left(1+\frac{r_A^2}{x_e^2\sin 2\theta}\right)} \tag{11.33}$$

Thus, Eqs. (11.32) and (11.33) give the closed-form expressions for $\sigma_{x'}$ and $\sigma_{z'}$ that maximize the collision probability P in terms of the collision parameters r_A, x_e, and θ. Substitution of Eqs. (11.29) and (11.33) into (11.18) yields

$$v = \frac{2x_e^2(1-\cos 2\theta)\ln\left(1+\frac{r_A^2}{x_e^2\sin 2\theta}\right)}{r_A^2\tan\theta} \tag{11.34}$$

$$e^{-v/2} = \left(e^{-u/2}\right)^{\frac{x_e^2(1-\cos 2\theta)}{r_A^2\tan\theta}} = \left(\frac{x_e^2\sin 2\theta}{r_A^2+x_e^2\sin 2\theta}\right)^{\frac{x_e^2(1-\cos 2\theta)}{r_A^2\tan\theta}} \tag{11.35}$$

Finally, by substituting Eqs. (11.30) and (11.35) into (11.16), we obtain the maximum probability that can be attained:

$$P_{\max}(r_A,x_e,\theta) = \left(\frac{r_A^2}{r_A^2+x_e^2\sin 2\theta}\right)\left(\frac{x_e^2\sin 2\theta}{r_A^2+x_e^2\sin 2\theta}\right)^{\frac{x_e^2(1-\cos 2\theta)}{r_A^2\tan\theta}} \tag{11.36}$$

This is the result we seek. In the process, we unexpectedly obtain a closed-form solution. Note that it is expressed in terms of r_A, x_e, and θ. More compactly, we may write this solution as

$$P_{\max}(r_A, x_e, \theta) = \left(\frac{\beta^2}{\beta^2 + \sin 2\theta} \right) \left(\frac{\sin 2\theta}{\beta^2 + \sin 2\theta} \right)^{\frac{(1-\cos 2\theta)}{\beta^2 \tan\theta}} \quad \text{where} \quad \beta \equiv \frac{r_A}{x_e} \tag{11.37}$$

Note that Eq. (11.37) involves only the ratio β and the angle θ. Equation (11.37) is used to compute the maximum probability when β and θ are specified.

Using L'Hospital's rule to obtain

$$\lim_{x \to 0} \left(\frac{x}{\ln x} \right) = 0 \tag{11.38}$$

$$\lim_{x \to 0} (x \ln x) = 0 \tag{11.39}$$

we can use Eqs. (11.32) and (11.33) to show that

$$\lim_{\theta \to 0} \sigma_{z'}^{2} = 0 \tag{11.40}$$

$$\lim_{\theta \to \pi/2} \sigma_{x'}^{2} = 0 \tag{11.41}$$

$$\lim_{\theta \to 0} \left(\frac{1}{\sigma_{x'}^{2}} \right) = 0 \tag{11.42}$$

$$\lim_{\theta \to \pi/2} \left(\frac{1}{\sigma_{z'}^{2}} \right) = 0 \tag{11.43}$$

That is, $\sigma_{z'}$ is equal to zero and $\sigma_{x'}$ becomes unbounded in the limit of $\theta = 0$. Similarly, $\sigma_{x'}$ is equal to zero and $\sigma_{z'}$ becomes unbounded in the limit of $\theta = \pi/2$. This behavior is expected because we can rewrite Eq. (11.33) in terms of the complementary angle $\theta^* \equiv \pi/2 - \theta$, which is the angle with respect to the z'-axis, and it then assumes a form identical to Eq. (11.32) with θ replaced by θ^*.

Next, we shall consider the case of

$$\theta \neq 0, \quad \theta \neq \pi/2 \quad \text{and} \quad \alpha \equiv \frac{r_A^{\,2}}{x_e^{\,2}\sin 2\theta} \equiv \frac{\beta^2}{\sin 2\theta} << 1 \tag{11.44}$$

Recalling the expansion for the natural logarithm

$$\ln(1+x) = x - \frac{1}{2}x^2 + \frac{1}{3}x^3 - \frac{1}{4}x^4 + \cdots \quad \text{for} \quad -1 < x \leq 1 \tag{11.45}$$

we may write

$$\ln\left(1 + \frac{r_A^{\,2}}{x_e^{\,2}\sin 2\theta}\right) \simeq \frac{r_A^{\,2}}{x_e^{\,2}\sin 2\theta} \tag{11.46}$$

It follows from Eqs. (11.32) and (11.33) that

$$\begin{aligned} \sigma_{x'} &\simeq x_e\left|\cos\theta\right| \\ \sigma_{z'} &\simeq x_e\left|\sin\theta\right| \end{aligned} \tag{11.47}$$

Note that Eq. (11.47) is in agreement with Eq. (11.11) obtained from the maximum likelihood approach.

We note that in Eq. (11.37), we may write

$$\frac{\beta^2}{\beta^2 + \sin 2\theta} = \frac{\alpha}{1+\alpha} \tag{11.48}$$

$$\frac{\sin 2\theta}{\beta^2 + \sin 2\theta} = \frac{1}{1+\alpha} \tag{11.49}$$

$$\frac{(1-\cos 2\theta)}{\beta^2 \tan\theta} = \left(\frac{2\sin^2\theta}{\beta^2}\right)\left(\frac{\sin 2\theta}{2\sin\theta\cos\theta}\right)\left(\frac{1}{\tan\theta}\right) \equiv \frac{1}{\alpha} \tag{11.50}$$

Hence, we obtain still another form of the maximum probability of collision:

$$P_{\max}(r_A, x_e, \theta) = \left(\frac{\alpha}{1+\alpha}\right)\left(\frac{1}{1+\alpha}\right)^{1/\alpha} \quad \text{where} \quad \alpha \equiv \frac{r_A^{\,2}}{x_e^{\,2}\sin 2\theta} \equiv \frac{\beta^2}{\sin 2\theta} \tag{11.51}$$

Recalling the definition

$$e = \lim_{\alpha \to 0} (1+\alpha)^{1/\alpha} \tag{11.52}$$

we see it follows that, for small α, Eq. (11.51) becomes

$$P_{max}(r_A, x_e, \theta) \simeq \frac{\alpha}{e} = \frac{\beta^2}{e \sin 2\theta} \quad \text{where} \quad \beta \equiv \left(\frac{r_A}{x_e}\right) \tag{11.53}$$

Note that Eq. (11.53) is precisely Eq. (11.13) obtained from the maximum likelihood approach. In that approach, in order to obtain the maximum probability, we assume that the pdf does not vary much over the combined circular collision cross-sectional area of radius r_A. A sufficient condition is that $r_A << \sigma_{x'}$ and $r_A << \sigma_{z'}$. In Eq. (11.11), if θ is not close to 0 or $\pi/2$, then $\sin\theta$ </< 1 and $\cos\theta$ </< 1. Thus, these conditions lead to $\beta \equiv r_A/x_e << 1$ and $\sin 2\theta$ </< 1. Hence, $\alpha \equiv \beta^2/\sin 2\theta << 1$. If we now apply this condition to Eq. (11.37), it is expected that we recover Eq. (11.13). This discussion is an attempt to tie the two methods, the maximum likelihood approach being a somewhat crude way of yielding the answer quickly in contrast to the "general" maximum probability approach.

The standard deviations $\sigma_{x'}$ and $\sigma_{z'}$ that yield the maximum collision probability $P_{max}(x', z')$ may also be written in terms of β and θ. Thus, Eq. (11.32) and (11.33) become

$$\left(\frac{\sigma_{x'}}{x_e}\right)^2 = \frac{\beta^2}{2 \tan\theta \ln\left(1 + \dfrac{\beta^2}{\sin 2\theta}\right)} \tag{11.54}$$

$$\left(\frac{\sigma_{z'}}{x_e}\right)^2 = \frac{\beta^2 \tan\theta}{2 \ln\left(1 + \dfrac{\beta^2}{\sin 2\theta}\right)} \tag{11.55}$$

For small values of α, these equations become Eq. (11.11) or (11.47) and we have

$$\left(\frac{\sigma_{x'}}{x_e}\right) \simeq |\cos\theta| \qquad \left(\frac{\sigma_{z'}}{x_e}\right) \simeq |\sin\theta| \tag{11.56}$$

11.3 Comparison of the Two Approaches

In Section 11.1, using the method of maximum likelihood, we multiplied $f_{max}(x', z')$ by the area $\pi r_A{}^2$ to obtain an approximation—shown in Eq. (11.13)—of the maximum probability. In Section 11.2, starting with the analytical expression Eq. (11.16) for the collision probability, we directly obtained the maximum probability $P_{max}(x', z')$ given by Eq. (11.37). In both analyses, we specified θ to be the angle measured from the principal x'-axis so that we have $0 \le |\theta| \le 90$ deg. However, we specifically did not impose the condition $\sigma_{x'} \ge \sigma_{z'}$. This allowed us to consider the complete first quadrant of the $(\sigma_{x'}, \sigma_{z'})$-plane to determine values of the two standard deviations $\sigma_{x'}$ and $\sigma_{z'}$ that would yield the maximum value of the pdf $f(x', z')$ or the probability $P(x', z')$. We took the partial derivatives and set them to zero in accordance with the standard procedure. This is the reason the resultant Eqs. (11.11) and (11.29) allow for $\sigma_{z'} > \sigma_{x'}$ when $|\theta| > 45$ deg. In this chapter, we consider the unconstrained problem for simplicity to avoid undue complications.

However, if we impose the constraint that $\sigma_{x'} \ge \sigma_{z'}$ by definition, then we insert the value of $|\theta| = 45$ deg into all the above results whenever $|\theta| > 45$ deg. This is to avoid the principal z'-axis from being associated with the larger standard deviation when yielding the maximum probability. It may be argued that this is the proper choice based more rigorously on the one-to-one transformation in Eq. (11.11), which relates x_e and θ to $\sigma_{x'}$ and $\sigma_{z'}$ for the maximum likelihood approach. Similarly, the same applies to the maximum probability approach by invoking Eqs. (11.29), (11.32), and (11.33), which relate x_e and θ to $\sigma_{x'}$ and $\sigma_{z'}$.

In Chapter 5, we showed that Eq. (11.16) for the collision probability is accurate to two or three significant figures (when compared to three other collision probability computation models) for a wide range of the collision parameters r_A, x_e, $\sigma_{x'}$, $\sigma_{z'}$, and θ. Moreover, this analytical expression is valid for the aspect ratio $\lambda \equiv \sigma_{x'}/\sigma_{z'} \lesssim 10$. Because $\tan^{-1}(0.1) = 5.7$ deg, it follows from Eq. (11.29) that we can apply this model whenever $|\theta| \gtrsim 5.7$ deg. The other condition for validity of this model is that $\beta \lesssim 0.3$. (We can relax this condition to $\beta \lesssim 1$ if we have $|\theta| \lesssim 10$ deg.) Numerical studies reveal that when 5.7 deg $\lesssim |\theta| \le 90$ deg and $\beta \lesssim 0.3$, the two models agree to two significant figures or approximately 1%. When $\beta = 1$ the second model based on Eq. (11.16) still yields valid answers for 10 deg $\le |\theta| \le 90$ deg; however, when $\beta = 1$ the first model, based on maximum likelihood, fails miserably for all values of θ. This is expected because one of the two basic conditions for using the maximum likelihood to obtain the maximum probability is that $\beta << 1$. When $\beta \lesssim 1$ and $|\theta| \lesssim 5.7$ deg, we shall use Eq. (11.15) for computing the maximum collision probability. Equation (11.15) computes the case of $\theta = 0$ deg.

11.4 Numerical Results

We recall that Eqs. (11.13) and (11.37) involve only the ratio β^2 and the angle θ whereas Eq. (11.15) involves only the ratio β and is applicable for $\theta = 0$. Thus, it suffices to compute the maximum probability in terms of only β and θ. Table 11.1 shows representative results of P_{max} obtained using the second model in terms of these two parameters. Figure 11.2 is a graphical display of the same results.

Table 11.2 compares the results obtained using the maximum likelihood approach and those obtained using the general approach based on Eq. (11.16). Both approaches yield identical results to four significant figures when 0 deg $\leq |\theta| \leq$ 90 deg and $\beta \leq 0.01$. However, for 10 deg $\leq |\theta| \leq$ 90 deg and $\beta \leq 0.1$, the results agree to two significant figures or approximately 1%. Finally, for 10 deg $\leq |\theta| \leq$ 90 deg and $\beta = 1$, the first model gives erroneous results whereas the second yields valid answers.

The standard deviations $\sigma_{x'}$ and $\sigma_{z'}$ given by Eqs. (11.54) and (11.55) that yield the maximum collision probability $P_{max}(x', z')$ in terms of β and θ are not tabulated nor plotted because they are not very different from the cosine and sine values given trivially by Eq. (11.56).

11.5 Discussion

In an encounter between a spacecraft and another orbiting object, the two trajectories are determined from tracking data. However, sometimes the covariances associated with orbit epoch elements are not revealed. Thus, the distance of closest approach x_e is generally known to a fair degree of confidence. Because we know that the largest uncertainties are in the intrack direction and to a lesser degree in the crosstrack and radial directions, it is possible to arrive at a rough estimate of the direction θ relative to the principal axes even though we may not know the standard deviations $\sigma_{x'}$ and $\sigma_{z'}$ along the principal axes.

Table 11.1. Maximum Probability of Collision (P_{max})

	β				
θ (deg)	1×10^{-4}	1×10^{-3}	1×10^{-2}	1×10^{-1}	1
0	4.84×10^{-05}	4.84×10^{-04}	4.84×10^{-03}	4.84×10^{-02}	4.84×10^{-01}
10	1.08×10^{-08}	1.08×10^{-06}	1.08×10^{-04}	1.06×10^{-02}	4.67×10^{-01}
20	5.72×10^{-09}	5.72×10^{-07}	5.72×10^{-05}	5.68×10^{-03}	3.33×10^{-01}
30	4.25×10^{-09}	4.25×10^{-07}	4.25×10^{-05}	4.22×10^{-03}	2.76×10^{-01}
40	3.74×10^{-09}	3.74×10^{-07}	3.74×10^{-05}	3.72×10^{-03}	2.53×10^{-01}
50	3.68×10^{-09}	3.68×10^{-07}	3.68×10^{-05}	3.66×10^{-03}	2.50×10^{-01}
60	3.68×10^{-09}	3.68×10^{-07}	3.68×10^{-05}	3.66×10^{-03}	2.50×10^{-01}
70	3.68×10^{-09}	3.68×10^{-07}	3.68×10^{-05}	3.66×10^{-03}	2.50×10^{-01}
80	3.68×10^{-09}	3.68×10^{-07}	3.68×10^{-05}	3.66×10^{-03}	2.50×10^{-01}
90	3.68×10^{-09}	3.68×10^{-07}	3.68×10^{-05}	3.66×10^{-03}	2.50×10^{-01}

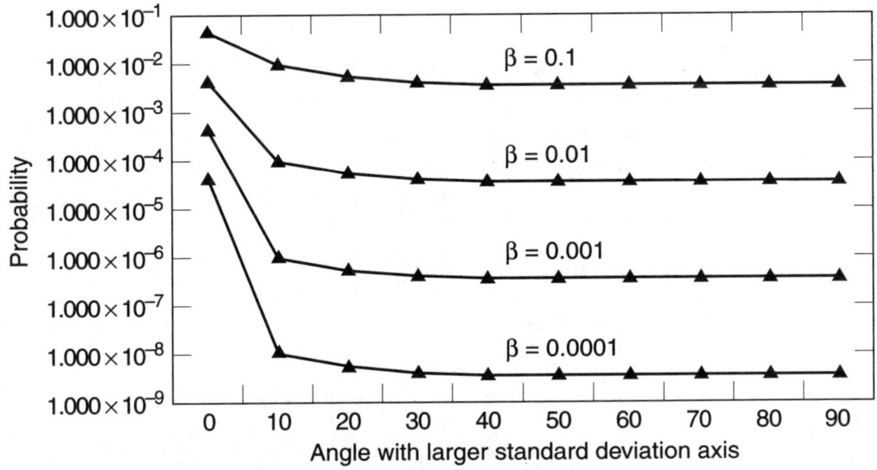

Figure 11.2. Maximum probability of collision; a graphical display of the computation results shown in Table 11.1. $\beta \equiv r_A/x_e$.

As discussed in Chapter 2, in a close encounter between two orbiting objects, the value of θ is usually in the range 10 deg $\leq |\theta| \leq$ 90 deg. Even if we naively assume a uniform distribution, the percentage for which we have 0 deg $\leq |\theta| \leq$ 10 deg is approximately 10%. Actually, if 0 deg $\leq |\theta| \leq$ 5 deg, then the miss distances in these cases are generally very large and are of the order of 100 km. The result is that the encounter is not a close one, and it is eliminated from consideration. The case of $\theta = 0$ deg is so rare or improbable that one has to construct an artificial example to illustrate when it can happen. Hence, we consider 10 deg $\leq |\theta| \leq$ 90 deg to be the relevant range for our consideration.

Let us take the example of a combined cross-sectional area of radius $r_A = 1$ m and a miss distance of $x_e = 10$ km, thus yielding $\beta = 10^{-4}$. From Table 11.1, we see that the maximum probability of collision is approximately 4×10^{-9} in the relevant range. However, if we take the case of $\theta = 0$ deg, we obtain a value of $P_{\max} \cong 4 \times 10^{-5}$, which is four orders of magnitude larger. As a second example, let us take $r_A = 10$ m and $x_e = 10$ km, thus yielding $\beta = 10^{-3}$. We see that $P_{\max} \cong 4 \times 10^{-7}$ in the relevant range compared to $P_{\max} \cong 4 \times 10^{-4}$ for the case of $\theta = 0$ deg, which is three orders of magnitude larger. Finally as a third example, let us take $r_A = 100$ m and $x_e = 10$ km, thus yielding $\beta = 10^{-2}$. We see that $P_{\max} \cong 4 \times 10^{-5}$ in the relevant range compared to $P_{\max} \cong 4 \times 10^{-3}$ for the case of $\theta = 0$ deg, which is two orders of magnitude larger.

Alfano[11.1] has also derived the maximum probability for spacecraft collision for the case of $\theta = 0$ deg only; however, in most cases of close encounter, the angle θ measured from the principal x'-axis associated with the larger standard deviation $\sigma_{x'}$ is not close to zero. Moreover, he has also arbitrarily specified the aspect ratio λ to be fixed so that he considered only one variable $\sigma_{z'}$ (instead of $\sigma_{x'}$ and $\sigma_{z'}$).

Table 11.2. Maximum Probability of Collision (P_{max}) Computed Using Maximum Likelihood Approach and General Approach

		θ (deg)									
	β	0	10	20	30	40	50	60	70	80	90
M[a]	1×10^{-4}	4.84×10^{-05}	1.08×10^{-08}	5.72×10^{-09}	4.25×10^{-09}	3.74×10^{-09}	3.68×10^{-09}	3.68×10^{-09}	3.68×10^{-09}	3.68×10^{-09}	3.68×10^{-09}
G[b]	1×10^{-4}	4.84×10^{-05}	1.08×10^{-08}	5.72×10^{-09}	4.25×10^{-09}	3.74×10^{-09}	3.68×10^{-09}	3.68×10^{-09}	3.68×10^{-09}	3.68×10^{-09}	3.68×10^{-09}
M	1×10^{-3}	4.84×10^{-04}	1.08×10^{-06}	5.72×10^{-07}	4.25×10^{-07}	3.74×10^{-07}	3.68×10^{-07}	3.68×10^{-07}	3.68×10^{-07}	3.68×10^{-07}	3.68×10^{-07}
G	1×10^{-3}	4.84×10^{-04}	1.08×10^{-06}	5.72×10^{-07}	4.25×10^{-07}	3.74×10^{-07}	3.68×10^{-07}	3.68×10^{-07}	3.68×10^{-07}	3.68×10^{-07}	3.68×10^{-07}
M	1×10^{-2}	4.84×10^{-03}	1.08×10^{-04}	5.72×10^{-05}	4.25×10^{-05}	3.74×10^{-05}	3.68×10^{-05}	3.68×10^{-05}	3.68×10^{-05}	3.68×10^{-05}	3.68×10^{-05}
G	1×10^{-2}	4.84×10^{-03}	1.08×10^{-04}	5.72×10^{-05}	4.25×10^{-05}	3.74×10^{-05}	3.68×10^{-05}	3.68×10^{-05}	3.68×10^{-05}	3.68×10^{-05}	3.68×10^{-05}
M	1×10^{-1}	4.84×10^{-02}	1.08×10^{-02}	5.72×10^{-03}	4.25×10^{-03}	3.74×10^{-03}	3.68×10^{-03}	3.68×10^{-03}	3.68×10^{-03}	3.68×10^{-03}	3.68×10^{-03}
G	1×10^{-1}	4.84×10^{-02}	1.06×10^{-02}	5.68×10^{-03}	4.22×10^{-03}	3.72×10^{-03}	3.66×10^{-03}	3.66×10^{-03}	3.66×10^{-03}	3.66×10^{-03}	3.66×10^{-03}
M	1	4.84×10^{-01}	$1.08\times10^{+00}$	5.72×10^{-01}	4.25×10^{-01}	3.74×10^{-01}	3.68×10^{-01}	3.68×10^{-01}	3.68×10^{-01}	3.68×10^{-01}	3.68×10^{-01}
G	1	4.84×10^{-01}	4.67×10^{-01}	3.33×10^{-01}	2.76×10^{-01}	2.53×10^{-01}	2.50×10^{-01}	2.50×10^{-01}	2.50×10^{-01}	2.50×10^{-01}	2.50×10^{-01}

[a]Max. likelihood
[b]General

Hence, he obtained the "maximum probability" $P_{max}(x', z')$ by solving only one equation $dP/d\sigma_{z'} = 0$. This methodology leaves something to be desired because a necessary condition for maximum probability is that $\sigma_{x'}$ and $\sigma_{z'}$ satisfy the condition in Eq. (11.29), which may not be the same as the specified aspect ratio λ. There is no doubt that the answers Alfano obtained are upper bounds, but they are often two to four orders of magnitude larger than the ones in the relevant range 10 deg $\leq |\theta| \leq$ 90 deg. Because of this overestimation, they may not serve as very good discriminators for filtering out many cases of miss distances for which the collision probability is low.

11.6 Conclusion

We formulated two approaches for computing the maximum probability of collision. The first approach relies on the method of maximum likelihood and is applicable when 10 deg $\leq |\theta| \leq$ 90 deg and $\beta \leq 0.1$. It computes maximum probability P_{max} using Eq. (11.13). The second approach is based on Eq. (11.16) as a starting point and is applicable when 10 deg $\leq |\theta| \leq$ 90 deg and $\beta \lesssim 1$. It computes P_{max} using Eq. (11.37). When $\beta \lesssim 1$ and $|\theta| \lesssim 5.7$ deg, we use Eq. (11.15) for computing P_{max}, which computes the case of $\theta = 0$ deg.

In the relevant range of application 10 deg $\leq |\theta| \leq$ 90 deg, the values of P increase by a factor of 100 if β is increased by a factor of 10. This is because P_{max} involves β^2 in Eqs. (11.13) and (11.37). However, for the case of $\theta = 0$ deg, the values of P increase by the same factor as β is increased because P_{max} involves β in Eq. (11.15).

The relevant range for applications is 10 deg $\leq |\theta| \leq$ 90 deg. The values of P_{max} obtained in this relevant range are four orders of magnitude smaller than those for $\theta = 0$ deg when $\beta = 10^{-4}$. They are three orders of magnitude smaller than those for $\theta = 0$ deg when $\beta = 10^{-3}$. They are two orders of magnitude smaller than those for $\theta = 0$ deg when $\beta = 10^{-2}$.

11.7 Summary

In this chapter, we considered the problem of finding the maximum probability of collision when we are not privileged to possess the covariances of the conjoining objects. All that we are given are the two trajectories of the primary and the secondary objects. From these orbital data, we showed in Chapter 2 how to derive the elevation angle at conjunction. It is quite amazing that we are able to obtain this upper bound.

In Section 11.1, we used the principle of maximum likelihood to obtain a quick estimate of the maximum probability when the pdf does not vary much over the combined circular collision cross-sectional area of radius.

In Section 11.2, we derived the maximum probability starting from first principles by equating to zero the two partial derivatives with respect to the standard deviations. Considering the complicated equations we had to solve, we were fortunate to obtain a closed-form solution to the problem.

In Section 11.3, we clarified a subtle point not quite apparent at first glance. We also discussed the differences in the two approaches and their respective limits of applicability.

In Section 11.4, we compared the results obtained from the two approaches. The numerical results agree to two significant figures or approximately 1% throughout much of the range of applications interest.

In Section 11.5, we discussed how the maximum collision probability P_{max} is very flat as a function of the angle $|\theta|$ with $\beta \equiv r_A/x_e$ as a parameter. For $|\theta|$ less than 5 deg, the curve rises very sharply. However, in this range, the miss distances are generally very large so that the encounters are not close. The case of $\theta = 0$ deg is so rare or improbable that one has to construct an artificial example to illustrate when it can happen.

In Section 11.6, we concluded that the relevant range for applications is 10 deg $\leq |\theta| \leq$ 90 deg. The values of P_{max} obtained in this relevant range are four orders of magnitude smaller than those for $\theta = 0$ deg when $\beta = 10^{-4}$. They are three orders of magnitude smaller than those for $\theta = 0$ deg when $\beta = 10^{-3}$. They are two orders of magnitude smaller than those for $\theta = 0$ deg when $\beta = 10^{-2}$.

11.8 Reference

[11.1.] S. Alfano, "Relating Position Uncertainty to Maximum Conjunction Probability," *J. Astronautical Sci.* **53** (2), 193–205 (2005).

Chapter 12: Close Encounters with Multiple Satellites

This chapter is concerned with a detailed calculation of the probability of collision between the primary spacecraft and numerous secondary orbiting objects over a period of time.[12.1] These secondary objects are grouped into different classes. The objects in each class lie within small tolerances about a specific altitude and inclination; the latter parameter can be different from that of the primary spacecraft. All the secondary objects in this class have ascending nodes uniformly distributed around the equator and have phase angles uniformly distributed within an orbital plane.

12.1 Transformation of pdf

In Chapter 5, we considered the probability density function (pdf)

$$f(x',z') = \frac{1}{2\pi\,\sigma_{x'}\sigma_{z'}} e^{-\frac{1}{2}\left[\left(\frac{x'}{\sigma_{x'}}\right)^2 + \left(\frac{z'}{\sigma_{z'}}\right)^2\right]} \tag{12.1}$$

After we transformed the bivariate Gaussian pdf to an isotropic pdf by a scale change, we replaced the resultant elliptical cross-sectional area by an equivalent circular cross-sectional area, meaning one with equal area and the same centroid. In this chapter, because we do not know a priori the angular direction with respect to the principal axes, we shall replace the elliptical pdf contours by equivalent circular pdf contours. This is accomplished by introducing the mean standard deviation σ:

$$\sigma^2 \equiv \sigma_{x'}\sigma_{z'} \tag{12.2}$$

Thus, we have the following isotropic pdf:

$$f(x, z) = \frac{1}{2\pi\,\sigma^2} e^{-\left(x^2 + z^2\right)/2\sigma^2} \tag{12.3}$$

Because our collision cross-section is a circle with radius r_A, we once again consider the Rician integral that involves one variable and whose analytical form we have already obtained. Note that the two problems are not tautologically the same. In the previous one, the elliptical cross-section was replaced by an equivalent circular cross-section. In the present one, the elliptical pdf contours were replaced by equivalent circular pdf contours; however, both are now handled by the same mathematics from this point onward.

Thus, we now have the probability of collision expressed with sufficient accuracy as

$$P = e^{-v/2}(1 - e^{-u/2}) \tag{12.4}$$

where the dimensionless variables u and v are defined in terms of the mean standard deviation σ, miss distance x_e, and the radius r_A of collision cross-sectional integration by

$$u \equiv \left(\frac{r_A}{\sigma}\right)^2 > 0 \tag{12.5}$$

$$v \equiv \left(\frac{x_e}{\sigma}\right)^2 > 0 \tag{12.6}$$

12.2 Number Density of Orbiting Objects

The main collision probabilities summarized here apply to the case of the primary satellite encountering a single secondary satellite when the angular direction is not known. In this section, the analysis is extended to the case of collision when there are many oncoming satellites whose angular directions are also not known. Thus, we invoke the concept of number density of orbiting objects. It is assumed that the oncoming satellites have circular orbits and can be grouped into classes, each class being characterized by the orbital inclination and orbital altitude. It is further assumed that, in a given orbital plane, the phase is statistically uniform; and the ascending node is also statistically uniform in the equatorial plane. This is already evident in the dispersion of the debris fragments from the Ariane-1 H-10 upper stage explosion on 13 November 1986. Figure 12.1 shows two stages of the dispersion one year apart.

Let $\rho(\theta)$ and $\rho_{eq}(\theta)$, respectively, denote the number density of ascending (or descending) satellites at latitude θ and at the equator. It is shown in Appendix C (see Eq. [C12]) that

$$\rho(\theta) = \frac{\rho_{eq}}{\cos\phi_s} \tag{12.7}$$

where ϕ_s is the "argument of latitude" of the secondary satellite (i.e., $\phi = \omega + \nu$, where ω is the argument of perigee and ν is the true anomaly). Note that the total number density $\rho_{eq,total}(\theta)$ of both ascending and descending satellites at the equator is

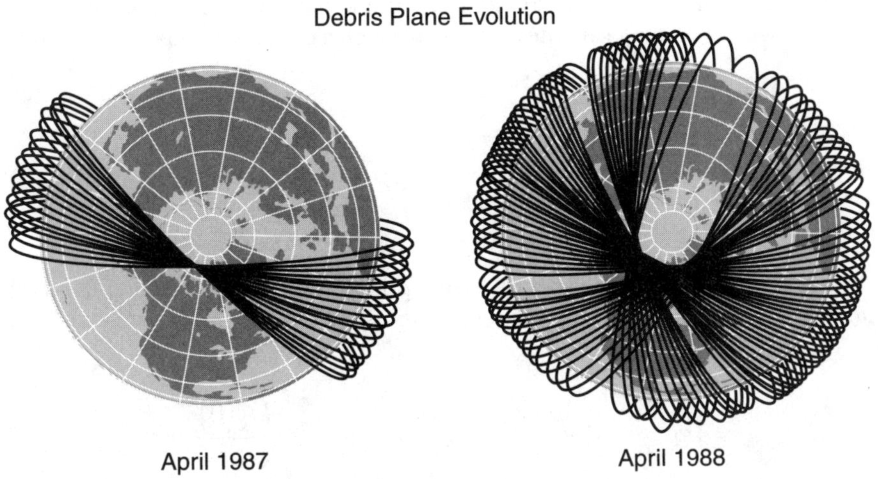

Figure 12.1. Dispersion of debris fragments from Ariane breakup.

$$\rho_{\text{eq}} = \frac{1}{2}\rho_{\text{eq,total}} \tag{12.8}$$

Consider satellites of a given class. Suppose the satellites of this class at latitude θ are uniformly distributed over a layer of thickness h. Let $\mathbf{V}_{\text{rel}}$ denote the average velocity of the oncoming secondary satellites relative to the primary satellite, defined within the region of interest. In the previous section, we had chosen the x-axis of the encounter coordinate system to be in the same direction as the relative position vector at closest approach and denoted that distance as x_e. In this section, it is more convenient to consider the position vector relative to the primary satellite at closest approach as random in direction in a plane perpendicular to the relative velocity vector. We shall denote this distance as r_e. Therefore, the number of oncoming satellites crossing an annulus of radius r_e and thickness dr_e in unit time is given by

$$dN^*(\theta) = 2\pi r_e \rho(\theta) V_{\text{rel}}(\theta)\, dr_e \tag{12.9}$$

12.3 Number of Collisions per Orbit (Part 1)

From Eqs. (12.1), (12.3), and (12.4), we know that the probability of collision with one oncoming satellite is approximately

$$P = e^{-\frac{1}{2}\left(\frac{r_e}{\sigma}\right)^2}\left[1 - e^{-\frac{1}{2}\left(\frac{r_A}{\sigma}\right)^2}\right] \tag{12.10}$$

Hence, from Eqs. (12.7) through (12.10), the number of collisions $N(\theta)$ per unit time with oncoming satellites passing through a circle of radius r_e'' at latitude θ is

$$N(\theta)=\pi\rho_{\text{eq,total}}\left[1-e^{-\frac{1}{2}\left(\frac{r_A}{\sigma}\right)^2}\right]\int_0^{r_e''} r_e e^{-\frac{1}{2}\left(\frac{r_e}{\sigma}\right)^2}\frac{V_{\text{rel}}(\theta)}{\cos\phi_s}dr_e \tag{12.11}$$

Let T denote the orbital period of the primary satellite. Therefore, the total number of collisions $N_{\text{total,orbit}}$ over an orbit is given by

$$N_{\text{total,orbit}}=4\pi\rho_{\text{eq,total}}\left[1-e^{-\frac{1}{2}\left(\frac{r_A}{\sigma}\right)^2}\right]\int_0^{T/4}\int_0^{r_e''} r_e e^{-\frac{1}{2}\left(\frac{r_e}{\sigma}\right)^2}\frac{V_{\text{rel}}(\theta)}{\cos\phi_s}dr_e dt \tag{12.12}$$

or, equivalently,

$$N_{\text{total,orbit}}=4\pi\rho_{\text{eq,total}}\left[1-e^{-\frac{1}{2}\left(\frac{r_A}{\sigma}\right)^2}\right]\int_0^{r_e''} r_e e^{-\frac{1}{2}\left(\frac{r_e}{\sigma}\right)^2}dr_e\int_0^{\theta''}\frac{V_{\text{rel}}(\theta)}{\dot{\theta}\cos\phi_s}d\theta \tag{12.13}$$

Let i_p and ϕ_p, respectively, denote the inclination and the argument of latitude of the primary satellite. Then, from spherical trigonometry, we have

$$\sin\theta=\sin i_p\sin\phi_p \tag{12.14}$$

$$\sin\theta=\sin i_s\sin\phi_s \tag{12.15}$$

Equation (12.14) yields on differentiation with respect to time

$$\dot{\theta}\cos\theta=\dot{\phi}_p\sin i_p\cos\phi_p \tag{12.16}$$

Because $d\phi_p/dt=2\pi/T$, therefore

$$\dot{\theta}\cos\phi_s=\frac{2\pi}{T}\sin i_p\frac{\cos\phi_p\cos\phi_s}{\cos\theta} \tag{12.17}$$

By substituting Eq. (12.17) into (12.13) and using (12.14) and (12.15), we obtain

$$N_{\text{total,orbit}} = \frac{2T\rho_{\text{eq,total}}}{\sin i_p}\left[1-e^{-\frac{1}{2}\left(\frac{r_A}{\sigma}\right)^2}\right]\int_0^{r_e''} r_e e^{-\frac{1}{2}\left(\frac{r_e}{\sigma}\right)^2} dr_e \int_0^{\theta''} \frac{V_{\text{rel}}(\theta)\cos\theta}{\cos\phi_p \cos\phi_s} d\theta \tag{12.18}$$

Hence,

$$N_{\text{total,orbit}} = K^* J^* I^* \tag{12.19}$$

where

$$K^* = 2T\sin i_s \rho_{\text{eq,total}}\left[1-e^{-\frac{1}{2}\left(\frac{r_A}{\sigma}\right)^2}\right] \tag{12.20}$$

$$J^* = \sigma^2\left[1-e^{-\frac{1}{2}\left(\frac{r_e''}{\sigma}\right)^2}\right] \tag{12.21}$$

$$I^* = \int_0^{\theta''} \frac{V_{rel}(\theta)\cos\theta}{\sqrt{\left[\left(\sin^2 i_p - \sin^2\theta\right)\left(\sin^2 i_s - \sin^2\theta\right)\right]}} d\theta \tag{12.22}$$

A little consideration of Eq. (12.22) reveals that the upper limit θ'' of integration is given by the minimum inclination in latitude, that is,

$$\sin\theta'' = \min\left\{\sin i_p,\ \sin i_s\right\} \tag{12.23}$$

where i_s denotes the inclination of the class of oncoming satellites.

12.4 Geometry of Encounters

Let ψ_p denote the acute angle between the orbit plane of the primary satellite and the meridian plane at latitude θ. Similarly, let ψ_s denote the corresponding acute angle for the class of oncoming secondary satellites. Fig. 12.2 shows these angles.

Then, from spherical trigonometry, we have

$$\cos i_p = \cos\theta \sin\psi_p \tag{12.24}$$

$$\cos i_s = \cos\theta \sin\psi_s \tag{12.25}$$

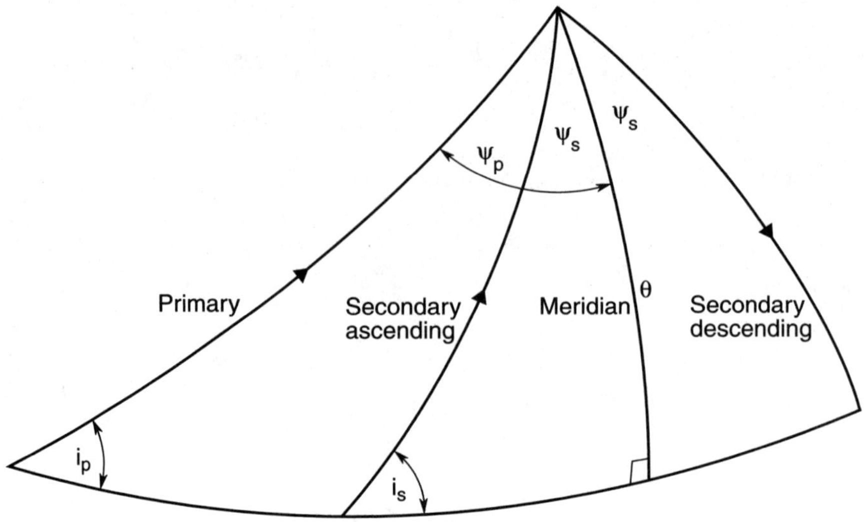

Figure 12.2. Orbital planes of primary spacecraft and secondary object.

so that

$$\psi_p = \sin^{-1}\left(\frac{\cos i_p}{\cos\theta}\right) \quad \text{where} \quad -\pi/2 \le \psi_p \le \pi/2 \tag{12.26}$$

$$\psi_s = \sin^{-1}\left(\frac{\cos i_s}{\cos\theta}\right) \quad \text{where} \quad -\pi/2 \le \psi_s \le \pi/2 \tag{12.27}$$

There are two cases to consider, approaching collisions and trailing collisions.

12.4.1 Approaching Collisions

This case has two subcases: (a) both orbits are direct or both orbits are retrograde, and one satellite is in ascending motion (relative to the equator) and the other satellite is descending; (b) one orbit is direct and the other is retrograde, while one is ascending and the other is descending. Let us assume that the magnitudes of the two velocity vectors are the same because the satellites are essentially at the same altitude. Let ψ_A and $V_{rel,A}$ denote the angle and magnitude of the relative velocity between these two velocity vectors. Then, we may show that, in general, ψ_A and $V_{rel,A}$ are respectively given by

$$\psi_A = \pi - \left(\psi_p + \psi_s\right) \tag{12.28}$$

$$V_{\text{rel},A} = 2V\cos\left(\frac{\psi_p + \psi_s}{2}\right) \tag{12.29}$$

12.4.2 Trailing Collisions

This case also has two subcases: (a) both orbits are direct or both orbits are retrograde, and both are ascending or both are descending; (b) one orbit is direct and the other is retrograde, while both are ascending or both are descending. Let ψ_T and $V_{\text{rel},T}$ denote the angle and the magnitude of the relative velocity between these two velocity vectors. Then, we may show that, in general, ψ_T and $V_{\text{rel},T}$ are respectively given by

$$\psi_T = \left|\psi_p - \psi_s\right| \tag{12.30}$$

$$V_{\text{rel},T} = 2V\sin\left|\frac{\psi_p - \psi_s}{2}\right| \tag{12.31}$$

12.5 Number of Collisions per Orbit (Part 2)

By substituting Eqs. (12.29) and (12.31) into (12.18), we obtain

$$N_{\text{total,orbit}} = K\,J\,I \tag{12.32}$$

where, for convenience, we define

$$K = 4VT\sigma^2 \sin i_s \rho_{\text{eq,total}}\left[1 - e^{-\frac{1}{2}\left(\frac{r_A}{\sigma}\right)^2}\right] \tag{12.33}$$

$$J = \left[1 - e^{-\frac{1}{2}\left(\frac{r_e''}{\sigma}\right)^2}\right] \tag{12.34}$$

$$I = \int_0^{\theta''} \frac{\left[\cos\left(\frac{\psi_p + \psi_s}{2}\right) + \sin\left|\frac{\psi_p - \psi_s}{2}\right|\right]\cos\theta}{\sqrt{\left[\left(\sin^2 i_p - \sin^2\theta\right)\left(\sin^2 i_s - \sin^2\theta\right)\right]}}\,d\theta \tag{12.35}$$

Equation (12.35) is applicable for all combinations of direct or retrograde orbits for the primary and secondary satellites. The cosine term corresponds to approaching collisions; the sine term corresponds to trailing collisions.

Let R denote the radial distance of the satellites of a given class, measured from Earth's center. Because the orbits are assumed to be circular, therefore the distance L traveled per orbit is

$$L = 2\pi R = VT \tag{12.36}$$

Let n_{total} denote the number of satellites in a given class. By statistically spreading the satellites over the equator, then over the satellite orbit, and finally over a layer of thickness h, then r_e'' in Eq. (12.34) may be taken as $h/2$. It is shown in Appendix C (see Eq. [C.10]) that

$$\rho_{\text{eq,total}} = \frac{2n_{\text{total}}}{L^2 h \sin i_s} \tag{12.37}$$

Substitution of Eqs. (12.36) and (12.37) into (12.33) yields

$$K = \frac{4\sigma^2 n_{\text{total}}}{\pi R h}\left[1 - e^{-\frac{1}{2}\left(\frac{r_A}{\sigma}\right)^2}\right] \tag{12.38}$$

Equations (12.32), (12.34), (12.35), and (12.38) constitute the basic equations for computing the total number of collisions per orbit. The K term given by Eq. (12.38) contains the collision cross section, the number of satellites of a given class, orbit determination uncertainties, orbital radius, and the thickness of the altitude band for that class. The J term given by Eq. (12.34) contains the orbit determination uncertainties and the maximum flux radius. Finally, the I term given by Eq. (12.35) contains only the effects of the orbital characteristics of both the primary satellite and the secondary orbiting object.

If $r_A << \sigma$, then Eq. (12.38) yields

$$K \cong \frac{2r_A^2 n_{\text{total}}}{\pi R h} \tag{12.39}$$

Next, in Eq. (12.34), we consider the case of $r_e'' > 4\sigma$. Then, we have

$$J \cong 1 \tag{12.40}$$

As an example, let $\sigma = 2.5$ km and $r_e = 10$ km. From Eq. (12.34), we obtain $J = 0.9997$.

Finally, in Eq. (12.35), it is observed that the integrand becomes infinite at the upper limit of integration where $\sin\theta'' = \sin i_p$ or $\sin\theta'' = \sin i_s$ as determined by Eq. (12.23). Detailed expressions for evaluating this integral are next derived to handle this situation. To do this, we have to consider two cases.

12.5.1 Case of $\sin i_p \neq \sin i_s$

12.5.1.1 Subcase of $\sin i_s < \sin i_p$

In this case, we have from Eq. (12.23)

$$\left.\begin{array}{ll}\theta'' = i_s & \text{for} \quad i_s < \pi/2 \\ \theta'' = (\pi - i_s) & \text{for} \quad i_s \geq \pi/2\end{array}\right\} \tag{12.41}$$

For convenience, let the integral Eq. (12.35) be written as

$$I = \int_0^{\theta''} \frac{Q(i_p,\, i_s;\, \theta)\cos\theta}{\sqrt{(\sin^2 i_s - \sin^2\theta)}}\, d\theta \tag{12.42}$$

where

$$Q(i_p,\, i_s;\, \theta) = \frac{\left[\cos\left(\dfrac{\psi_p + \psi_s}{2}\right) + \sin\left|\dfrac{\psi_p - \psi_s}{2}\right|\right]}{\sqrt{(\sin^2 i_p - \sin^2\theta)}} \tag{12.43}$$

Note that the numerator on the right-hand side of Eq. (12.43) is symmetrical in i_p and i_s. However, the denominator contains only i_p. We observe that $Q(i_p, i_s; \theta)$ is an analytic function in a neighborhood of $\theta = \theta''$. However, the integrand in Eq. (12.42) is not an analytic function in a neighborhood of $\theta = \theta''$ because it tends to infinity as $\theta \to \theta''$. Let ε be an arbitrary small positive number compared to θ''; and let θ' be defined by

$$\theta' = \theta'' - \varepsilon \tag{12.44}$$

Then, we may write Eq. (12.42) in terms of two integrals

$$I = \int_0^{\theta'} \frac{Q(i_p,\, i_s;\, \theta)\cos\theta}{\sqrt{(\sin^2 i_s - \sin^2\theta)}}\, d\theta + \int_{\theta'}^{\theta''} \frac{Q(i_p,\, i_s;\, \theta)\cos\theta}{\sqrt{(\sin^2 i_s - \sin^2\theta)}}\, d\theta \tag{12.45}$$

Note that the first integral in Eq. (12.45) is free of singularities. To show that the second integral exists (by showing that it is bounded), we let Q_{max} denote the maximum value of Q in the interval $\theta' \le \theta \le \theta''$. Then we obtain

$$\int_{\theta'}^{\theta''} \frac{Q(i_p, i_s; \theta)\cos\theta}{\sqrt{(\sin^2 i_s - \sin^2\theta)}} d\theta < Q_{max} \int_{\theta'}^{\theta''} \frac{\cos\theta}{\sqrt{(\sin^2 i_s - \sin^2\theta)}} d\theta = Q_{max} \cos^{-1}\left(\frac{\sin\theta'}{\sin i_s}\right) \tag{12.46}$$

in which we have used Eq. (12.41) for θ''.

To evaluate this integral, we note that

$$Q(i_p, i_s; \theta) = Q(i_p, i_s; \theta_{ave}) + O(\varepsilon) \quad \text{for} \quad \theta' \le \theta \le \theta'' \tag{12.47}$$

where

$$\theta_{ave} = \frac{1}{2}(\theta' + \theta'') \tag{12.48}$$

It follows that

$$\int_{\theta'}^{\theta''} \frac{Q(i_p, i_s; \theta)\cos\theta}{\sqrt{(\sin^2 i_s - \sin^2\theta)}} d\theta = \left[Q(i_p, i_s; \theta_{ave}) + O(\varepsilon)\right]\cos^{-1}\left(\frac{\sin\theta'}{\sin i_s}\right) \tag{12.49}$$

From Eqs. (12.41) and (12.44), we obtain

$$\sin\theta' = \sin(\theta'' - \varepsilon) = \sin i_s \cos\varepsilon - |\cos i_s|\sin\varepsilon = \sin i_s - \varepsilon|\cos i_s| + O(\varepsilon^2) \tag{12.50}$$

or, equivalently,

$$\frac{\sin\theta'}{\sin i_s} = 1 - \varepsilon|\cot i_s| + O(\varepsilon^2) \tag{12.51}$$

Let γ be defined by

$$\cos\gamma = \frac{\sin\theta'}{\sin i_s} \tag{12.52}$$

Then, we also have

$$\cos\gamma = 1 - \frac{\gamma^2}{2} + O\left(\gamma^4\right) \tag{12.53}$$

From Eqs. (12.51) through (12.53), we obtain

$$\cos^{-1}\left(\frac{\sin\theta'}{\sin i_s}\right) = \sqrt{\left[2\varepsilon\left|\cot i_s\right|\right]} + O\left(\varepsilon^{3/2}\right) \tag{12.54}$$

Therefore, the integral Eq. (12.45) and hence (12.35) may be written as

$$I = \int_0^{\theta'} \frac{Q\left(i_p,\, i_s;\, \theta\right)\cos\theta}{\sqrt{\left(\sin^2 i_s - \sin^2\theta\right)}} d\theta + Q\left(i_p,\, i_s;\, \theta_{\text{ave}}\right)\cos^{-1}\left(\frac{\sin\theta'}{\sin i_s}\right) + O\left(\varepsilon^{3/2}\right) \tag{12.55}$$

12.5.1.2 Subcase of sin i_p < sin i_s

In this case, we have from Eq. (12.23)

$$\left.\begin{aligned} \theta'' &= i_p \quad \text{for} \quad i_p \le \pi/2 \\ \theta'' &= \left(\pi - i_p\right) \quad \text{for} \quad i_p \ge \pi/2 \end{aligned}\right\} \tag{12.56}$$

If we proceed as before, we obtain the integral Eq. (12.35) as

$$I = \int_0^{\theta'} \frac{Q\left(i_p,\, i_s;\, \theta\right)\cos\theta}{\sqrt{\left(\sin^2 i_p - \sin^2\theta\right)}} d\theta + Q\left(i_s,\, i_p;\, \theta_{\text{ave}}\right)\cos^{-1}\left(\frac{\sin\theta'}{\sin i_p}\right) + O\left(\varepsilon^{3/2}\right) \tag{12.57}$$

Note that in Eq. (12.57), the arguments i_p and i_s are in reverse order compared to that in Eq. (12.55). That is, we have

$$Q\left(i_s,\, i_p;\, \theta\right) = \frac{\left[\cos\left(\frac{\psi_p + \psi_s}{2}\right) + \sin\left|\frac{\psi_p - \psi_s}{2}\right|\right]}{\sqrt{\left(\sin^2 i_s - \sin^2\theta\right)}} \tag{12.58}$$

Note that the first integral in Eq. (12.55) or (12.57) may be evaluated numerically. The second integral has been reduced to an explicit term as shown and is accurate to order $\varepsilon^{3/2}$. From the analysis given here, we note that for the case of $\sin i_p \neq \sin i_s$, the integral Eq. (12.35) exists even though the integrand tends to infinity as $\theta \to \theta''$.

12.5.2 Case of $\sin i_1 = \sin i_2$

In this case, the integral Eq. (12.35) becomes

$$I = \int_0^{\theta''} \frac{\left[\cos\left(\frac{\psi_p + \psi_s}{2}\right) + \sin\left|\frac{\psi_p - \psi_s}{2}\right|\right]\cos\theta}{\left(\sin^2 i_p - \sin^2\theta\right)} d\theta \qquad (12.59)$$

It may be easily shown that this integral does not exist. A priori, we know that the approximation of uniform area density (where the normal to the area is in the direction of $\mathbf{V}_{\text{rel}}$) leading to Eq. (12.9) is no longer valid. This is because at latitude i_p, the primary satellite is moving in the same direction as the secondary satellites when $i_s = i_p$, or moving in the opposite direction when $i_s = \pi - i_p$. The density of the secondary satellites is infinite at latitude i_p. Thus, if we assume a uniform area density normal to $\mathbf{V}_{\text{rel}}$, we would have infinite density in some neighborhood containing $\theta = i_p$.

(Note that this situation does not arise in the case of $\sin i_p \neq \sin i_s$. The explanation is as follows: In the subcase of $\sin i_s < \sin i_p$, the secondary satellite density is infinite at latitude $\theta'' = i_p$ (or $\pi - i_s$), but the relative velocity $\mathbf{V}_{\text{rel}}$ is not parallel to that latitude. In the subcase where $\sin i_p < \sin i_s$, the secondary satellite density is finite at latitude $\theta'' = i_p$ (or $\pi - i_p$); however, the integrand in Eq. (12.35) is infinite because $\sin i_p - \sin\theta'' = 0$, which yields $\phi_p = \pi/2$ by Eq. (12.14) so that $d\theta/dt = 0$ by Eq. (12.16). This leads to a singularity in the integrand in Eq. (12.13) but not in the integrand in Eq. (12.12). That is, the singularity in Eq. (12.13) is nonessential and can be removed by a change of integration variable from latitude θ to time t.)

To analyze the present case of $\sin i_p = \sin i_s$, we have to consider a (small) finite latitude band from θ' to θ'' and obtain an average density $\rho(\theta', \theta'')$ in this band. This is in contrast to the previous formulation, which relied on a density $\rho(\theta)$ at a given latitude θ. Let us consider a toroidal ring bounded by latitudes θ' and θ'' where $0 \leq \theta' < \theta''$, and shells of radii R and $(R + h)$. It is shown in Appendix C (see Eq. [C.19]) that the average total density of both ascending and descending satellites in this toroidal ring is given by

$$\bar{\rho}_{\text{total}}\left(\theta', \theta''\right) = \frac{3n_{\text{total}} \cos^{-1}\left(\frac{\sin\theta'}{\sin i_s}\right)}{2\pi^2\left[\left(R+h\right)^3 - R^3\right]\left(\sin\theta'' - \sin\theta'\right)} \qquad (12.60)$$

To compute the total number of collisions from the equator to θ'', we analyze up to θ' as before using Eq. (12.13). But from latitudes θ' to θ'', we proceed in Subsection 12.5.2.1 as follows.

12.5.2.1 Subcase of Different Quadrants ($i_p < \pi/2$ and $i_s > \pi/2$ or vice versa)

In this case, the primary satellite encounters the secondary satellites essentially head-on with relative velocity

$$V_{\text{rel}} = 2V + O(\varepsilon) \tag{12.61}$$

Therefore, the number of oncoming satellites crossing an annulus (perpendicular to $\mathbf{V}_{\text{rel}}$) of radius r_e and thickness dr_e in unit time is given by

$$dN(\theta',\theta'') = 2\pi\, \mathrm{r_e}\, \bar{\rho}_{\text{total}}(\theta',\theta'') V_{\text{rel}}\, dr_e \tag{12.62}$$

which is the analog of Eq. (12.9). Proceeding as before, we find that therefore the number of collisions $N(\theta',\theta'')$ per unit time with oncoming satellites passing a circle radius of r_e'' is

$$\begin{aligned} N(\theta', \theta'') &= 2\pi\bar{\rho}_{\text{total}}(\theta',\theta'') V_{\text{rel}} \left[1 - e^{-\frac{1}{2}\left(\frac{r_A}{\sigma}\right)^2}\right] \int_0^{r_e''} r_e e^{-\frac{1}{2}\left(\frac{r_e}{\sigma}\right)^2} dr_e \\ &= 2\pi\bar{\rho}_{\text{total}}(\theta',\theta'') V_{\text{rel}} \left[1 - e^{-\frac{1}{2}\left(\frac{r_A}{\sigma}\right)^2}\right] \sigma^2 \left[1 - e^{-\frac{1}{2}\left(\frac{r_e''}{\sigma}\right)^2}\right] \end{aligned} \tag{12.63}$$

Let τ denote the time spent by the primary satellite in the toroidal ring from latitudes θ' to θ''. Let ϕ_p' and ϕ_p'' denote its argument of latitude corresponding to latitudes θ' and θ''. Because $\theta'' = i_p$, therefore $\phi_p'' = \pi/2$. The value of ϕ_p' is obtained from Eq. (12.14), which yields

$$\phi_p' = \sin^{-1}\left(\frac{\sin\theta'}{\sin i_p}\right) \tag{12.64}$$

Hence

$$\Delta\phi_p = \phi_p'' - \phi_p' = \frac{\pi}{2} - \sin^{-1}\left(\frac{\sin\theta'}{\sin i_p}\right) = \cos^{-1}\left(\frac{\sin\theta'}{\sin i_p}\right) \tag{12.65}$$

Because $d\phi_p/dt = 2\pi/T$, therefore

$$\tau = \frac{\Delta\phi_1}{\dot{\phi}_p} = \frac{T}{2\pi}\cos^{-1}\left(\frac{\sin\theta'}{\sin i_p}\right) \tag{12.66}$$

Therefore, the total number of collisions $N_{\text{total}}(\theta', \theta'')$ during the passage of the primary satellite through the toroidal ring from latitude θ' to θ'' is given by

$$N_{\text{total}}(\theta',\theta'') = N(\theta',\theta'')\tau \tag{12.67}$$

Substitution of Eqs. (12.60), (12.61), (12.63), and (12.66) into (12.67) yields (note that $\sin i_p = \sin i_s$)

$$N_{\text{total}}(\theta',\theta'') = J\left[1 - e^{-\frac{1}{2}\left(\frac{r_A}{\sigma}\right)^2}\right] \frac{3VT\sigma^2 n_{\text{total}}\left[\cos^{-1}\left(\frac{\sin\theta'}{\sin i_p}\right)\right]^2}{\pi^2\left[(R+h)^3 - R^3\right](\sin\theta'' - \sin\theta')} \tag{12.68}$$

where J is defined by Eq. (12.34). Furthermore, if we assume that h is small compared to R, then Eq. (12.68) becomes (note that $VT = 2\pi R$)

$$N_{\text{total}}(\theta',\theta'') = K\,J\frac{\left[\cos^{-1}\left(\frac{\sin\theta'}{\sin i_p}\right)\right]^2}{2(\sin\theta'' - \sin\theta')} \tag{12.69}$$

where K is defined by Eq. (12.38). In view of Eq. (12.54) (note that $\sin i_p = \sin i_s$), therefore

$$N_{\text{total}}(\theta',\theta'') = K\,J\left[\csc\, i_p + O(\varepsilon)\right] \tag{12.70}$$

Because $N_{\text{total}}(\theta',\theta'')$ denotes the total number of collisions experienced by the primary satellite passing from latitudes θ' to θ'', therefore from the foregoing analysis the total number of collisions $N_{\text{total,orbit}}$ over an orbit is still given by Eq. (12.32), but I is now given by

$$I = \int_0^{\theta'} \frac{Q(i_1,\, i_1;\, \theta)\cos\theta}{\sqrt{(\sin^2 i_1 - \sin^2\theta)}}\,d\theta + \csc\, i_1 + O(\varepsilon) \tag{12.71}$$

12.5.2.2 Subcase of Same Quadrant (i_p and $i_s < \pi/2$ or i_p and $i_s > \pi/2$)

In this case, the relative velocity is zero at latitude $\theta'' = i_p$. Moreover, for trailing collisions, the trailing velocity is zero at all latitudes because we have $i_p = i_s$. However, at latitude θ', the relative velocity for approaching collisions is given by Eq. (12.29). Hence, the average velocity for approaching collisions in the toroidal ring between latitudes θ' and θ'' is

$$V_{\text{rel},A} = V\left[\cos\left(\frac{\psi_p + \psi_s}{2}\right)\right]_{\theta=\theta'} \tag{12.72}$$

Because $i_p = i_s$, therefore $\psi_p = \psi_s$ by Eqs. (12.26) and (12.27). Hence,

$$V_{\text{rel},A} = V\cos\left[\sin^{-1}\left(\frac{\cos i_p}{\cos\theta'}\right)\right] = V\sin\left[\cos^{-1}\left(\frac{\cos i_p}{\cos\theta'}\right)\right] \tag{12.73}$$

Proceeding as before, with Eq. (12.73) replacing (12.61), we obtain

$$dN(\theta',\theta'') = 2\pi r_e \frac{1}{2}\bar{\rho}_{\text{total}}(\theta',\theta'')V_{\text{rel},A}dr_e \tag{12.74}$$

which is the analog of Eq. (12.62), and

$$N_{\text{total}}(\theta',\, \theta'') = KJ\frac{\left[\cos^{-1}\left(\dfrac{\sin\theta'}{\sin i_p}\right)\right]^2}{8(\sin\theta'' - \sin\theta')}\sin\left[\cos^{-1}\left(\frac{\cos i_p}{\cos\theta'}\right)\right] \tag{12.75}$$

which is the analog of Eq. (12.69). In a way similar to that used in deriving Eq. (12.54), we may easily show that

$$\cos^{-1}\left(\frac{\cos i_p}{\cos\theta'}\right) = \sqrt{[2\varepsilon\tan\theta']} + O(\varepsilon^{3/2}) \tag{12.76}$$

Then, substitution of Eqs. (12.54) and (12.76) into (12.75) yields

$$N_{\text{total}}(\theta',\theta'') = \mathrm{K\,J}\frac{1}{2}\sqrt{\left(\frac{\varepsilon}{\sin 2i_p}\right)} + 0(\varepsilon^{3/2}) \tag{12.77}$$

Because $N_{total}(\theta',\theta'')$ denotes the total number of collisions experienced by the primary satellite passing from latitudes θ' to θ'', therefore from the foregoing analysis, the total number of collisions $N_{total,orbit}$ over an orbit is still given by Eq. (12.32), but I is now given by

$$I = \int_0^{\theta'} \frac{Q\left(i_p,\, i_p;\, \theta\right)\cos\theta}{\sqrt{\left(\sin^2 i_p - \sin^2\theta\right)}} d\theta + \frac{1}{2}\sqrt{\left(\frac{\varepsilon}{\sin 2i_p}\right)} + O\left(\varepsilon^{3/2}\right) \qquad (12.78)$$

12.6 Numerical Results

The main results are given by Eq. (12.32) for the total number of collisions $N_{total,orbit}$ per orbit. The expression for K, given by Eq. (12.38), involves the number n_{total} of secondary objects of a particular class, the orbital radius R, the layer thickness h, the collision cross-sectional radius r_A, and the combined standard deviation σ of the isotropic Gaussian distribution. The expression for J, given by Eq. (12.34), involves σ and the maximum flux radius r_e'', which is bounded by h. The expression for I, given by Eq. (12.35) in general and by Eqs. (12.55), (12.57), (12.71), or (12.78) for specific cases, involves only the inclinations i_p of the primary spacecraft and i_s of the secondary objects. Furthermore, as indicated by Eq. (12.35), the integral I comprises two terms: the first term I_A for the approaching collisions and the second I_T for the trailing collisions. Thus, we may compute I for various combinations of i_p and i_s, independent of altitude, which appears only through R in Eq. (12.38) for K.

Using the foregoing equations, we obtain the results shown in Tables 12.1 and 12.2, which pertain to the Iridium constellation of satellites.

Table 12.1. Evaluation of Improper Integral *I* Defined by Eq. (12.35)[a]

Satellite Class	Inclination i_s (deg)	Approaching Collision Integral $I_A(0,\theta')+I_A(\theta',\theta'')=I_A$	Trailing Collision Integral $I_T(0,\theta')+I_T(\theta',\theta'')=I_T$	Total Integral $I_A + I_T = I$
1	33	1.094 + 0.287 = 1.381	0.665 + 0.244 = 0.909	2.290
2	53	1.437 + 0.283 = 1.720	0.612 + 0.223 = 0.834	2.554
3	63	1.680 + 0.309 = 1.989	0.562 + 0.230 = 0.791	2.780
4	74	2.080 + 0.169 = 2.249	0.461 + 0.022 = 0.483	2.731
5	81	2.506 + 0.503 = 3.009	0.317 + 0.251 = 0.568	3.577
6	90	3.113 + 0.841 = 3.954	0.356 + 0.406 = 0.762	4.716
7	98	2.696 + 0.691 = 3.387	0.697 + 0.502 = 1.199	4.586
8	106	2.156 + 0.446 = 2.603	0.696 + 0.338 = 1.034	3.637

[a] Remarks: (1) The upper limit of integration θ'' is defined by Eq. (12.23). Because i_p = 86.4 deg, therefore θ'' is given by the minimum of 86.4 and i_s (if i_s is acute) or the minimum of 86.4 and the supplement of i_s (if i_s is obtuse). (2) The value of θ' is chosen to be 2 deg less than θ'' (i.e., ε in Eq. (12.44) is equal to 2 deg (0.0349 rad)).

Table 12.2. Expected Number of Collisions Experienced by Primary Spacecraft Computed Using Eq. (12.32)[a]

Satellite Class	Inclination i_s (deg)	Number of Space Objects[b]	Value of K for Each Class	Number of Collisions per Orbit	Number of Collisions per Year
1	33	20	5.634×10^{-10}	1.290×10^{-9}	6.991×10^{-6}
2	53	30	8.451×10^{-10}	2.158×10^{-9}	11.695×10^{-6}
3	63	30	8.451×10^{-10}	2.349×10^{-9}	12.729×10^{-6}
4	74	150	42.255×10^{-10}	11.540×10^{-9}	62.526×10^{-6}
5	81	160	45.072×10^{-10}	16.122×10^{-9}	87.345×10^{-6}
6	90	10	2.817×10^{-10}	1.329×10^{-9}	7.198×10^{-6}
7	98	80	22.536×10^{-10}	10.335×10^{-9}	55.998×10^{-6}
8	106	10	2.817×10^{-10}	1.025×10^{-9}	5.551×10^{-6}
		490		46.148×10^{-9}	250.042×10^{-6}

[a]The orbital radius R = 6996.6 km, the layer thickness h = 323 km, and the collision cross-sectional radius r_A = 10 m are used in Eq. (12.39) for computing K.

[b]Data was current as of May 1996.

12.7 Discussion

Table 12.1 gives the values for I_A, I_T, and I for $i_p = 86.4$ deg and $i_s = 33, 53, 63, 74, 81, 90, 98$, and 106 deg. In turn, the integrals I_A and I_T are each decomposed into two terms as indicated in Eqs. (12.55) and (12.57). The first term corresponds to integration from 0 to $(\theta'' - \varepsilon)$, the second from $(\theta'' - \varepsilon)$ to θ''. The value of ε is chosen to be 2 deg, which is 0.0349 rad. The general expression for J is given by Eq. (12.34) and is shown by Eq. (12.40) to be very close to unity when $r_e'' > 4\sigma$. This inequality is certainly satisfied for reasonable values of σ and the values of h because we can take r_e up to be $h/2$. It is safe to take σ up to be 5 km; for this, we need to choose h to be at least 40 km. In column 3 of Table 12.1, note that the contribution of the last 2 deg to the value of the approaching-collision integral I_A is substantially larger in proportion to the rest of the contribution. The same statement holds for the trailing-collision integral I_T shown in column 4. For most of these cases, this contribution is approximately 25%. However, for satellite class 6, column 4 shows that this contribution even exceeds the remaining part. This larger contribution means that there is a greater probability of collision near the inclination latitude.

Table 12.2 shows the inclination and total number of secondary objects having perigee and/or apogee between 457 and 780 km altitude. Thus, we have R = (6378.1 + 618.5) = 6996.6 km and h = 323 km. The collision cross-sectional radius r_A is taken to be (5 + 5) = 10 m. These values are used to compute K, via Eq. (12.39), for each class of objects. Together with the values of I in Table 12.1 and the assumption $J = 1$, Eq. (12.32) is used to compute the number of collisions per orbit and per year for each of the eight classes. We conclude that the total number of collisions per year experienced by the primary spacecraft is approximately 2×10^{-4}.

This result is in agreement with those obtained using time-consuming Monte Carlo simulations. If the input parameters are changed, these simulations have to be repeated. On the other hand, by using Eqs. (12.34), (12.35), and (12.38), we need only recompute some or all of the three terms I, J, and K as necessary. Moreover, we can also observe the dependence of the input parameters analytically.

12.8 Conclusion

For collisions of the primary spacecraft with all the secondary objects of a given class, computations reveal that the predominant contribution to the collision integral comes from encounters near the inclination latitude. (The inclination latitude is defined to be the highest or the lowest latitude reached during an orbit.) An example is worked out for the case of a primary spacecraft orbit with a semimajor axis of 7000 km and an inclination of 86.4 deg encountering presently orbiting objects within ±160 km and belonging to the inclination classes of 33, 53, 63, 74, 81, 90, 98, and 106 deg. The number of collisions per year is found to be approximately 2×10^{-4}. This result is in agreement with those obtained using time-consuming Monte Carlo simulations.

12.9 Summary

In this chapter, we formulated the collision probability between a primary spacecraft encountering a host of secondary orbiting objects over an extended period of time. These secondary objects are assumed to have circular orbits and can be grouped into classes, each class being characterized by the orbital inclination and the altitude.

In Section 12.1, we approximated the bivariate Gaussian pdf by an isotropic pdf because the angular direction with respect to the principal axes is not known. The problem is again reduced to that involving the Rician integral.

In Section 12.2, we introduced the concept of number density in dealing with the orbiting objects of any given class.

In Section 12.3, we formulated the equation giving the number of collisions per orbit for each class of secondary objects in terms of its equatorial density, inclination, orbital period, relative velocity, and other collision parameters.

In Section 12.4, we considered the geometry of the encounters in terms of the inclinations of the primary and secondary objects and the latitude of the encounter. We also categorized the collisions into approaching and trailing.

In Section 12.5, we continued discussion on the number of collisions per orbit and separated the contributions of orbital geometric factors from nongeometric parameters.

In Section 12.6, we presented tabular results of the collision probabilities of the Iridium space vehicles with eight classes of secondary objects within 161.5 km altitude.

In Section 12.7, we pointed out the two contributions to the approaching and trailing collision integrals. The second contribution covers only the last two degrees of the latitude and is substantially larger (25% or more) in proportion to the first contribution, which covers the rest of the range.

In Section 12.8, we reaffirmed the predominant contribution to the collision integral from encounters near the inclination latitude. We also noted the agreement of the results with those obtained using Monte Carlo simulations.

12.10 Reference

[12.1] F. K. Chan, "Close Encounters with Multiple Satellites," *AAS/AIAA Space Flight Mechanics Meeting* (San Antonio, TX, 27–30 January 2002).

Chapter 13: Instantaneous Probability of Collision

In Chapters 2 through 12, we considered whether the probability of collision between two orbiting objects over a time interval is a case of short-term or long-term encounter. The probability integral was evaluated over a volume of the random variable space correspondingly swept out by the motion of a sphere of combined radius $r_A = (r_p + r_s)$ in the physical three-dimensional space. (See Chapters 3 and 8.) In the case of short-term encounters, the volume of integration was an infinitely long, circular cylinder. In the case of long-term encounters, the volume was more complicated, being contained in the enveloping surface traced out by a time-varying ellipsoid. We used a torus and an elliptical doughnut as simple illustrative examples.

In certain other applications, we may be required to determine the probability of collision at a specific instant of time. In this case, the volume of integration is a sphere of radius R, which may be the combined radius r_A or some other parameter, such as an effective event radius r_E. This event may be the explosion of an orbiting object producing many fragments. Inside a sphere of radius r_E, an object can be considered as being struck by the exploding fragments within a very short time interval containing the instant of explosion. Three approaches come to mind to compute this instantaneous probability. Obviously, the first is the brute-force method of evaluating a three-dimensional integral of a Gaussian pdf over a sphere. The second, based on considerations that will be addressed separately in the discussion of spherical error probability computation in Chapter 14, is the direct problem, which uses approximating probability density distributions. The third is the method of equivalent areas in Chapter 5, generalized to three dimensions so that we have the method of equivalent volume.

13.1 Method of Approximating Distributions

The present discussion on instantaneous probability of collision does not assume a detailed knowledge of the direct problem. In Chapter 14, which elaborates that concept, the problem is to evaluate the integral of dimension three (or higher) within a sphere displaced from the center of a Gaussian pdf. The methodology is to convert that integral to a cumulative noncentral chi-square distribution. In turn, the problem is "converted" to the evaluation of a cumulative central chi-square distribution. Finally, this is "converted" to the evaluation of a cumulative Gaussian distribution of one variable.

The reader will find more details within Chapter 14; however, the main results are summarized in this discussion. (*Note*: For the reader who wishes to associate the present discussion with the computations in that chapter, the following text references equation numbers from Chapter 14.)

In Eqs. (14.13) through (14.15) of Chapter 14, the mean, variance, and third moment of the noncentral chi-square distribution ψ^2 will be shown to be given by:

$$m \equiv \mu = \sum_{j=1}^{3}\left[\sigma_j^2 + b_j^2\right] \tag{13.1}$$

$$v \equiv \mu_2 = 2\sum_{j=1}^{3}\left[\sigma_j^4 + 2\sigma_j^2 b_j^2\right] \tag{13.2}$$

$$\mu_3 = 8\sum_{j=1}^{3}\left[\sigma_j^6 + 3\sigma_j^4 b_j^2\right] \tag{13.3}$$

where the biases b_j are now associated with the center of the sphere of radius R at the instant of interest. Eq. (14.39) yields the degree n' of the desired central chi-square distribution χ^2:

$$n' = \frac{8v^3}{\mu_3^2} \tag{13.4}$$

When $\psi^2 = R^2$, let $\chi^2 = X^2$. Eq. (14.25) yields

$$X^2 = n' + \sqrt{\frac{2n'}{v}}\left(R^2 - m\right) \tag{13.5}$$

When $\chi^2 = X^2$, let $t = T$ where t denotes the normal variable in the Gaussian pdf $N(0,1)$. Eq. (14.41) yields

$$T = \left[\sqrt[3]{\frac{X^2}{n'}} - \left(1 - \frac{2}{9n'}\right)\right] \Big/ \sqrt{\frac{2}{9n'}} \tag{13.6}$$

From Eq. (14.46), we obtain the instantaneous probability of collision

$$P = \frac{1}{2}\left[1 + erf\left(\frac{T}{\sqrt{2}}\right)\right] \tag{13.7}$$

where $erf(x)$ denotes the error function. It is imperative that a very good algorithm be available for evaluating this function with an accuracy of at least five significant figures, that is, 0.001% relative error.

The error function *erf*(*x*) is defined by either one of the following two equivalent forms:

$$erf(x) \equiv \frac{2}{\sqrt{\pi}} \int_0^x e^{-\tau^2} d\tau \qquad (13.8)$$

$$erf(x) \equiv \sqrt{\frac{2}{\pi}} \int_0^{\sqrt{2}x} e^{-t^2/2} dt \qquad (13.9)$$

This is the definition given in standard references,[13.1-13.4] and it is currently used by most authors. (Laplace[13.5] used the definition in Eq.(13.8), but with 1 as the coefficient before the integral. Other authors—Papoulis,[13.6] for example—used the definition in Eq. (13.9) but with the coefficient $1/\sqrt{2\pi}$ before the integral and x as the upper limit of integration. It is not crucial which definition is used, but extreme caution must be exercised to ensure that consistency is maintained.) An important point about the definitions in Eqs. (13.8) and (13.9) is that the error function does not give exactly the area under the normalized Gaussian pdf $N(0, 1)$ between $-x$ and $+x$. This is because the probability that the normal variable x lies in this range is given by

$$P\{-x \le \xi \le +x\} = \frac{1}{\sqrt{2\pi}} \int_{-x}^{+x} e^{-\xi^2/2} d\xi \qquad (13.10)$$

whereas, by Eq. (13.9), we have

$$erf\left(\frac{x}{\sqrt{2}}\right) = \sqrt{\frac{2}{\pi}} \int_0^x e^{-t^2/2} dt = \frac{2}{\sqrt{2\pi}} \int_0^x e^{-t^2/2} dt = \frac{1}{\sqrt{2\pi}} \int_{-x}^x e^{-t^2/2} dt \qquad (13.11)$$

Therefore, it is worth remembering that the relation between the two is

$$P\{-x \le \xi \le +x\} = erf\left(\frac{x}{\sqrt{2}}\right) \qquad (13.12)$$

so that

$$P\{-\sqrt{2}x \le \xi \le +\sqrt{2}x\} = erf(x) \qquad (13.13)$$

The discussion by Margenau and Murphy[13.1] on random errors gives a physical explanation of the mathematical rationale of the definitions in Eqs. (13.8) and (13.9).

By expanding the integrand in a power series and integrating termwise, we can show that the error function in (13.8) or (13.9) can be represented by the following convergent infinite series:[13.3]

$$erf(x) = \frac{2}{\sqrt{\pi}} \sum_{n=0}^{\infty} \frac{(-1)^n x^{2n+1}}{n!(2n+1)} = \frac{2}{\sqrt{\pi}} \sum_{n=0}^{\infty} t_n \tag{13.14}$$

We may compute it efficiently using the recursive relation

$$t_0 = x; \quad t_{n+1} = -t_n \frac{x^2(2n+1)}{(n+1)(2n+3)} \quad for \quad n = 0,1,2,\cdots \tag{13.15}$$

The series in Eq. (13.14) converges rapidly for small values of the argument x. Moreover, the successive partial sums of this series lie on alternate sides of the function and thus provide upper and lower bounds. However, for large values of the argument, the series converges slowly and the bounds are not very helpful. As an alternative, we turn to the complementary function *erfc*(x) defined by the equation

$$erfc(x) \equiv 1 - erf(x) = \sqrt{\frac{2}{\pi}} \int_{\sqrt{2}x}^{\infty} e^{-t^2/2} dt \tag{13.16}$$

By performing repeated integration by parts, we observe that this complementary error function has the following asymptotic expansion as x tends to infinity:[13.3]

$$erfc(x) \sim \frac{e^{-x^2}}{\sqrt{\pi}x} \left[1 + \sum_{n=1}^{\infty} (-1)^n \frac{1 \cdot 3 \cdot 5 \cdots (2n-1)}{\left(2x^2\right)^n} \right] \tag{13.17}$$

We can show that this series does not converge. However, if we take only the first term, we can obtain a very good approximation. That is, for large values of x, we have

$$erf(x) \simeq 1 - \frac{e^{-x^2}}{\sqrt{\pi}x} \tag{13.18}$$

By numerical evaluation, we find that the expressions on the right-hand side of Eqs. (13.14) and (13.18) are approximately equal when $x = 4$. Thus, when $x \leq 4$, we use Eq. (13.14) and when $x > 4$, we use Eq. (13.18). At the transition point $x =$ 4.000357371, the values obtained from both expressions agree to ten significant figures, being that *erf*(x) = 0.99999999844.

When $x \cong 6$, $erf(x)$ differs from unity in the 17th decimal place. This corresponds to the limit of accuracy of a computer using double-precision arithmetic. Thus, we need not exceed $x \cong 8.5$ in Eq. (13.13) when evaluating a one-dimensional integral of the normalized Gaussian pdf $N(0,1)$. Any contribution to the integral beyond this integration limit will not appear in the displayed numerical results of the integral. This is the rationale for the discussion in Section 3.2 of Chapter 3.

13.2 Method of Equivalent Volume

This analysis follows the formulation discussed in Chapter 5. There, we considered the integration of a two-dimensional pdf over a circle displaced from the center of the two-dimensional bivariate Gaussian pdf. We introduced a transformation so that the Gaussian pdf assumed an isotropic form. In this process, we automatically changed the region of integration into an ellipse. To apply our knowledge of the Rician integral, we transformed this ellipse into a circle of equal area with the same centroid. The accuracy of this approximation was generally in the third significant figure for a wide range of collision parameters such as the two standard deviations σ_x and σ_z, the radius of the collision cross-section r_A, and the miss distance x_e.

In the present case, we must integrate a three-dimensional pdf over a sphere displaced from the center of a three-dimensional Gaussian pdf. Again, we can introduce a transformation so that the Gaussian pdf assumes an isotropic form. In this process, we automatically change the region of integration into a general triaxial ellipsoid, that is, an ellipsoid with three unequal axes. The most obvious generalization is that we transform this ellipsoid into a sphere of equal volume with the same centroid. We can certainly do this, but it is not advisable, for this approach will not yield a good approximation as shown in Appendix D. Rather, it is much better to transform this triaxial ellipsoid into an ellipsoid with axial symmetry having the same volume.

In the (x, y, z) coordinate system, let the combined covariance C describing the relative position uncertainties be defined by

$$C = \begin{bmatrix} \sigma_x^2 & \rho_{xy}\sigma_x\sigma_y & \rho_{xz}\sigma_x\sigma_z \\ \rho_{xy}\sigma_x\sigma_y & \sigma_y^2 & \rho_{yz}\sigma_y\sigma_z \\ \rho_{xz}\sigma_x\sigma_z & \rho_{yz}\sigma_y\sigma_z & \sigma_z^2 \end{bmatrix} \qquad (13.19)$$

As in Chapter 5, we shall take the origin to be at the secondary object; hence, the instantaneous probability of collision at time t is given by

$$P = \iiint_V \frac{1}{\sqrt{(2\pi)^3 |C|}} e^{-\frac{1}{2}\mathbf{r}^T C^{-1}\mathbf{r}} \, dx \, dy \, dz \qquad (13.20)$$

where V is a sphere of radius R centered at the primary object whose coordinates are $\mathbf{r}_p \equiv (x_p, y_p, z_p)$. Let A denote the circle obtained by the intersection of the sphere V and a plane, with $y =$ constant, where $(y_p - R) \le y \le (y_p + R)$. Let us rotate the (x, y, z) axes to principal axes (x', y', z'). Let T denote the transformation matrix that accomplishes this. Then, the covariance in the principal system is

$$C' = T^T C T = \begin{bmatrix} \sigma_{x'}^{\ 2} & 0 & 0 \\ 0 & \sigma_{y'}^{\ 2} & 0 \\ 0 & 0 & \sigma_{z'}^{\ 2} \end{bmatrix} \tag{13.21}$$

In general, the covariance ellipsoid given by Eq. (13.21) is triaxial. For the best computational results to be presented later, we choose the y'-axis to be in the direction of the smallest or largest standard deviation so that the cross section of the covariance ellipsoid will have the least aspect ratio. For simplicity, we choose $\sigma_{x'} \ge \sigma_{z'}$. Then, the collision probability in Eq. (13.20) becomes

$$P = \frac{1}{(2\pi)^{3/2}\sigma_{x'}\sigma_{y'}\sigma_{z'}} \iiint_{V'} e^{-\frac{1}{2}\mathbf{r}'^T (C')^{-1}\mathbf{r}'} dx'\, dy'\, dz' \tag{13.22}$$

where V' is a sphere of radius R' centered at the primary object. Let $\mathbf{r}_p' \equiv (x_p', y_p', z_p')$ denote the coordinates of the center of mass of the primary in the (x', y', z') system. Let A' denote the circle obtained by the intersection of the sphere V' and a plane, with $y' =$ constant, where $(y_p' - R) \le y' \le (y_p' + R)$ and $y' = y$. Let r_A' denote the radius of this circle A'. Therefore, we have

$$V' = V, \qquad A' = A, \qquad R' = R, \qquad R^2 = r_{A'}^{\ 2} + (y' - y_p')^2, \qquad \mathbf{r}_p' = T\mathbf{r}_p \tag{13.23}$$

In Eq. (13.23), we mean that V maps into V' having the same volume, but that the areas of A and A' are equal even though the circle A does not necessarily map into the circle A' unless the y-axis is already the principal y'-axis. We next wish to map the triaxial covariance ellipsoids of constant pdf,

$$\frac{x'^2}{\sigma_{x'}^2} + \frac{z'^2}{\sigma_{z'}^2} + \frac{y'^2}{\sigma_{y'}^2} = k^2 \tag{13.24}$$

into axially symmetrical ellipsoids of constant pdf having the equation

$$\frac{x''^2}{\sigma_{z'}^{\ 2}} + \frac{z''^2}{\sigma_{z'}^{\ 2}} + \frac{y''^2}{\sigma_{y'}^{\ 2}} = k^2 \tag{13.25}$$

Note that Eq. (13.25) has symmetry about the y'-axis so that the second set of ellipsoids has circular cross-sectional areas. The constant k in Eqs. (13.24) and (13.25) is a label for the corresponding ellipsoids in the two sets. This mapping is accomplished by the following transformation:

$$x'' = \frac{\sigma_{z'}}{\sigma_{x'}} x', \qquad z'' = z', \qquad y'' = y' \tag{13.26}$$

In the (x'', y'', z'') system, the collision probability (13.22) is

$$P = \frac{1}{\sqrt{2\pi}\sigma_{y'}} \int_{y_p''-R}^{y_p''+R} e^{-y''^2/2\sigma_{y''}^2} \left[\frac{1}{2\pi\,\sigma_{z'}^2} \iint_{A''} e^{-\left(x''^2 + z''^2\right)/2\sigma_{z'}^2}\, dx''\, dz'' \right] dy'' \tag{13.27}$$

where $\mathbf{r}_p'' \equiv (x_p'', y_p'', z_p'')$ denotes the coordinates of the center of mass of the primary in the (x'', y'', z'') system. Let A'' denote the ellipse obtained from the circle A' as a result of the transformation in Eq. (13.26). That is, A'' is the ellipse obtained by the intersection of the ellipsoid V'' and a plane, with y'' = constant, where $(y_p'' - R) \le y'' \le (y_p'' + R)$ and $y'' = y'$. It is an ellipse with semimajor axis α and semiminor axis β respectively defined to be along the z'' and x'' axes. Let V'' denote the ellipsoid derived from V' by using Eq. (13.26). Therefore, we have

$$V'' = \frac{\sigma_{z'}}{\sigma_{x'}} V', \quad A'' = \frac{\sigma_{z'}}{\sigma_{x'}} A', \quad \alpha = r_{A'}, \quad \beta = \frac{\sigma_{z'}}{\sigma_{x'}} r_{A'}, \quad x_p'' = \frac{\sigma_{z'}}{\sigma_{x'}} x_p', \quad z_p'' = z_p', \quad y_p'' = y_p' \tag{13.28}$$

In Eq.(13.28), we mean that V' maps into V'' having the same volume and that A' maps into A'' having the same area.

Up to this step, we have not made any approximations. Suppose we now approximate the elliptical cross section A'' with a circular cross section A''' of the same area with radius r_A'''. That is, the ellipsoid V'' is transformed into another ellipsoid V''' of equal volume and the same centroid, and that V''' has symmetry about the y''-axis. For convenience, let us use d to denote the perpendicular distance of the primary from the y''-axis. Then, we have

$$V''' = V'', \qquad A''' = A'', \qquad r_{A'''} = \sqrt{\alpha\beta} = \sqrt{\frac{\sigma_{z'}}{\sigma_{x'}}} r_{A'}, \qquad d^2 = x_p''^2 + z_p''^2 \tag{13.29}$$

In Eq. (13.29), we mean that V'' maps into V''' having the same volume and that A'' maps into A''' having the same area. Thus, the collision probability (13.27) is approximated by

$$P = \frac{1}{\sqrt{2\pi}\sigma_{y'}} \int_{y_p''-R}^{y_p''+R} e^{-y''^2/2\sigma_{y'}^2} \left[\frac{1}{2\pi\,\sigma_{z'}^2} \iint_{A'''} e^{-\left(x''^2+z''^2\right)/2\sigma_{z'}^2} dx''\, dz'' \right] dy'' \tag{13.30}$$

We note that the double integral I defined by

$$I \equiv \frac{1}{2\pi\sigma_{z'}^2} \iint_{A'''} e^{-(x''^2+z''^2)/2\sigma_{z'}^2} dx''\, dz'' \tag{13.31}$$

represents the integral of a two-dimensional isotropic Gaussian pdf over a circle with center at the point (x_p'', z_p'') in the (x'', z'')-plane. It is identical to Eq. (5.17) in Chapter 5 and may be expressed in the form of the convergent infinite series seen in Eq. (5.21):

$$I = e^{-v/2} \sum_{m=0}^{\infty} \frac{v^m}{2^m m!} \left[1 - e^{-u/2} \sum_{k=0}^{m} \frac{u^k}{2^k k!} \right] \tag{13.32}$$

As discussed in Chapter 5, we truncate after the first ten terms ($m = 10$) in this infinite series for our computational purposes. In this sense, in computing the integral I, we essentially perform three exponential evaluations. By using Eqs. (13.23), (13.26), (13.28), and (13.29), we may express the two dimensionless parameters u and v—see Eqs. (5.22) and (5.23)—as

$$u \equiv \left(\frac{r_{A'''}}{\sigma_{z'}} \right)^2 = \left(\frac{r_{A'}^{\;2}}{\sigma_{x'}\sigma_{z'}} \right) = \left(\frac{R^2 - (y'' - y_p'')^2}{\sigma_{x'}\sigma_{z'}} \right) > 0 \tag{13.33}$$

$$v \equiv \left(\frac{d}{\sigma_{z'}} \right)^2 = \frac{x_p'^{\,2}}{\sigma_{x'}^2} + \frac{z_p'^{\,2}}{\sigma_{z'}^2} > 0 \tag{13.34}$$

Equations (13.32) through (13.34) are substituted into (13.30), and the integration with respect to y'' is performed numerically. Thus, we have what can be referred to as a "semianalytical" formulation of the collision probability.

13.3 Comparison of the Two Approaches

We have presented two approaches to obtain the probability integral of a three-dimensional Gaussian pdf within a sphere displaced from the center of the pdf. The first approach of approximating distributions is based on concepts from Chapter 14 that transform the volume integral into the noncentral chi-square cumulative distribution. In turn, by appropriately matching moments, we transformed this into the central chi-square cumulative distribution. Finally, by appropriately matching moments again, we transformed it into the Gaussian cumulative distribution. The second approach judiciously invoked the Rician pdf and the conversion of an ellipsoid to an axially symmetrical ellipsoid of equivalent volume. In the first approach, the end result was an analytical expression of the probability integral. In the second approach, the end result was a semianalytical formulation of the collision integral that required numerical integration in one variable. The general philosophy of these approaches is a far cry from the brute-force method of performing numerical evaluation of a three-dimensional integral wherein one has no feel for the qualitative nature of the answer.

From the discussions in Sections 13.2, it was of paramount importance to compute the error function accurately (to at least five significant figures) over a large portion of the entire range of the argument from 0 to ∞. We developed an algorithm that achieves this objective with ample room to spare. It remains now to examine the accuracy of the fitting process of the distributions in the first case and of the conversion to equivalent volume in the second case. These two processes respectively determine the usefulness of the two methods.

In Section 14.2 of Chapter 14, the noncentral chi-square distribution is fitted to the central chi-square distribution by appropriately matching the first three moments of the two distributions to ensure consistency so that we have n' for the mean, $2n'$ for the variance and $8n'$ for the third moment about the mean. (This is not to say that we equate respectively the two sets of moments, one from the central chi-square distribution and the other from the noncentral chi-square distribution.) Matching the first three moments was performed by Pearson[13.7] because he was interested in the upper and lower tail end 5% of the cumulative distribution for hypothesis testing and goodness of fit. The central chi-square distribution was then fitted to a Gaussian distribution using the Wilson-Hilferty[13.8] transformation by appropriately matching the first two moments of the two distributions. We note that the chi-square pdf is defined from 0 to ∞ whereas the Gaussian pdf is defined from $-\infty$ to $+\infty$. Because of this, we expect the method of approximating distributions (AD) to yield good results at the upper tail end, but not at the lower. Even for the two-dimensional case of circular error probability, the results have relative errors of approximately 2% when the probability of containment is 0.5 and above, and approximately 50% when the probability of containment is 0.1. (See Table 14.3 in Chapter 14.)

On the other hand, in the method of equivalent volume (EV), we noted that we expect to have at least two or three significant figures of accuracy over a wide range of parameters as evidenced in the numerical results of Chapters 4 and 5.

13.4 Numerical Results

The brute-force (BF) method of evaluating a three-dimensional integral of a Gaussian pdf over a sphere is based on the generalization of Eq. (5.30) in Chapter 5.

There, we evaluated a two-dimensional integral over a circle using r and θ as the integration variables. We now augment this by integrating along the y''-axis. (For sufficient fidelity, a three-dimensional integral needs approximately 1000 steps in each of the Cartesian variables (x, y, z).) Thus, we will retain the angle step size in Chapter 5 to be 0.5 deg so that we have 720 steps. However, we increase the radial step size to $R/120$. In essence, this means that we divide the diameter into 240 steps. For the y'' integration, we will choose 200 steps. Thus, we have $720 \times 120 \times 200 = 1.728 \times 10^7$ integration steps. Numerical testing reveals that we achieve approximately five or six significant figures of accuracy with this choice. This makes it sufficiently accurate to be used as a standard for comparison for the general case of a sphere offset from the center of a three-dimensional Gaussian pdf. Because there are two trigonometric evaluations (evals) and one exponential eval in the inner (r, θ) loop and one exponential eval in the outer y'' loop, there are approximately 5.18×10^7 evals in the integration.

For computing the instantaneous collision probability using the AD method, we conclude from Eqs. (13.5) through (13.7) that there are two square root evals and one error function eval, thus only three evals altogether. For the EV method, we conclude from Eqs. (13.30) and (13.32) that there are essentially three exponential evals in the Rician integral and one exponential eval in the y'' integration. To be consistent with the BF method, we will choose 200 steps in the y″ integration. Thus, there are a total of $200 \times 4 = 800$ evals in the integration. Based on the number of function evals, which is an indication of computing time, the BF method takes approximately 1.7×10^7 times longer than the AD method and approximately 65,000 times longer than the EV method. On a computer with a Pentium 4 processor with 1.9 GHz processing speed, BF takes approximately 2.5 min or 150 sec. In comparison, AD takes an estimated 9 μsec and EV takes 2 msec.

For the special case of a sphere concentric with a three-dimensional isotropic Gaussian pdf, we have the following exact solution:

$$P = P\left\{r^2 \le R^2\right\} = erf\left(\frac{R}{\sqrt{2}\sigma}\right) - \sqrt{\frac{2}{\pi}}\frac{R}{\sigma}e^{-R^2/2\sigma^2} \tag{13.35}$$

Table 13.1 shows the accuracies of the AD and EV results compared to the exact solution. The standard deviation σ is set equal to unity and the radius R of the spherical volume of integration is varied from 10 to 0.0001 so as to enable us to study the transition from large to small collision probabilities. For collision probabilities larger than 0.2, from the first three cases, it is seen that AD yields answers with less than 1% error. However, for collision probabilities smaller than 0.03 in the remaining eight cases, the answers deviate noticeably from the exact solution, and the errors become excessively large, being 10^9 times larger than the true values when $R = 0.0001\sigma$. Thus, this approach completely fails if we need to compute small collision probabilities. This observation does not come as a surprise and has

Table 13.1. Comparison of AD and EV with Exact Solution for Concentric Isotropic Gaussian pdf

Case	Radius of Sphere	Probability (Exact)	Probability (Approx. Distributions)	Percent Error for Approx. Distributions	Probability (Equivalent Volume)	Percent Error for Equivalent Volume
1	10	1.00×10^{00}	1.00×10^{00}	0	1.00×10^{00}	0
2	5	1.00×10^{00}	1.00×10^{00}	0	1.00×10^{00}	0
3	1	1.99×10^{-01}	1.96×10^{-01}	–1	1.99×10^{-01}	0
4	0.5	3.09×10^{-02}	3.62×10^{-02}	17	3.09×10^{-02}	0
5	0.1	2.65×10^{-04}	2.16×10^{-03}	716	2.65×10^{-04}	0
6	0.05	3.32×10^{-05}	1.12×10^{-03}	3273	3.32×10^{-05}	0
7	0.01	2.66×10^{-07}	5.12×10^{-04}	1.92×10^{5}	2.66×10^{-07}	0
8	0.005	3.32×10^{-08}	4.38×10^{-04}	1.32×10^{6}	3.32×10^{-08}	0
9	0.001	2.66×10^{-10}	3.67×10^{-04}	1.38×10^{8}	2.66×10^{-10}	0
10	0.0005	3.32×10^{-11}	3.55×10^{-04}	1.07×10^{9}	3.32×10^{-11}	0
11	0.0001	2.66×10^{-13}	3.41×10^{-04}	1.28×10^{11}	2.66×10^{-13}	0

already been expected from the discussion in Section 13.3. In contrast, the EV approach yields practically the same values as the exact answers with at least three significant figures of agreement for all 11 cases shown. That is, it can be used successfully to compute small collision probabilities.

Table 13.2 shows the accuracies of the AD results compared with the high-precision solution for the case of the sphere offset from an isotropic Gaussian pdf. The standard deviation σ is set equal to unity and the radius R of the spherical

Table 13.2. Comparison of AD with Numerical Solution for Displaced Isotropic Gaussian pdf

Case	$\sigma_x, \sigma_y, \sigma_z$	Displacement x_0, y_0, z_0 of Sphere	Radius of Sphere	Probability (Numerical Integration)	Probability (Approx. Distributions)	Percent Error for Approx. Distributions
1	1,1,1	0.5,0,0	0.5	2.74×10^{-02}	3.38×10^{-02}	23.46
2	1,1,1	1,0,0	0.5	1.92×10^{-02}	3.11×10^{-02}	62.03
3	1,1,1	0.5,0,0	1	1.80×10^{-01}	1.78×10^{-01}	–1.00
4	1,1,1	1,0,0	1	1.32×10^{-01}	1.33×10^{-01}	0.28
5	1,1,1	1,0,0	2	6.02×10^{-01}	6.00×10^{-01}	–0.43
6	1,1,1	2,0,0	1	3.85×10^{-02}	4.56×10^{-02}	18.42
7	1,1,1	2,0,0	2	3.01×10^{-01}	2.92×10^{-01}	–2.80
8	1,1,1	5,0,0	1	4.91×10^{-06}	7.67×10^{-05}	1464.16
9	1,1,1	10,0,0	1	1.01×10^{-20}	4.91×10^{-14}	4.87×10^{8}

volume of integration is varied from 0.5 to 2 to enable us to study the transition from large to small collision probabilities. The displacement of the center of the sphere is varied from 0.5 to 10 to investigate the effects of large offsets. For collision probabilities larger than 0.1, from the third, fourth, fifth, and seventh cases, AD yields answers with less than 3% error. However, for collision probabilities smaller than 0.04 in the other cases, the answers deviate noticeably from the numerical solution, and the errors become excessively large and are 5×10^6 times larger than the true values when the offset $x_0 = 10\sigma$. This reinforces the evidence that this approach fails miserably if we need to compute small collision probabilities.

Table 13.3 shows the accuracies of the EV results compared to the same high-precision solution under the same conditions. In contrast to the AD formulation, the EV approach yields practically the same values as the numerical answers with at least three significant figures of agreement for all nine cases shown, having discrepancies of less than 0.02% error. Again, this approach can be used for computing small collision probabilities.

Table 13.4 shows the accuracies of the AD results compared with the high-precision solution for the case of the sphere with offset from a general Gaussian pdf. The standard deviation $\sigma_{y'}$ is set equal to 1 or 10; $\sigma_{x'}$ and $\sigma_{z'}$ are set equal to 3 and 2 respectively to yield the smallest aspect ratio, as discussed in Section 13.2. The radius R of the spherical volume of integration is varied from 1 to 10 so as to include large integration volumes. The displacement of the center of the sphere is varied from 1 to 10 to study the effects of large offsets of the sphere from the center of the Gaussian pdf. For collision probabilities larger than 0.6 because the volume of integration is large, as in the third and seventh cases, AD yields answers with less than 0.6% error. However, for collision probabilities smaller than 0.04,

Table 13.3. Comparison of EV with Numerical Solution for Displaced Isotropic Gaussian pdf

Case	$\sigma_x, \sigma_y, \sigma_z$	Displacement x_0, y_0, z_0 of Sphere	Radius of Sphere	Probability (Numerical Integration)	Probability (Equivalent Volume)	Percent Error for Equivalent Volume
1	1,1,1	0.5,0,0	0.5	2.74×10^{-02}	2.74×10^{-02}	0.00
2	1,1,1	1,0,0	0.5	1.92×10^{-02}	1.92×10^{-02}	–0.02
3	1,1,1	0.5,0,0	1	1.80×10^{-01}	1.80×10^{-01}	–0.02
4	1,1,1	1,0,0	1	1.32×10^{-01}	1.32×10^{-01}	–0.30
5	1,1,1	1,0,0	2	6.02×10^{-01}	6.01×10^{-01}	–0.20
6	1,1,1	2,0,0	1	3.85×10^{-02}	3.84×10^{-02}	–0.28
7	1,1,1	2,0,0	2	3.01×10^{-01}	3.00×10^{-01}	–0.12
8	1,1,1	5,0,0	1	4.91×10^{-06}	4.90×10^{-06}	–0.13
9	1,1,1	10,0,0	1	1.01×10^{-20}	1.01×10^{-20}	–0.02

Table 13.4. Comparison of AD with Numerical Solution for Displaced General Gaussian pdf

Case	$\sigma_x, \sigma_y, \sigma_z$	Displacement x_0, y_0, z_0 of Sphere	Radius of Sphere	Probability (Numerical Integration)	Probability (Approx. Distributions)	Percent Error for Approx. Distributions
1	3,1,2	1,0,0	1	3.68×10^{-02}	5.56×10^{-04}	–98.49
2	3,1,2	10,0,0	1	1.70×10^{-04}	3.75×10^{-03}	2106.94
3	3,1,2	1,0,0	10	9.98×10^{-01}	9.98×10^{-01}	–0.01
4	3,10,2	1,0,0	1	4.05×10^{-03}	3.36×10^{-03}	–17.09
5	3,10,2	10,0,0	1	1.86×10^{-05}	3.50×10^{-06}	–81.20
6	3,10,2	1,0,0	1	4.05×10^{-03}	3.36×10^{-03}	–17.09
7	3,10,2	1,0,0	10	6.41×10^{-01}	6.41×10^{-01}	–0.11

as in the other cases, the answers deviate noticeably from the numerical solution, and the errors become excessively large—20 times larger than the true values when the offset $x_0 = 10\sigma$, demonstrating that this approach fails dreadfully for computing small collision probabilities.

Table 13.5 shows the accuracies of the EV results compared to the same high-precision solution under the same conditions. In contrast to the AD formulation, the EV approach yields practically the same values as the numerical answers with at least two significant figures of agreement for five of the seven cases shown, having discrepancies of less than 0.4% error. For cases 2 and 5, corresponding to large offsets $x_0 = 10\sigma$, the discrepancies are approximately 6% error. Again, the EV method can be used without encountering severe difficulties for computing small collision probabilities; however, caution must be exercised if we displace the spherical volume of integration more than 100σ away from the center of the Gaussian pdf. Such a case probably would not be of interest.

Table 13.5. Comparison of EV with Numerical Solution for Displaced General Gaussian pdf

Case	$\sigma_x, \sigma_y, \sigma_z$	Displacement x_0, y_0, z_0 of Sphere	Radius of Sphere	Probability (Numerical Integration)	Probability (Equivalent Volume)	Percent Error for Equivalent Volume
1	3,1,2	1,0,0	1	3.68×10^{-02}	3.69×10^{-02}	0.34
2	3,1,2	10,0,0	1	1.70×10^{-04}	1.81×10^{-04}	6.35
3	3,1,2	1,0,0	10	9.98×10^{-01}	$1.00 \times 10^{+00}$	0.17
4	3,10,2	1,0,0	1	4.05×10^{-03}	4.06×10^{-03}	0.33
5	3,10,2	10,0,0	1	1.86×10^{-05}	1.98×10^{-05}	6.19
6	3,10,2	1,0,0	1	4.05×10^{-03}	4.06×10^{-03}	0.33
7	3,10,2	1,0,0	10	6.41×10^{-01}	6.47×10^{-01}	0.87

13.5 Discussion

In Section 13.4, we noted that the EV method yields better results than the AD method for low probabilities. Hence, it will be used to compute the probabilities for a wide range of values of the standard deviations $\sigma_{x'}$, $\sigma_{y'}$, and $\sigma_{z'}$; event radius r_E; and distance d. (We recall from Section 13.2 that $\mathbf{r}_p'' \equiv (x_p'', y_p'', z_p'')$ are the coordinates of the primary object in the principal axes system in which the secondary object is at the origin and the volume V'' of integration has a circular cross section A''. Then d is the perpendicular distance of the primary from the y''-axis.) Because we now consider the instantaneous collision probability at any relative position $\mathbf{r}_p \equiv (x_p, y_p, z_p)$ at any time t, we can no longer use the concept of distance of closest approach or miss distance x_e, as we did in Chapters 4 and 5 where we considered integration over an infinitely long circular cylinder for the case of short-term encounters.

For the sake of simplicity, we shall consider the case of an isotropic Gaussian pdf so that we have a common standard deviation σ. With this choice, there is no need to distinguish d from the separation r_p at time t. The standard deviation σ is set equal to unity and the separation d is varied from 5 to 15. The event radius r_E, which is also the radius R of the spherical volume of integration, is varied from 5 to 10. Table 13.6 shows collision probabilities as a function of the separation and the event radius. Figure 13.1 depicts the instantaneous probability P as a function of the separation d with R as a parameter.

If we wish to determine the separation distance for specified values of the probability and the event radius, we would have to resort to interpolation using Fig. 13.1. This is a rather cumbersome procedure. Because we are also interested

Table 13.6. Collision Probability as as Function of Separation and Event Radius

Radius, R	Distance, d: 5	6	7	8	9	10
5	4.20×10^{-01}	7.93×10^{-01}	9.66×10^{-01}	9.98×10^{-01}	$1.00\times10^{+00}$	$1.00\times10^{+00}$
6	1.18×10^{-01}	4.34×10^{-01}	8.01×10^{-01}	9.68×10^{-01}	9.98×10^{-01}	$1.00\times10^{+00}$
7	1.50×10^{-02}	1.24×10^{-01}	4.43×10^{-01}	8.07×10^{-01}	9.70×10^{-01}	9.98×10^{-01}
8	7.96×10^{-04}	1.60×10^{-02}	1.28×10^{-01}	4.50×10^{-01}	8.11×10^{-01}	9.71×10^{-01}
9	1.68×10^{-05}	8.57×10^{-04}	1.68×10^{-02}	1.32×10^{-01}	4.56×10^{-01}	8.14×10^{-01}
10	1.38×10^{-07}	1.83×10^{-05}	9.07×10^{-04}	1.74×10^{-02}	1.34×10^{-01}	4.60×10^{-01}
11	4.34×10^{-10}	1.51×10^{-07}	1.95×10^{-05}	9.47×10^{-04}	1.78×10^{-02}	1.37×10^{-01}
12	5.19×10^{-13}	4.80×10^{-10}	1.63×10^{-07}	2.05×10^{-05}	9.81×10^{-04}	1.83×10^{-02}
13	2.26×10^{-16}	5.77×10^{-13}	5.19×10^{-10}	1.72×10^{-07}	2.14×10^{-05}	1.01×10^{-03}
14	$0.00\times10^{+00}$	1.30×10^{-16}	6.27×10^{-13}	5.53×10^{-10}	1.80×10^{-07}	2.21×10^{-05}
15	$0.00\times10^{+00}$	$0.00\times10^{+00}$	4.36×10^{-16}	6.71×10^{-13}	5.82×10^{-10}	1.88×10^{-07}

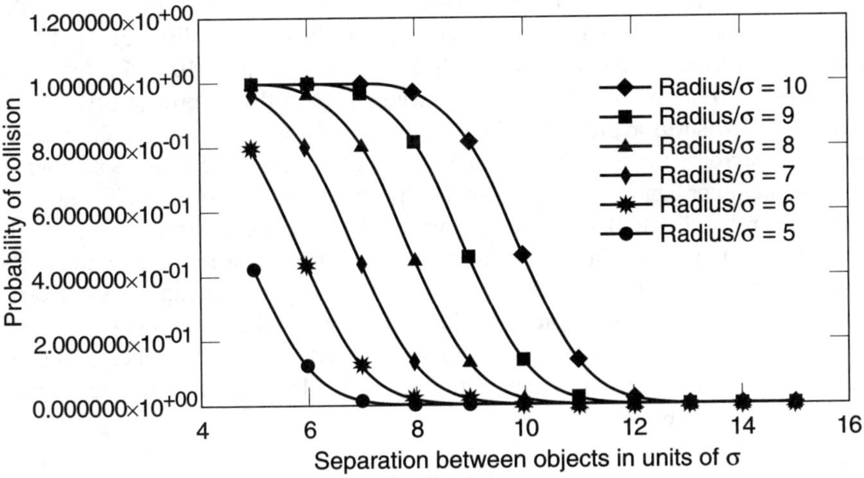

Figure 13.1. Instantaneous collision probability *P* as a function of separation distance and event radius.

in high collision probabilities, therefore, we may find a solution by means of the inverse problem, which will be discussed in more depth in Chapter 14. Again, we set the standard deviation equal to unity and vary the separation from 0 to 12. Also, we specify the probability to be 0.1, 0.5, 0.9, and 0.99. Figure 13.2 depicts the radius R as a function of the separation d with the probability P as a parameter. Usually, we are interested in the necessary separation when the event radius and the probability are specified. This information may be obtained by rotating the graph 90 deg.

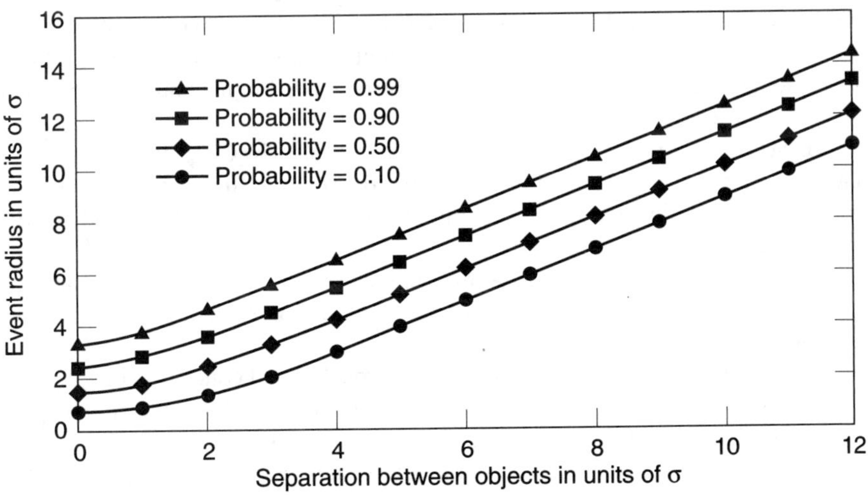

Figure 13.2. Event radius as a function of separation and probability.

For example, consider the case where the standard deviation $\sigma = 10$ m, the effective event radius $R = 100$ m, and the primary object is at a distance $d = 100$ m from the exploding secondary object. Thus, we have $(R/\sigma) = 10$ and $(d/\sigma) = 10$. From the last column of Table 13.6, we see that the collision probability is 0.46. Thus, if we wish to avoid any exploding fragments, we increase the distance to 150 m to decrease the probability to 1.88×10^{-7}, which is 2×10^{6} times smaller.

On the other hand, if we decrease the distance to 70 m, we would increase the collision probability to 0.998. In doubling that distance, we go from almost certain impact to virtual safety. Table 13.6 may illustrate other scenarios of collision probability as a function of the effective event radius and the separation distance for the special case of the isotropic Gaussian pdf. If we have a general Gaussian pdf, then we have more parameters to consider and recall that d is no longer defined to be the separation distance but now as the perpendicular distance from the primary object to the y''-axis.

13.6 Conclusion

Figures 13.1 and 13.2 are applicable to the case of the isotropic Gaussian pdf. In Fig. 13.1, we see that, in the range of separation shown, the probability curves are similar in shape and they are approximately regularly spaced in terms of the parameter (R/σ). In Fig. 13.2, we see that the probability curves for $P = 0.1$, 0.5, 0.9, and 0.99 are essentially linear in the range of (d/σ) from 2 to 12.

13.7 Summary

In this chapter, we considered the probability of collision between two objects at an instant of time. It was assumed that the uncertainty of their relative position is described by a three-dimensional Gaussian pdf. A little consideration will reveal that the analysis given here is not restricted just to the probability of collision between two objects in orbit. It is equally applicable to the case of other three-dimensional phenomena, such as the explosion of a fragmentation bomb near Earth's surface.

In Section 13.1, a method that will be elaborated in Chapter 14 is used to match moments of approximating probability distribution functions in succession to obtain an analytical expression giving the collision probability in terms of the error function.

In Section 13.2, we generalized the approach used in Chapter 5 by using the transformation of a Gaussian pdf to a Rician pdf and introducing the concept of equivalent volume.

In Section 13.3, we compared the two approaches and concluded that the first method yields good results when the collision probability is greater than 0.1, whereas the second method is accurate over a much wider range.

In Section 13.4, we presented numerical results using both methods for the cases of the spherical volume of integration with zero as well as nonzero offset from the center of the Gaussian pdf that may be isotropic and nonisotropic.

In Section 13.5, we discussed the particular case of an isotropic Gaussian pdf offset from the spherical volume of integration.

In Section 13.6, we concluded that the probability curves as a function of (d/σ), in the range of at least 5 to 10, are essentially similar in shape and are regularly spaced in terms of (R/σ). Moreover, the probability curves for values of P from 0.1 to 0.99 are essentially linear in the range of (d/σ) from 2 to 12.

13.8 References

13.1. H. Margenau and G. M. Murphy, *The Mathematics of Physics and Chemistry*, 2nd ed. (Van Nostrand, Princeton, 1956), pp. 504–506.

13.2. G. A. Korn and T. M. Korn, *Mathematical Handbook for Scientists and Engineers* (McGraw-Hill, New York, 1961), p. 630.

13.3. M. Abramowitz and I. A. Stegun, *Handbook of Mathematical Functions* (National Bureau of Standards, Washington, D.C., 1964), p. 297.

13.4. C. E. Pearson, ed., *Handbook of Applied Mathematics* (Van Nostrand, New York, 1983), p. 351.

13.5. P. S. de Laplace, *Theorie analytique des probabilities* (Paris, 1820), pp. 88–108.

13.6. A. Papoulis, *Probability, Random Variables, and Stochastic Processes* (McGraw-Hill, New York, 1965), p. 65.

Chapter 14: Spherical Error Probability Computation

In Chapters 2 through 12, we determined the probability of collision between a pair of orbiting objects under various circumstances. Now, we turn our attention to a slightly different scenario. Suppose we are given a probability density function (pdf) and a spherical volume of a certain radius. We can determine the collision probability by evaluating a three-dimensional integral either analytically or numerically, as we did in Chapter 13. This is known as the *direct problem*.

However, we may be given the *inverse problem*: We need to determine the radius of the spherical region when the collision probability is specified. There are applications in spacecraft encounters of both the short-term and long-term types that require this knowledge. This problem first arose in the location of an object in three dimensions (latitude, longitude, and altitude).

The inverse problem (the determination of the size of a sphere with a specified probability of containment) is also known as the "spherical error probability" (SEP) problem. Specifically, it is required to determine the radius of the sphere for which there exists an arbitrary, user-specified probability that a certain point will lie within it. (The probability is not necessarily 50%, though that is the usual default value used in defining SEP.)

Six parameters are input to the problem: three standard deviations of the Gaussian pdf, and the three components of the displacement vector of the center of the sphere of consideration. The most obvious approach to determining SEP is to perform time-consuming numerical evaluation of three-dimensional integrals and interpolation involving five dimensionless parameters obtained by dividing any one of the parameters into the remaining five.

The approach in this chapter, however, is based on first formulating the problem in terms of the cumulative noncentral chi-square distribution; then appropriately choosing the degree n' of a central chi-square distribution to approximate the noncentral one; and last, in a second approximation, transforming the central distribution to a Gaussian distribution. The degree n' is chosen so that the first three moments are satisfied. The transformation from central chi-square to Gaussian distribution is accomplished using an expression derived by Wilson and Hilferty.[14.1] The radius of the sphere is obtained by using an efficient algorithm for the inverse error function.

For a wide range of aspect ellipsoidal axis ratios and displacement vectors, the answer when computed by this method is found to be within 1% of the exact answer for several special known cases. This level of accuracy meets the requirements of most applications.

14.1 Historical Background

There is no known closed-form solution to the direct problem of determining the integral of a Gaussian pdf within a sphere of a specified radius displaced from the origin. The easiest approach is numerical evaluation of a three-dimensional integral, but that can be rather time-consuming for the small integration step-sizes required for accurate answers. An alternative approach is to obtain the answer in the form of a convergent infinite series. Proceeding in this direction, however, one soon finds that the expressions become unwieldy. Moreover, the convergence is slow, except for instances where small values of the expansion parameters are used, with the consequence that numerous terms have to be used for moderate or large values of the parameters. Furthermore, the presence of factorials means the computations are subject to numerical overflow unless special caution is exercised.

Even more troublesome is the inverse problem of determining the radius of the sphere when the probability of containment is specified. The solution of this problem would involve the iterative procedure of the direct problem, using Newton's root-finding method. Thus, an approach in this direction is not recommended because of convergence problems when the starting point of the iteration process is not close to the answer.

The groundwork leading to a radically different approach was laid in 1949 by Patnaik,[14.2] who approximated a noncentral chi-square distribution by a central chi-square distribution, expressing the degree n for the latter in terms of the first two moments of the former. In this process, he satisfied the first two moments, but not the third, of the latter. He then transformed the central chi-square distribution into a Gaussian distribution by using the result Fisher[14.3] obtained in 1925. However, Patnaik was interested in the statistical aspects of hypothesis testing and the goodness of fit (i.e., the upper and lower tail-end 5% of the cumulative distribution).

In 1959, Pearson[14.4] studied the asymptotic behavior of the noncentral chi-square distribution in the limits of small and large displacement parameters for the case of equal variances in all the variables. By using heuristic arguments, he expressed the degree n' of a central chi-square distribution in terms of the second and third moments of the noncentral chi-square distribution. In this process, he satisfied the first three moments of the desired central chi-square distribution. His results for the upper and lower tail-end 5% of the noncentral cumulative distribution were more accurate, as reported by Johnson[14.5] and by Imhof.[14.6]

In 1964, Grubbs[14.7] extended the usefulness of Patnaik's analysis by employing the more accurate Wilson-Hilferty[14.1] transformation, originally derived in 1931, from central chi-square distribution to Gaussian distribution. He performed his study using both Patnaik's representation of the degree n and Pearson's representation of the degree n'.

All these investigators, as well as Grad and Solomon,[14.8] Pachares,[14.9] and Shah and Khatri,[14.10] were essentially interested in the direct problem—not the inverse one, which was easily within reach, in view of the efforts by Patnaik. Finally, in 1974, making use of Grubbs's work, Terzian[14.11] considered the inverse problem. He only considered explicitly the case of 50% circular error probability (CEP), because it did not invoke the inverse error function. However, his equations contained a high rate of typographical errors (three errors in six equations), and he quoted two equations from Grubbs's paper that are erroneous, off by a factor of σ^2 (more about this problem later).

Moreover, Terzian seemed to imply that the first two moments of the central chi-square distribution were matched with the first two moments of the noncentral distribution. This is not true. What Grubbs did (and what Patnaik had done much earlier) was to express the degree $n = 2m^2/v$, where m is the mean and v the variance of the noncentral distribution. As Patnaik[14.2] said (on both pp. 206 and 231), "fit [the central distribution] from the first two moments [of the noncentral distribution]." It is easy to verify that the first two moments of these distributions are not correspondingly equal.

Another point to note is that, by the choice of n in terms of the first two moments as given by Patnaik and Grubbs, the third moment of the fitted central chi-square distribution is not automatically satisfied. Note that for consistency we should have n for the first moment, $2n$ for the variance, and $8n$ for the third moment about the mean. One particular case in which the third moment is satisfied is that of the isotropic Gaussian pdf with zero mean, which may easily be proven.

The analysis in the next section of this chapter derives the general form of the degree n' of the central chi-square distribution to ensure that the first three moments are satisfied (i.e., for consistency we should have n' for the first moment, $2n'$ for the variance, and $8n'$ for the third moment about the mean). We obtain $n' = 8v^3/\mu_3{}^2$, where μ_3 is the third moment about the mean of the noncentral chi-square distribution. This is the same expression as that derived by Pearson, except that there is no resort to the asymptotic behavior of the noncentral chi-square distribution in the limits of small and large displacement parameters, and also equal variances are not required in all the variables.

For Pearson's case, the first three moments of the chi-square distribution are satisfied a posteriori after the form for n' has been obtained. Moreover, the fourth moment of the fitted central chi-square distribution is not automatically satisfied; for consistency we should have $(48n' + 12n'^2)$ for the fourth moment about the mean. Again, the reader should verify if the fourth moment is satisfied for the particular case of the isotropic Gaussian pdf with zero mean.

14.2 Formulation in Terms of Noncentral Chi-Square Distribution

The following analysis is applicable to any number of variables. Let $\{\xi_j; j = 1, 2, \ldots n\}$ denote n independent Gaussian random variables with biases $\{b_j; j = 1, 2, \ldots n\}$ and variances $\{v_j \equiv \sigma_j^2; j = 1, 2, \ldots n\}$. For a three-dimensional space, $\{\xi_j; j = 1, 2, 3\} = \{x, y, z\}$. The biases are the coordinates of the symmetrical point of the Gaussian pdf displaced from the origin. We are interested in determining the probability P that the distance $r^2 \equiv x^2 + y^2 + z^2 \leq R^2$, where R is a specified value. We have noted that this probability may be obtained by evaluating the three-dimensional integral of the Gaussian pdf within a sphere of radius R. If we define y^2 by

$$\psi^2 = \sum_{j=1}^{n} \xi_j^{\,2} \tag{14.1}$$

then we wish to calculate the probability $P\{\psi^2 \leq R^2\}$. Note that Eq. (14.1) may be written as

$$\psi^2 = \sum_{j=1}^{n} v_j (q_j + a_j)^2 \tag{14.2}$$

where q_j and a_j are defined by

$$q_j = (\xi_j - b_j)/\sigma_j \tag{14.3}$$

$$a_j = b_j / \sigma_j \tag{14.4}$$

Thus, the q_j are Gaussian variables with zero mean and unit standard deviation, that is, the normal distribution $N(0,1)$. Thus, ψ^2 is a noncentral chi-square statistic (random variable). Hence, we have written the n-dimensional integral within a hypersphere as the probability that the noncentral chi-square statistic is less than or equal to the value R^2 (i.e., the cumulative distribution of ψ^2). That is,

$$P = P\left\{r^2 \leq R^2\right\} = P\left\{\psi^2 \leq R^2\right\} \tag{14.5}$$

Because the Gaussian random variables ξ_j are independent, the characteristic function $\phi(t)$ of ψ^2 is given by

$$\phi(t) = \left[\prod_{j=1}^{n} \phi_j(t)\right] = \left[\prod_{j=1}^{n} (1 - 2it\sigma_j^{\,2})^{-1/2}\right] \exp\left\{\sum_{j=1}^{n} (it\sigma_j^{\,2} a_j^{\,2}) / (1 - 2it\sigma_j^{\,2})\right\} \tag{14.6}$$

where $i^2 = -1$. (Except for a factor of $1/2\pi$ and a negative sign in the exponent, the characteristic function of a random variable x is the Fourier transform of the probability density function $f(x)$. It is used instead of the moment-generating function because the latter may not exist for certain pdfs.) This is the corrected form of Eq. (4) in the appendix to Patnaik's paper, where a typographical error appeared in the terms under the summation sign on the right-hand side (RHS). If $\phi(t)$ is expanded in powers of t, the rth moment μ_r' (about $t = 0$) is given by the coefficient of $(it)^r/r!$

in the expansion. The first moment μ_1' is the mean and is simply denoted by μ. The first few moments about the mean are easily obtained and are given by Kendall, Stuart, and Ord:[14.12]

$$\mu_2 = \mu_2' - \mu_1'^2 \tag{14.7}$$

$$\mu_3 = \mu_3' - 3\mu_2'\mu_1' + 2\mu_1'^3 \tag{14.8}$$

$$\mu_4 = \mu_4' - 4\mu_3'\mu_1' + 6\mu_2'\mu_1'^2 - 3\mu_1'^4 \tag{14.9}$$

We may easily compute the first three moments of the characteristic function $\phi(t)$ by using the characteristic function $\phi_j(t)$ for each value j to obtain the first three moments and then invoking the following relations, which are easily proved for any two independent random variables u and v:

$$E(u+v) = E(u) + E(v) \tag{14.10}$$

$$V(u+v) = V(u) + V(v) \tag{14.11}$$

$$T(u+v) = T(u) + T(v) \tag{14.12}$$

where $E(\cdot)$, $V(\cdot)$, and $T(\cdot)$ respectively denote the operators yielding the mean, variance, and third moment about the mean. That is, the individual means, variances, and third moments are merely summed to obtain the total mean, variance, and third moment. Thus,

$$m \equiv \mu = \sum_{j=1}^{n}\left[v_j + v_j a_j^2\right] = \sum_{j=1}^{n}\left[\sigma_j^2 + b_j^2\right] \tag{14.13}$$

$$v \equiv \mu_2 = 2\sum_{j=1}^{n}\left[v_j^2 + 2v_j^2 a_j^2\right] = 2\sum_{j=1}^{n}\left[\sigma_j^4 + 2\sigma_j^2 b_j^2\right] \tag{14.14}$$

$$\mu_3 = 8\sum_{j=1}^{n}\left[v_j^3 + 3v_j^3 a_j^2\right] = 8\sum_{j=1}^{n}\left[\sigma_j^6 + 3\sigma_j^4 b_j^2\right] \tag{14.15}$$

These results were originally obtained by Patnaik. Note with caution, however, that Grubbs incorrectly used Patnaik's results in his equations numbered (10), (11), and (21); his ψ^2 is defined with a factor of $\sigma^2 \equiv \Sigma\sigma_j^2$. However, he eventually used the ratio $2\mu^2/\mu_2$ in his analysis so that this multiplicative factor cancelled out by virtue of his equations numbered (30) and (31).

For the higher moments about the mean, we no longer have the simple additive relation exemplified by Eqs. (14.10) through (14.12). For the fourth moment, $Q(\cdot)$, it may be shown that

$$Q(u+v)=Q(u)+Q(v)+6V(u)V(v) \tag{14.16}$$

By using the characteristic function $\phi_j(t)$ for each value j to obtain the fourth moment, and invoking the relation in Eq. (14.16), we obtain

$$\mu_4=\sum_{j=1}^{n}\mu_{j,4}+6\sum_{k=2}^{n}\mu_{k,2}\sum_{i=1}^{k-1}\mu_{i,2} \tag{14.17}$$

where $\mu_{j,4}$ denotes the fourth moment about the mean obtained using the characteristic function $\phi_j(t)$. For the cases of $n = 2$ and 3,

$$\mu_4=(\mu_{1,4}+\mu_{2,4})+6\mu_{2,2}\mu_{1,2} \tag{14.18}$$

$$\mu_4=(\mu_{1,4}+\mu_{2,4}+\mu_{3,4})+6\mu_{3,2}(\mu_{1,2}+\mu_{2,2})+6\mu_{2,2}\mu_{1,2} \tag{14.19}$$

Having derived the expressions for the first four moments about the mean for the noncentral chi-square distribution (ψ^2), we next consider the corresponding moments for the central chi-square distribution (χ^2). We may simply set $a_j = 0$ and $\sigma_j = 1$ in these equations. However, these moments are well known and have already been obtained using the simple characteristic function

$$\phi(t)=(1-2it)^{-n/2} \tag{14.20}$$

where n is the number of degrees of freedom. Thus, we have (see Kendall et al.[14.12])

$$\mu=n \tag{14.21}$$

$$\mu_2=2n \tag{14.22}$$

$$\mu_3=8n \tag{14.23}$$

$$\mu_4=48n+12n^2 \tag{14.24}$$

14.3 Formulation in Terms of Central Chi-Square Distribution

Let us next obtain a central chi-square distribution by requiring that the first three moments be consistent by using the moments of the noncentral chi-square distribution. We know that when the biases are zero and the standard deviations are equal, the latter become the former. Let n' denote the degree of the desired chi-square distribution. Then, from Eq. (14.21), its mean, variance, and third moment should be respectively n', $2n'$, and $8n'$. To avoid confusion, let m and v denote the expressions on the RHS of Eqs. (14.13) and (14.14) for the mean and variance of the ψ^2 distribution. The "fit" should satisfy the condition

$$\frac{\chi^2 - n'}{\sqrt{2n'}} = \frac{\psi^2 - m}{\sqrt{v}} \tag{14.25}$$

If $E(\cdot)$, $V(\cdot)$, and $T(\cdot)$ respectively denote the operators for the mean, variance, and third moment about the mean, it follows that

$$E\left(\frac{\chi^2 - n'}{\sqrt{2n'}}\right) = E\left(\frac{\psi^2 - m}{\sqrt{v}}\right) \tag{14.26}$$

However, from Eqs. (14.10) through (14.12), we know that if c is a constant, then

$$E(u+c) = E(u) \tag{14.27}$$

$$V(u+c) = V(u) \tag{14.28}$$

$$T(u+c) = T(u) \tag{14.29}$$

Moreover, it is easily proved that

$$E(cu) = cE(u) \tag{14.30}$$

$$V(cu) = c^2V(u) \tag{14.31}$$

$$T(cu) = c^3T(u) \tag{14.32}$$

From Eqs. (14.26), (14.27), and (14.30), it follows that

$$E\left(\chi^2\right) = n' \tag{14.33}$$

so that Eq. (14.25) yields consistently the desired first moment. Next, we have

$$V\left(\frac{\chi^2 - n'}{\sqrt{2n'}}\right) = V\left(\frac{\psi^2 - m}{\sqrt{v}}\right) \tag{14.34}$$

From Eqs. (14.28), (14.31), and (14.34), it follows that

$$V\left(\chi^2\right) = 2n' \tag{14.35}$$

so that Eq. (14.25) yields consistently the desired second moment. Next, we have

$$T\left(\frac{\chi^2 - n'}{\sqrt{2n'}}\right) = T\left(\frac{\psi^2 - m}{\sqrt{v}}\right) \tag{14.36}$$

From Eq. (14.29), (14.32), and (14.36), it follows that

$$T\left(\chi^2\right) = \left(\frac{2n'}{v}\right)^{3/2} \mu_3 \tag{14.37}$$

For Eq. (14.25) to yield consistently the desired third moment

$$T\left(\chi^2\right) = 8n' \tag{14.38}$$

we equate the two expressions on the RHS so that n' is given by

$$n' = \frac{8v^3}{\mu_3^{\ 2}} \tag{14.39}$$

where v and μ_3 are given by Eqs. (14.14) and (14.15).

Only the second and third moments of the noncentral chi-square distribution (ψ^2) are used to determine the degree of freedom n' of the desired central chi-square distribution (χ^2). The first moment appears only in Eq. (14.25). By using the condition in Eqs. (14.25) and (14.39), one consistently satisfies the mean, variance, and third moment of the latter. Thus, we have approximated the noncentral chi-square distribution by a central chi-square distribution whose first three moments are consistent.

When $\psi^2 = R^2$, let $\chi^2 = X^2$. Eq. (14.25) gives the relation between R^2 and X^2. Hence, Eq. (14.5) now becomes

$$P = P\{r^2 \le R^2\} = P\{\psi^2 \le R^2\} = P\{\chi^2 \le X^2\} \tag{14.40}$$

Thus, we have transformed the evaluation of a multidimensional integral to the determination of the probability when χ^2 is less than or equal to the value X^2 (i.e., the cumulative distribution of χ^2).

14.4 Formulation in Terms of Gaussian Distribution

We shall next approximate this central chi-square distribution by a normal distribution. Fisher[14.3] obtained the first approximation in 1925. Wilson and Hilferty[14.1] improved on it in 1931. Even though Cornish and Fisher,[14.13] Peizer and Pratt,[14.14] and Pratt[14.15] derived better approximations, their methods are however more cumbersome to use and are not amenable to solving the inverse probability problem of interest here. The Wilson-Hilferty transformation to the $N(0,1)$ normal variable t is

$$t = \left[\sqrt[3]{\chi^2/n'} - (1 - 2/9n')\right] \Big/ \sqrt{2/9n'} \tag{14.41}$$

That is, $(\chi^2/n')^{1/3}$ is a normally distributed variable with mean $(1 - 2/9n')$ and variance $2/9n'$.

When $\chi^2 = X^2$, let $t = T$. Eq. (14.41) gives the relation between X^2 and T. Hence, Eq. (14.5) now becomes

$$P = P\{r^2 \le R^2\} = P\{\psi^2 \le R^2\} = P\{\chi^2 \le X^2\} = P\{t \le T\} \tag{14.42}$$

Thus, we have transformed the evaluation of a multidimensional integral to the determination of the probability when t is less than or equal to the value T (i.e., the cumulative distribution of the Gaussian variable t).

For the inverse problem, the probability P is given and one must determine the radius R of the sphere such that the probability of containment is P. Thus, we are led to the inverse of the error function that is defined by the equation

$$erf(\eta) = \sqrt{\frac{2}{\pi}} \int_0^{\sqrt{2}\eta} e^{-t^2/2} dt \tag{14.43}$$

Because the probability P that the normal variable t is less than or equal to some specified value T is given by the cumulative distribution

$$P = P\{t \le T\} = \frac{1}{\sqrt{2\pi}} \int_{-\infty}^{0} e^{-t^2/2} dt + \frac{1}{\sqrt{2\pi}} \int_0^T e^{-t^2/2} dt \tag{14.44}$$

or, equivalently,

$$P = \frac{1}{2} + \frac{1}{2}\sqrt{\frac{2}{\pi}}\int_0^T e^{-t^2/2}dt \tag{14.45}$$

therefore we determine T from the inverse error function accordingly:

$$T = \sqrt{2}\,erf^{-1}(2P-1) \tag{14.46}$$

We then obtain X^2 using Eq. (14.41), which yields

$$X^2 = n'\left[T\sqrt{2/9n'} + (1-2/9n')\right]^3 \tag{14.47}$$

Similarly, by using Eq. (14.25), we obtain R^2:

$$R^2 = m + \sqrt{\frac{v}{2n'}}\left(X^2 - n'\right) \tag{14.48}$$

Equations (14.13) through (14.15), (14.39), and (14.46) through (14.48) form the basis for the computation of the radius R when the probability P of containment is specified. The remaining topic of discussion is the evaluation of the inverse error function for T. Let y equal the error function of the argument x. That is,

$$y = erf(x) = \frac{2}{\sqrt{\pi}}\sum_{n=0}^{\infty}\frac{(-1)^n x^{2n+1}}{n!(2n+1)} \tag{14.49}$$

Chan[14.16] has derived the following very simple formula:

$$x \simeq z + \frac{1}{3}z^3 + \frac{7}{30}z^5 + \frac{53}{250}\frac{z^7}{(1-z^2)} \quad \text{where} \quad z \equiv \frac{\sqrt{\pi}}{2}y \tag{14.50}$$

This formula yields a value of x that is accurate to 0.1% for $|y| \le 0.9$ and 2.0% for $|y| \le 0.95$. In Eq. (14.46), note that $y = 2P - 1$. Hence, we may use this for P in the range $0.05 \le P \le 0.95$ with 0.1% accuracy and in the range $0.025 \le P \le 0.975$ with 2.0% accuracy. However, the actual software implementation only uses this formula as an initial value for an iterative process based on Eq. (14.49) and is accurate to 14 significant figures. This evaluation of the inverse error function is thus very accurate.

14.5 Numerical Results

An algorithm based on this formulation was developed to run as an Excel macro and is available as "Spherical Error Probability Calculation.xls," described in Chapter 15, Computer Programs. More than 200 benchmark runs are included for reference. In the data input and output, all lengths (σ values, biases, and radii) are assumed to be measured in consistent units (meters, kilometers, feet, miles, etc.); thus no physical units are attached to them.

The four tables in this section contain data extracted from the sheets in the Excel workbook. Table 14.1 compares the results obtained with this algorithm and the exact values for the known case of three-dimensional isotropic Gaussian pdf with center of symmetry at the origin. This special solution with all three equal variances of σ is given by

$$P = P\left\{r^2 \le R^2\right\} = erf\left(\frac{R}{\sqrt{2}\sigma}\right) - \sqrt{\frac{2}{\pi}}\frac{R}{\sigma}e^{-R^2/2\sigma^2} \tag{14.51}$$

The percent error is seen to be generally less than 0.5% in the range of probability of containment studied. For comparison, we will consider the case of the two-dimensional isotropic Gaussian pdf with center of symmetry at the origin. Table 14.2 compares the results obtained with this algorithm and the exact values for this known case. This special solution with both equal variances of σ is given by the equation

$$P = P\left\{r^2 \le R^2\right\} = 1 - e^{-R^2/2\sigma^2} \tag{14.52}$$

Table 14.1. Comparison for the Spherical Case (σ = 1)

Probability of Containment	Computed SEP Radius	Exact SEP Radius	Percent Error
0.1	0.759	0.764	–0.66
0.2	1.008	1.003	0.50
0.3	1.201	1.193	0.62
0.4	1.374	1.367	0.50
0.5	1.543	1.538	0.33
0.6	1.719	1.716	0.14
0.7	1.913	1.914	–0.05
0.8	2.150	2.154	–0.21
0.9	2.493	2.500	–0.30
0.95	2.788	2.795	–0.25
0.99	3.372	3.368	0.11
0.995	3.594	3.583	0.32

Table 14.2. Comparison for the Circular Case ($\sigma = 1$)

Probability of Containment	Computed CEP Radius	Exact CEP Radius	Percent Error
0.1	0.444	0.459	–3.35
0.2	0.671	0.668	0.45
0.3	0.853	0.845	1.04
0.4	1.020	1.011	0.95
0.5	1.185	1.177	0.66
0.6	1.358	1.354	0.32
0.7	1.551	1.552	–0.02
0.8	1.788	1.794	–0.32
0.9	2.135	2.146	–0.50
0.95	2.437	2.448	–0.46
0.99	3.037	3.035	0.06
0.995	3.267	3.255	0.36

The percent error for the CEP is seen to be generally larger than that in the previous case for SEP in the range of probability of containment studied. In some cases, it is even slightly smaller. Note that the spherical case directly leads to a central chi-square distribution with 3 degrees of freedom, and the circular case directly leads to a central chi-square distribution with 2 degrees of freedom from the very beginning. The observation that, in some cases, the circular case yields slightly better results does not contradict the well-known fact that the central chi-square distribution becomes $N(0, 1)$ as the number of degrees of freedom tends to infinity.

At issue here is that, for a particular probability of containment, one must deal with the lower tail-end of the chi-square distribution. In general, with biases and unequal variances, we have to consider the whole process of approximating the noncentral chi-square distribution by a central one and then approximating this by a normal distribution. We cannot categorically state that when we deal with a three-dimensional Gaussian pdf, we always obtain a better approximation than we do with a two-dimensional Gaussian pdf.

Because exact solutions are only available for a few cases, we shall next consider the two-dimensional case of Gaussian pdf with unequal variances but with zero biases. Chan[14.17] has obtained an analytical solution in the form of a convergent series. This solution yields as accurate an answer as desired and is best obtained by the following recursive process to circumvent numerical overflow in the computations:

$$P = P\left\{r^2 \le R^2\right\} = 1 - e^{\beta}\sum_{n=0}^{\infty} T_n(\varepsilon,\beta) \tag{14.53}$$

$$\beta \equiv -\frac{R^2}{2\sigma_y^{\ 2}}, \quad \varepsilon \equiv 1 - \frac{\sigma_x^{\ 2}}{\sigma_y^{\ 2}}, \quad \sigma_x^{\ 2} \le \sigma_y^{\ 2}, \quad T_0 = 1, \quad T_1 = \frac{1}{2}\varepsilon\beta \tag{14.54}$$

$$T_n = \frac{\varepsilon}{n}\left(\frac{2n-1}{2n}\right)\left[(\beta + 2n - 2)T_{n-1} - \varepsilon(n-2)\left(\frac{2n-3}{2n-2}\right)T_{n-2}\right] \tag{14.55}$$

Table 14.3 compares the three-moment consistency of the present fit with the two-moment consistency fit used by Patnaik and Grubbs. It considers elliptical aspect ratios from 1 to 12 for the three cases of 10, 50, and 90% probability of containment. Even though the percent error is not small, the three-moment method is seen to be far superior to the two-moment method for the case of 10% CEP. The results are slightly better with the three-moment method for the case of 50% CEP, and they are comparable for the case of 90% CEP.

Another case for which an exact solution is available is that of the two-dimensional Gaussian pdf with equal variances but with nonzero biases. From Eq. (14.17),

$$P = P\{r^2 \le R^2\} = e^{-v/2} \sum_{m=0}^{\infty} \frac{v^m}{2^m m!}\left[1 - e^{-u/2} \sum_{k=0}^{m} \frac{u^k}{2^k k!}\right] \tag{14.56}$$

$$u \equiv R^2/\sigma^2 \ \text{ and } \ v \equiv (b_x^{\ 2} + b_y^{\ 2})/\sigma^2 \tag{14.57}$$

Table 14.4 compares the three-moment consistency of the present fit with the two-moment consistency fit. It considers biases from 1 to 6 for the three cases of 10, 50, and 90% probability of containment. Except for an isolated case, the three-moment method is far superior to the two-moment method for the case of 10% CEP. The error is generally less than 0.5% for the former and 5% for the latter. The results are definitely better with the three-moment method for the case of 50% CEP, and they are comparable for the case of 90% CEP.

14.6 Application to Other Problems

By invoking concepts from other fields, we have circumvented the excessive computation time required by the straightforward numerical integration. This method is also applicable to the evaluation of integrals of much higher dimensions (probably exceeding even 100) that are of use in other areas such as statistical analysis and signal detection. This has been the motivation behind the analysis presented in this chapter.

Table 14.3. Comparison for the Elliptical Case with No Biases

$(\sigma_x, \sigma_y, \sigma_z)$	(Bias x_0, Bias y_0, Bias z_0)	Exact 10% CEP Radius	3 Moments 10% CEP Radius	Percent Error	2 Moments 10% CEP Radius	Percent Error
(1, 1, 0)	(0, 0, 0)	0.459	0.444	–3.35	0.444	–3.35
(1, 2, 0)	(0, 0, 0)	0.654	0.789	20.70	0.464	–28.93
(1, 3, 0)	(0, 0, 0)	0.809	0.924	14.14	0.445	–44.97
(1, 4, 0)	(0, 0, 0)	0.946	0.986	4.16	0.463	–51.11
(1, 5, 0)	(0, 0, 0)	1.072	1.029	–4.07	0.501	–53.31
(1, 6, 0)	(0, 0, 0)	1.191	1.067	–10.46	0.550	–53.84
(1, 7, 0)	(0, 0, 0)	1.305	1.104	–15.41	0.606	–53.60
(1, 8, 0)	(0, 0, 0)	1.416	1.143	–19.30	0.666	–53.00
(1, 9, 0)	(0, 0, 0)	1.525	1.184	–22.38	0.728	–52.25
(1, 10, 0)	(0, 0, 0)	1.633	1.227	–24.86	0.793	–51.44
(1, 11, 0)	(0, 0, 0)	1.740	1.272	–26.88	0.859	–50.63
(1, 12, 0)	(0, 0, 0)	1.847	1.320	–28.54	0.926	–49.85
$(\sigma_x, \sigma_y, \sigma_z)$	(Bias x_0, Bias y_0, Bias z_0)	Exact 50% CEP Radius	3 Moments 50% CEP Radius	Percent Error	2 Moments 50% CEP Radius	Percent Error
(1, 1, 0)	(0, 0, 0)	1.177	1.185	0.66	1.185	0.66
(1, 2, 0)	(0, 0, 0)	1.741	1.705	–2.06	1.749	0.46
(1, 3, 0)	(0, 0, 0)	2.305	2.291	–0.60	2.339	1.46
(1, 4, 0)	(0, 0, 0)	2.902	2.922	0.69	2.963	2.13
(1, 5, 0)	(0, 0, 0)	3.529	3.573	1.25	3.609	2.26
(1, 6, 0)	(0, 0, 0)	4.175	4.236	1.46	4.267	2.20
(1, 7, 0)	(0, 0, 0)	4.830	4.905	1.55	4.932	2.11
(1, 8, 0)	(0, 0, 0)	5.490	5.578	1.60	5.602	2.04
(1, 9, 0)	(0, 0, 0)	6.154	6.254	1.63	6.276	1.98
(1, 10, 0)	(0, 0, 0)	6.820	6.932	1.64	6.952	1.93
(1, 11, 0)	(0, 0, 0)	7.487	7.611	1.66	7.629	1.89
(1, 12, 0)	(0, 0, 0)	8.156	8.292	1.66	8.308	1.87
$(\sigma_x, \sigma_y, \sigma_z)$	(Bias x_0, Bias y_0, Bias z_0)	Exact 90% CEP Radius	3 Moments 90% CEP Radius	Percent Error	2 Moments 90% CEP Radius	Percent Error
(1, 1, 0)	(0, 0, 0)	2.146	2.135	–0.50	2.135	–0.50
(1, 2, 0)	(0, 0, 0)	3.474	3.459	–0.44	3.496	0.63
(1, 3, 0)	(0, 0, 0)	5.043	4.995	–0.96	5.042	–0.03
(1, 4, 0)	(0, 0, 0)	6.658	6.583	–1.13	6.627	–0.48
(1, 5, 0)	(0, 0, 0)	8.287	8.188	–1.18	8.226	–0.73
(1, 6, 0)	(0, 0, 0)	9.921	9.801	–1.21	9.834	–0.87
(1, 7, 0)	(0, 0, 0)	11.558	11.417	–1.22	11.446	–0.96
(1, 8, 0)	(0, 0, 0)	13.197	13.036	–1.23	13.062	–1.03
(1, 9, 0)	(0, 0, 0)	14.838	14.655	–1.23	14.679	–1.07
(1, 10, 0)	(0, 0, 0)	16.479	16.276	–1.23	16.298	–1.10
(1, 11, 0)	(0, 0, 0)	18.121	17.898	–1.23	17.917	–1.12
(1, 12, 0)	(0, 0, 0)	19.764	19.520	–1.23	19.538	–1.14

Table 14.4. Comparison for the Circular Case with Biases

$(\sigma_x, \sigma_y, \sigma_z)$	(Bias x_0, Bias y_0, Bias z_0)	Exact 10% CEP Radius	3 Moments 10% CEP Radius	Percent Error	2 Moments 10% CEP Radius	Percent Error
(1, 1, 0)	(1, 0, 0)	0.587	0.540	–7.96	0.610	3.88
(1, 1, 0)	(2, 0, 0)	1.091	1.092	0.13	1.195	9.58
(1, 1, 0)	(3, 0, 0)	1.931	1.942	0.55	2.016	4.40
(1, 1, 0)	(4, 0, 0)	2.868	2.875	0.27	2.928	2.11
(1, 1, 0)	(5, 0, 0)	3.833	3.839	0.14	3.878	1.17
(1, 1, 0)	(6, 0, 0)	4.812	4.816	0.08	4.847	0.72
(1, 1, 0)	(7, 0, 0)	5.809	5.800	–0.15	5.825	0.28
(1, 1, 0)	(8, 0, 0)	7.565	6.789	–10.27	6.810	–9.99
$(\sigma_x, \sigma_y, \sigma_z)$	(Bias x_0, Bias y_0, Bias z_0)	Exact 50% CEP Radius	3 Moments 50% CEP Radius	Percent Error	2 Moments 50% CEP Radius	Percent Error
(1, 1, 0)	(1, 0, 0)	1.475	1.496	1.37	1.482	0.43
(1, 1, 0)	(2, 0, 0)	2.246	2.260	0.62	2.226	–0.87
(1, 1, 0)	(3, 0, 0)	3.165	3.171	0.18	3.136	–0.94
(1, 1, 0)	(4, 0, 0)	4.124	4.127	0.07	4.095	–0.71
(1, 1, 0)	(5, 0, 0)	5.100	5.101	0.03	5.073	–0.52
(1, 1, 0)	(6, 0, 0)	6.086	6.084	–0.03	6.059	–0.43
(1, 1, 0)	(7, 0, 0)	7.462	7.072	–5.23	7.050	–5.52
$(\sigma_x, \sigma_y, \sigma_z)$	(Bias x_0, Bias y_0, Bias z_0)	Exact 90% CEP Radius	3 Moments 90% CEP Radius	Percent Error	2 Moments 90% CEP Radius	Percent Error
(1, 1, 0)	(1, 0, 0)	2.602	2.585	–0.65	2.579	–0.88
(1, 1, 0)	(2, 0, 0)	3.473	3.457	–0.47	3.451	–0.65
(1, 1, 0)	(3, 0, 0)	4.420	4.409	–0.24	4.408	–0.26
(1, 1, 0)	(4, 0, 0)	5.390	5.383	–0.13	5.386	–0.07
(1, 1, 0)	(5, 0, 0)	6.371	6.366	–0.08	6.371	0.00
(1, 1, 0)	(6, 0, 0)	7.494	7.353	–1.87	7.359	–1.80

14.7 Discussion

The three-moment consistency fit yields results with approximately 1% error throughout a wide range of input parameters. This level of accuracy meets the requirements of most applications. The method is simple to implement, which is evident from the computer code that is provided. The execution time for each run is definitely superior to the time required for the direct numerical evaluation of a three-dimensional integral and the subsequent requisite iterations to determine the SEP radius.

For example, if we choose 1000 integration steps for each dimension, three dimensions will require 1 billion integration steps. The whole process is then repeated until the desired probability of containment is obtained—whether 10, 50, 90, or any other percent. It is not unreasonable to expect 5 such iterations.

Hence, there are a total of 5 billion integration steps. Each SEP computation devised in this chapter is equivalent to approximately 5 integration steps. Consequently, performing a three-dimensional integral with 5 iterations is 1 billion times as long as the SEP evaluation. If we have 100 integration steps for each dimension, then the numerical evaluation will be 1 million times as long. However, it is felt that this coarse grid will not yield an answer as accurate as the analytical solution.

14.8 Conclusion

This method is also applicable to the case of two-dimensional integrals by merely setting $n = 2$ in Eqs. (14.13) through (14.15). For this, we have the general case of circular error probability (CEP) for the 3-moment consistency fit (not the inferior 2-moment consistency fit used by Patnaik and Grubbs). It is easy to see that we have four input parameters: two standard deviations of the Gaussian pdf and two components of the displacement vector of the center of the circle of consideration. Most formulations of CEP are restricted to the special case of CEP with zero displacement vector.

14.9 Summary

In this chapter, we used concepts from statistics to derive a method for rapidly computing the direct problem (determine the probability when the spherical region is given) and also the inverse problem (determine the spherical region when the probability is specified).

In Section 14.1, we reviewed the pertinent historical background of a radically different approach based on approximations by the sequential use of noncentral chi-square, then central chi-square, and finally the Gaussian distributions for dealing with the direct problem. The inverse problem was solved by reversing the sequence of transformations.

In Section 14.2, we discussed the formulation in terms of the noncentral chi-square distribution.

In Section 14.3, we described the reduction to central chi-square distribution.

In Section 14.4, we formulated the computation in terms of the Gaussian distribution.

In Section 14.5, we presented numerical results for more than 200 benchmark cases. Comparison with several cases of known exact analytical solutions indicates that this method is accurate to two significant figures.

In Section 14.6, we recommended that this analytical approximation be used when we have to evaluate very high-dimension integrals of this nature arising in statistical analysis and signal detection.

In Section 14.7, we compared the computation times between a straightforward numerical evaluation of a three-dimensional integral and the present method for the inverse problem. It is estimated that the numerical integration is 1 billion times longer if we have 1000 integration steps for each dimension.

In Section 14.8, we pointed out that by letting $n = 2$, we have the solution for the general case of CEP.

14.10 References

14.1. E. B. Wilson and M. M. Hilferty, "The Distribution of Chi Square," *Proc. Nat. Acad. Sci.*, Washington, D. C., **17**, 684–688 (1931).

14.2. P. B. Patnaik, "The Non-Central χ^2 and F Distributions and Their Applications," *Biometrika* **36**, 202–232 (1949).

14.3. R. A. Fisher, *Statistical Methods for Research Workers*, 12th ed. (Hafner Publishing Company, New York, 1954), p. 81.

14.4. E. S. Pearson, "Note on an Approximation to the Distribution of Non-Central χ^2," *Biometrika* **46**, 364 (1959).

14.5. N. L. Johnson, "On an Extension of the Connexion Between Poisson and χ^2 Distributions," *Biometrika* **46**, 352–363 (1959).

14.6. J. P. Imhof, "Computing the Distribution of Quadratic Forms in Normal Variables," *Biometrika* **48**, 419–426 (1961).

14.7. F. E. Grubbs, "Approximate Circular and Non-Circular Probabilities of Hitting," *Operations Research* **12**, 51–61 (1964).

14.8. A. Grad and H. Solomon, "Distribution of Quadratic Forms and Some Applications," *Ann. Math. Stat.* **26**, 464–477 (1955).

14.9. J. Pachares, "Note on the Distribution of a Definite Quadratic Form," *Ann. Math. Stat.* **26**, 128–131 (1955).

14.10. B. K. Shah and C. G. Khatri, "Distribution of a Definite Quadratic Form for Non-Central Normal Variables," *Ann. Math. Stat.* **32**, 883–887 (1961).

14.11. R. C. Terzian, "Discussion of a Note on CEPs," *IEEE Trans. Aerospace and Electronic Systems* (September 1974).

14.12. M. Kendall, A. Stuart, and J. K. Ord, *Kendall's Advanced Theory of Statistics*, 5th ed. (Oxford University Press, New York, 1987), pp. 73, 507.

14.13. E. A. Cornish and R. A. Fisher, "Moments and Cumulants in the Specification of Distributions," *Rev. Int. Stat. Inst.* **5**, 307 (1937).

14.14. D. B. Peizer and J. W. Pratt, "A Normal Approximation for Binomial, F, Beta, and Other Common Related Tail Probabilities I," *J. Amer. Stat. Assoc.* **63**, 1416 (1968).

14.15. J. W. Pratt, "A Normal Approximation for Binomial, F, Beta, and Other Common Related Tail Probabilities II," *J. Amer. Stat. Assoc.* **63**, 1457 (1968).

14.16. F. K. Chan, "Analytical Expression for the Inverse Error Function," 2002 (unpublished).

14.17. F. K. Chan, "Circular Error Probability with Zero Displacement," 2002 (unpublished).

Chapter 15: Computer Programs

15.1 Introduction

This chapter gives an overview of the Excel macros that were used to generate all numerical tables, graphical plots, and other supporting information in this book. As expected, most of these computer programs are devoted to the computation of the probability of short-term collisions for operational spacecraft and also for the International Space Station (ISS). However, they are not restricted to just these topics. Many additional programs have been developed for other topics, such as the computation of the error function and its inverse, the transition from small to large arguments, the Rician integral and its inverse, and the circular error probability and the spherical error probability for use in geolocation. The algorithm for computing the sun vector is made available for the reader to use for the years 1961 to 2060.

The following sections correspond to chapters with the same numbers.

15.2 Spacecraft Encounters

15.2.1 Combined Covariance General.xls

This algorithm computes the combined covariance for the "general simplified model." The alignment of the covariance ellipsoid with the coordinate axes for both the objects is referred to as the general simplified model if the velocity magnitudes and the covariances of the primary and the secondary are not assumed to be equal as depicted in Fig. 2.2 of Chapter 2. The algorithm computes the components C_{11}, C_{12}, C_{22}, and C_{33} according to Eq. (2.22) and also the aspect ratio of the ellipse in the encounter plane as a function of the angle between the velocities $\mathbf{v}_p$ and $\mathbf{v}_s$. Sample results are shown in Figs. 2.14 and 2.15 and also Table 2.3.

15.2.2 Combined Covariance Special.xls

This algorithm computes the combined covariance for the "special simplified model." The alignment of the covariance ellipsoid with the coordinate axes for both the objects is referred to as the special simplified model if the velocity magnitudes and the covariances of the primary and the secondary are assumed to be equal as depicted in Fig. 2.3 of Chapter 2. The algorithm computes the components C_{11}, C_{22}, and C_{33} (note that $C_{12} = 0$) according to Eq. (2.26) and also the aspect ratio of the ellipse in the encounter plane as a function of the angle between the velocities $\mathbf{v}_p$ and $\mathbf{v}_s$. Sample results are shown in Figs. 2.7 and 2.8 and also Table 2.1.

15.2.3 Minimum Separation Special.xls

This algorithm computes the minimum separation x_e and the elevation angle θ. It considers the case for which the primary P and the secondary S approach each other with equal speeds v at an angle $\phi = 90$ deg in the projection (X, Y)-plane as depicted in Fig. 2.10 of Chapter 2. It computes the minimum separation and the elevation according to Eqs. (2.35) and (2.36) as a function of the vertical separation H of an overhead encounter, the speed v, and the time offset from overhead encounter T. Sample results are shown in Fig. 2.11 and Table 2.2.

15.2.4 Combined Covariance General Ultra Regime for $\mathbf{v_p} > \mathbf{v_s}$.xls

This algorithm computes the ultrasmall regime combined covariance for the general simplified model for the case of $\mathbf{v}_p > \mathbf{v}_s$. It computes the components C_{11}, C_{12}, C_{22}, and C_{33} according to Eq. (2.22) and also the aspect ratio of the ellipse in the encounter plane as a function of the angle between the velocities $\mathbf{v}_p$ and $\mathbf{v}_s$. It is similar to Combined Covariance General.xls except that the angle lies within the ultrasmall region from 0 to 0.2 deg instead of the region from 0 to 180 deg. Sample results are shown in Figs. 2.16 and 2.17.

15.2.5 Combined Covariance General Ultra Regime for $\mathbf{v_p} < \mathbf{v_s}$.xls

This algorithm computes the ultrasmall regime combined covariance for the general simplified model for the case of $\mathbf{v}_p < \mathbf{v}_s$. It computes the components C_{11}, C_{12}, C_{22}, and C_{33} according to Eq. (2.22) and also the aspect ratio of the ellipse in the encounter plane as a function of the angle between the velocities $\mathbf{v}_p$ and $\mathbf{v}_s$. It is similar to Combined Covariance General.xls except that the angle lies within the ultrasmall region from 0 to 0.2 deg instead of the region from 0 to 180 deg. Sample results are shown in Figs. 2.18 and 2.19.

15.3 The Encounter Region

15.3.1 Spacecraft Linear Motion Approximation LEO1.xls

This algorithm computes the accuracy of the spacecraft linear motion approximation in the encounter region. The angle ϕ between the two velocities ranges from 5 to 30 deg and the radial error D ranges from 10 to 100 m. The algorithm computes the linear path length L, the error $E \equiv (L - C)$ between L and the actual curved path length C, and the ingress separation distance S between the two spacecraft according to Eqs. (3.6) through (3.13) as functions of ϕ and the radial error D. Sample results are shown in Table 3.1.

15.3.2 Spacecraft Linear Motion Approximation LEO2.xls

This algorithm computes the accuracy of the spacecraft linear motion approximation in the encounter region. The angle ϕ between the two velocities ranges from 5 to 30 deg and the radial error D ranges from 100 to 1000 m. The algorithm computes the linear path length L, the error $E \equiv (L - C)$ between L and the actual curved path length C, and the ingress separation distance S between the two spacecraft according to Eqs. (3.6) through (3.13) as functions of ϕ and the radial error D. Sample results are shown in Table 3.1.

15.3.3 Spacecraft Linear Motion Approximation LEO3.xls

This algorithm computes the accuracy of the spacecraft linear motion approximation in the encounter region. The angle ϕ between the two velocities ranges from 30 to 180 deg and the radial error D ranges from 10 to 100 m. The algorithm computes the linear path length L, the error $E \equiv (L - C)$ between L and the actual curved path length C, and the ingress separation distance S between the two spacecraft according to Eqs. (3.6) through (3.13) as functions of ϕ and the radial error D. Sample results are shown in Table 3.1.

15.3.4 Spacecraft Linear Motion Approximation LEO4.xls

This algorithm computes the accuracy of the spacecraft linear motion approximation in the encounter region. The angle ϕ between the two velocities ranges from 30 to 180 deg and the radial error D ranges from 100 to 1000 m. The algorithm computes the linear path length L, the error $\mathrm{E} \equiv (L - C)$ between L and the actual curved path length C, and the ingress separation distance S between the two spacecraft according to Eqs. (3.6) through (3.13) as functions of ϕ and the radial error D. Sample results are shown in Table 3.1.

15.3.5 Spacecraft Linear Motion Approximation GEO1.xls

This algorithm computes the accuracy of the spacecraft linear motion approximation in the encounter region. The angle ϕ between the two velocities ranges from 1 to 6 deg and the radial error D ranges from 1 to 10 km. The algorithm computes the linear path length L, the error $E \equiv (L - C)$ between L and the actual curved path length C, and the ingress separation distance S between the two spacecraft according to Eqs. (3.6) through (3.13) as functions of ϕ and the radial error D. Sample results are shown in Table 3.2.

15.3.6 Spacecraft Linear Motion Approximation GEO2.xls

This algorithm computes the accuracy of the spacecraft linear motion approximation in the encounter region. The angle ϕ between the two velocities ranges from 1 to 6 deg and the radial error D ranges from 10 to 100 km. The algorithm computes the linear path length L, the error $E \equiv (L - C)$ between L and the actual curved path length C, and the ingress separation distance S between the two spacecraft according to Eqs. (3.6) through (3.13) as functions of ϕ and the radial error D. Sample results are shown in Table 3.2.

15.4 The Isotropic Problem

15.4.1 Rician PDF.xls

This algorithm computes the Rician probability density function (pdf) as a function of the radius R when σ and x_e are given as parameters. It computes the pdf according to Eq. (4.5). Sample results are shown in Fig. 4.3.

15.4.2 Spacecraft Collision Probability for Circle Rician Strips.xls

This algorithm computes the probability of collision between two orbiting objects as a function of σ, x_e, and r_A. It determines the order m of the series by using rectangular strips of $u \equiv (r_A/\sigma)^2$ and $v \equiv (x_e/\sigma)^2$ as follows: If $u \leq 10$ or $v \leq 10$, then $m = 10$; else $m = 100$. The algorithm computes the collision probability according to Eqs. (4.34) through (4.39). It is used in constructing Tables 4.1 through 4.3.

15.4.3 Spacecraft Collision Probability for Circle Rician Square Root.xls

This algorithm computes the probability of collision between two orbiting objects as a function of σ, x_e, and r_A. It determines the order m of the series by using the square root of the product uv where $u \equiv (r_A/\sigma)^2$ and $v \equiv (x_e/\sigma)^2$ as follows: Let $M = \text{Int}[\sqrt{(uv)} + 1]$. If $M \leq 100$, then $m = M$; else $m = 101$. The algorithm computes the collision probability according to Eqs. (4.34) through (4.39). It is used in constructing Tables 4.1 through 4.3.

15.4.4 Spacecraft Collision Probability for Circle Rician Combined.xls

This algorithm computes the probability of collision between two orbiting objects as a function of σ, x_e, and r_A. It determines the order m of the series by combining the features in the algorithms of Sections 16.4.2 and 16.4.3 through the use of Table 4.2 and $u \equiv (r_A/\sigma)^2$ and $v \equiv (x_e/\sigma)^2$ as follows: If $u \leq 0.01$ or $v \leq 1$, then $m = 3$; if $0.01 < u \leq 1$ or $1 < v \leq 9$, then $m = 10$; if $1 < u \leq 25$ or $9 < v \leq 25$, then $m = 30$; else $m = 60$. The algorithm computes the collision probability according to Eqs. (4.34) through (4.39). Henceforth, it is used as the basic algorithm described in Section 16.5.1 to compute the collision probability in Chapters 5, 6, and 13.

15.5 Analytical Expressions for Short-Term Encounters

15.5.1 Spacecraft Collision Probability for Circle Rician Cartesian.xls

This algorithm computes the probability of collision between two orbiting objects as a function of σ, x_e, and r_A. It is structurally the same as the algorithm described in Section 16.4.4 except that it is generalized, by the introduction of equivalent area, to compute the collision probability for the case of nonisotropic Gaussian pdf in the encounter plane. The inputs are Cartesian coordinates of the primary object in the encounter plane. The coordinate axes (x', z') coincide with the principal axes of the covariance ellipses in the encounter plane. The algorithm computes the collision probability according to Eqs. (5.21), (5.22), and (5.25).

15.5.2 Spacecraft Collision Probability for Circle Rician Polar.xls

This algorithm computes the probability of collision between two orbiting objects as a function of σ, x_e, and r_A. It is essentially the same as the algorithm described in Section 16.5.1 except that the inputs are polar coordinates of the primary object in the encounter plane. The coordinate axes (x', z') coincide with the principal axes of the covariance ellipses in the encounter plane. The algorithm computes the collision probability according to Eqs. (5.21) through (5.24).

15.5.3 Spacecraft Collision Probability for Circle Contour Integral.xls

This algorithm computes the probability of collision between two orbiting objects as a function of σ, x_e, and r_A. The inputs are in Cartesian coordinates of the primary object in the encounter plane. The coordinate axes (x', z') coincide with the principal axes of the covariance ellipses in the encounter plane. The algorithm uses polar coordinates for numerical integration to compute the collision probability. It computes the collision probability according to Eqs. (5.33) through (5.34).

15.5.4 Spacecraft Collision Probability for Circle Error Function Simpson.xls

This algorithm computes the probability of collision between two orbiting objects as a function of σ, x_e, and r_A. The inputs are in Cartesian coordinates of the primary object in the encounter plane. The coordinate axes (x', z') coincide with the principal axes of the covariance ellipses in the encounter plane. The algorithm uses Simpson's rule for numerical integration to compute the collision probability. It computes the collision probability according to Eq. (5.35).

15.5.5 Spacecraft Collision Probability for Circle Error Function Trapezoidal.xls

This algorithm computes the probability of collision between two orbiting objects as a function of σ, x_e, and r_A. The inputs are in Cartesian coordinates of the primary object in the encounter plane. The coordinate axes (x', z') coincide with the principal axes of the covariance ellipses in the encounter plane. The algorithm uses the trapezoidal rule for numerical integration to compute the collision probability. It computes the collision probability according to Eq. (5.35).

15.5.6 Spacecraft Collision Probability for Circle NASA Simpson.xls

This algorithm computes the probability of collision between two orbiting objects as a function of σ, x_e, and r_A. The inputs are in "polar" coordinates (referenced to the z'-axis) in the encounter plane. The coordinate axes (x', z') coincide with the principal axes of the covariance ellipses in the encounter plane. The algorithm uses Euler's method for the inner loop (angle integration) and Simpson's rule for the outer loop (radius integration) for numerical integration to compute the collision probability. It computes the collision probability according to Eq. (5.30).

15.5.7 Spacecraft Collision Probability for Circle Compare Algorithms.xls

This algorithm computes the probability of collision between two orbiting objects as a function of σ, x_e, and r_A. It compares the probability of collision for the NASA, Patera, Alfano, and Chan models using the NASA model as the basis of comparison. Sample results on Sheet 1 are shown in Tables 5.1 through 5.3.

15.5.8 Spacecraft Collision Probability for Rectangle Rician.xls

This algorithm computes the probability of collision between two orbiting objects as a function of σ, x_e, and dimensions of the rectangle. The inputs are in Cartesian coordinates of the primary object in the encounter plane. The coordinate axes (x', z') coincide with the principal axes of the covariance ellipses in the encounter plane. The algorithm computes the collision probability according to Eqs. (5.21), (5.22), and (5.25). Sample results on Sheet 2 are shown in Tables 5.4, 5.5, and 5.8.

15.5.9 Spacecraft Collision Probability for Rectangle Contour Integral.xls

This algorithm computes the probability of collision between two orbiting objects as a function of σ, x_e, and dimensions of the rectangle. The inputs are in Cartesian coordinates of the primary object in the encounter plane. The coordinate axes (x', z') coincide with the principal axes of the covariance ellipses in the encounter plane. The algorithm uses polar coordinates for numerical integration to compute the collision probability. Sample results on Sheet 2 are shown in Tables 5.4, 5.5, and 5.8.

15.5.10 Spacecraft Collision Probability for Rectangle Error Function.xls

This algorithm computes the probability of collision between two orbiting objects as a function of σ, x_e, and dimensions of the rectangle. The inputs are in Cartesian coordinates of the primary object in the encounter plane. The coordinate axes (x', z') coincide with the principal axes of the covariance ellipses in the encounter plane. The algorithm uses the trapezoidal rule for numerical integration to compute the collision probability. Sample results on Sheet 2 are shown in Tables 5.4, 5.5, and 5.8.

15.5.11 Spacecraft Collision Probability for Triangle Rician.xls

This algorithm computes the probability of collision between two orbiting objects as a function of σ, x_e, and dimensions of the triangle. The inputs are in Cartesian coordinates of the primary object in the encounter plane. The coordinate axes (x', z') coincide with the principal axes of the covariance ellipses in the encounter plane. The algorithm computes the collision probability according to Eqs. (5.21), (5.22), and (5.25). Sample results on Sheet 3 are shown in Tables 5.6, 5.7, and 5.8.

15.5.12 Spacecraft Collision Probability for Triangle Contour Integral.xls

This algorithm computes the probability of collision between two orbiting objects as a function of σ, x_e, and dimensions of the triangle. The inputs are in Cartesian coordinates of the primary object in the encounter plane. The coordinate axes (x', z') coincide with the principal axes of the covariance ellipses in the encounter plane. The algorithm uses polar coordinates for numerical integration to compute the collision probability. Sample results on Sheet 3 are shown in Tables 5.6, 5.7, and 5.8.

15.5.13 Spacecraft Collision Probability for Triangle Error Function.xls

This algorithm computes the probability of collision between two orbiting objects as a function of σ, x_e, and dimensions of the triangle. The inputs are in Cartesian coordinates of the primary object in the encounter plane. The coordinate axes (x',

z') coincide with the principal axes of the covariance ellipses in the encounter plane. The algorithm uses the trapezoidal rule for numerical integration to compute the collision probability. Sample results on Sheet 3 are shown in Tables 5.6, 5.7, and 5.8.

15.6 International Space Station Collision Probability

15.6.1 ISS Collision Probability

This algorithm computes the probability of collision between the ISS and a secondary orbiting object as a function of σ and miss distance. The secondary is assumed to be small compared to the ISS or its components. The miss distance is measured from the center of the secondary to the origin of the ISS body coordinate system. The offset of the ISS center of mass from the origin can be included in the detailed computations as necessary. The time of the encounter is used to compute the sun vector, which determines the directional pointing of the huge (70 m × 110 m) solar panels. Details of the formulation are given in Chapter 6. Sample results on Sheets 1, 2, and 3 are shown in Tables 6.3, 6.4, and 6.5.

15.6.2 Sun Vector Computation Custom Fitted Coefficients Averaged.xls

This spreadsheet displays the coefficients obtained by custom-fitting the sun vector for the years 1989 to 2007. The results are shown in Table A.1 of Appendix A. The average/linear fits to these coefficients are shown in Figs. A.5 through A.9. They are given in Eq. (A.11) to be used for computing the sun vector for the years 1961 to 2060.

15.6.3 Sun Vector Computation 2008.xls

This spreadsheet computes the sun vector for the year 2008. Use Sheet 0 to enter inputs for cells B3 and B4. Enter the desired (Day + Fraction of Day) into cell B31. Read the right ascension and declination in cells F31 and G31.

15.6.4 Sun Vector Cone Angle Computation 2007.xls

This spreadsheet computes the sun vector cone angle for the year 2007. Sample results are shown in Fig. 6.8.

15.7 Maneuvers to Mitigate Potential Collision Threats

15.7.1 Intrack Thrusting Maneuvers.xls

This algorithm computes the amount of thrust ($\Delta v_{\text{intrack}}$) necessary to reduce an unacceptable collision probability (P) to an acceptable threshold value (P') when only intrack thrusting is performed. The details are given in Chapter 7. Sample results are given on Sheet 2.

15.8 Analytical Expressions for Long-Term Encounters

15.8.1 Spacecraft Collision Probability for Long-Term Encounters 1-Term.xls

This algorithm computes and compares the one-term analytical and numerical long-term probability of collision between two orbiting objects in which the secondary executes a nominal circular Clohessy-Wiltshire orbit whose center may be offset from the primary. The inputs are the combined σ, the offset distance, the circular orbit radius R, and the combined radii r of the primary and the secondary. The algorithm computes the collision probability according to Eqs. (8.65) and (8.58). Sample results are shown on Sheet 2.

15.8.2 Spacecraft Collision Probability for Long-Term Encounters 20-Term.xls

This algorithm computes and compares the 20-term analytical and numerical long-term probability of collision between two orbiting objects in which the secondary executes a nominal circular Clohessy-Wiltshire orbit whose center may be offset from the primary. The inputs are the combined σ, the offset distance, the circular orbit radius R, and the combined radii r of the primary and the secondary. The algorithm computes the collision probability according to Eqs. (8.65) and (8.58). Sample results are shown on Sheet 2.

15.9 Short-Term vs. Long-Term Spacecraft Encounters

15.9.1 Shortest Distance.xls

This algorithm computes the shortest distance between two orbiting objects in which the secondary executes a nominal elliptic Clohessy-Wiltshire relative orbit whose center may be offset from the primary. The inputs are the semimajor axis A of the ellipse, the aspect ratio of the ellipse, and the displacement C of the primary from the center of the ellipse. It computes the shortest distance according to Eqs. (9.11), (9.13), and (9.14). Sample results are shown in Fig. 9.2 and on Sheet 2.

15.9.2 Spacecraft Collision Probability for Long-Term vs Short-Term Analytical.xls

This algorithm computes the probability of collision between two orbiting objects in which the secondary executes a nominal elliptic Clohessy-Wiltshire relative orbit whose center may be offset from the primary. The inputs are the semimajor axis A of the ellipse and the displacement C of the primary from the center of the ellipse. The aspect ratio of the ellipse is implicitly set equal to 2. The algorithm computes the short-term collision probability computation according to Eqs. (4.19), (9.15), and (9.16) and the long-term collision probability computation according to Eq. (9.29).

Three case studies were considered. For Case Study I (Concentric Ellipses, Primary at Center), sample results are shown in Figs. 9.4 and 9.5 and on Sheet 2. For Case Study II (Fixed Size Ellipses, Variable Apsidal Distances), sample results are shown in Figs. 9.7 and 9.8 and on Sheet 3A. For Case Study III (Variable Size Ellipses, Fixed Apsidal Distances), sample results are shown in Figs. 9.10 and 9.11 and on Sheet 5A.

15.9.3 Spacecraft Collision Probability for Long-Term vs Short-Term Enhanced.xls

This algorithm computes the probability of collision between two orbiting objects in which the secondary executes a nominal elliptic Clohessy-Wiltshire relative orbit whose center may be offset from the primary. The inputs are the semimajor axis A of the ellipse and the displacement C of the primary from the center of the ellipse. The aspect ratio of the ellipse is implicitly set equal to 2. The algorithm is essentially the same as the one in Section 16.9.2 except that it computes the short-term collision probability computation according to Eqs. (9.15), (9.16), and (4.19) and the long-term collision probability computation according to Eqs. (B.1) through (B.32) of Appendix B.

Three case studies were considered. For Case Study I (Concentric Ellipses, Primary at Center), sample results are shown in Figs. 9.4 and 9.5 and on Sheet 2. For Case Study II (Fixed Size Ellipses, Variable Apsidal Distances), sample results are shown in Figs. 9.7 and 9.8 and on Sheet 3A. For Case Study III (Variable Size Ellipses, Fixed Apsidal Distances), sample results are shown in Figs. 9.10 and 9.11 and on Sheets 5A1 and 5A2. Note that Sheet 5A of the algorithm in Section 16.9.2 has been replaced by Sheets 5A1 and 5A2, which collectively cover a larger range of values for the semimajor axis. It is recommended that this algorithm be used preferentially.

15.10 Formation Flying

No algorithm has been developed for this section. However, as pointed out in Chapter 10, serious consideration should be given to the implementation of an algorithm based on Eqs. (10.1) and (10.2) for the computation of the relative motion of a spacecraft referenced to a general elliptic orbit in a general gravitational field with drag and solar radiation effects. In this formulation, we have an algorithm for obtaining a whole slew of high-precision orbits with perturbations in terms of *only one numerical high-precision orbit and the difference between two analytical J_2 orbits* (one with perturbations and the other with no perturbations) by using the analytical theories of Kozai and Brouwer for the main problem of artificial satellite theory. For more discussion, see Section 10.3 of Chapter 10.

15.11 Maximum Probability of Collision

15.11.1 Gaussian Probability Density Function.xls

This algorithm computes the Gaussian pdf. The inputs are the range of the argument and the standard deviation. The algorithm computes the pdf according to Eq. (11.1). Sample results are given in Fig. 11.1 and Sheet 2.

15.11.2 Maximum Probability.xls

This algorithm computes the maximum probability. The first method uses the maximum likelihood based on Eq. (11.13) of Chapter 11. It is valid for all values of θ between 10 and 90 deg if $r_A/x_e \leq 0.1$. The second method is based only on the first term of the Rician integral given by Eq. (4.19) of Chapter 4. It is valid for all values of θ between 0 and 90 deg if $r_A/x_e \leq 0.3$ and for θ between 10 and 90 deg if $0.3 \leq r_A/x_e \leq 1$. Eq. (11.15) is used for values of θ between 0 and 10 deg if $r_A/x_e \leq 1$. The inputs are r_A, x_e, and θ. Sample results are shown in Figs. 11.2 and Tables 11.1 and 11.2 of Chapter 11.

15.12 Close Encounters with Multiple Satellites

15.12.1 Spacecraft Collision Probability with Multiple Satellites.xls

This algorithm computes the expected number of collisions per orbit $N_{\text{total,orbit}}$ for a spacecraft moving in a circular orbit within a spherical layer of debris of a specified thickness. The debris are classified according to the interval containing the inclination of their orbits. The algorithm computes $N_{\text{total,orbit}}$ according to Eqs. (12.32) through (12.35). Sample results are shown in Tables 12.1 and 12.2.

15.13 Instantaneous Probability of Collision

15.13.1 Error Function.xls

This algorithm computes the error function and the inverse error function. For the error function, the input argument is X. For the inverse error function, the input argument is Y. The algorithm will automatically return the appropriate answer. It computes the error function according to Eq. (13.14) or (13.18), and computes the inverse error function using Eq. (14.50) as the seed for Newton's iterative method. Sample results are shown on Sheet 2.

15.13.2 Error Function Comparison.xls

This algorithm computes and compares the values of the error function using the convergent series and the asymptotic series. Sample results are shown on Sheets 2 and 3 and in Chart 1.

15.13.3 Error Function Transition.xls

This algorithm computes the transition point for the error function between the convergent series and the asymptotic series. Sample results are shown on Sheet 2.

15.13.4 Error Function Accuracy Test.xls

This algorithm tests the accuracy of the computation of the error function as a function of the argument and the number of terms used in computing the series. Sample results are shown on Sheet 2.

15.13.5 Instantaneous Collision Probability Analytical.xls

This algorithm computes the probability within a sphere of radius R by the method of approximating distributions and the method of equivalent volume. The order m in the Rician series is determined by the combined method (see the algorithm in Section 16.4.4). Sample results are shown in Tables 13.1 through 13.5, which are derived from Sheet 2; Table 13.6, from Sheet 6; and Fig. 13.1, from Chart 1.

15.13.6 Instantaneous Collision Probability Numerical.xls

This algorithm computes the probability within a sphere of radius R by numerical integration. Sample results are shown on Sheets 2 through 4, which are used in Tables 13.2 through 13.5.

15.14 Spherical Error Probability Computation

15.14.1 CEP Algorithm.xls

This circular error probability (CEP) algorithm computes the radius of the circle when σ_x, σ_y (both in the same units) and the probability (between 0 and 1) are specified. The result is accurate to approximately 14 significant figures for aspect ratios of the ellipse up to 100 and probability values up to 0.999.

15.14.2 Inverse Rician Algorithm.xls

This algorithm computes the radius of integration of the Rician integral when given the probability, bias, and σ. Sample results are shown on Sheet 2.

15.14.3 CEP Algorithm with Plots.xls

This algorithm is basically the same as the algorithm of Section 16.14.1, except that it executes and plots a batch of runs instead of a single run. Sample results are shown on Sheet 2 and in Chart 1.

15.14.4 Spherical Error Probability 2D Isotropic PDF.xls

This algorithm computes the spherical error probability (SEP) for the special case of an isotropic two-dimensional Gaussian pdf. Sample results are shown on Sheet 2.

15.14.5 Spherical Error Probability 3D Isotropic PDF.xls

This algorithm computes the SEP for the special case of an isotropic three-dimensional Gaussian pdf. Sample results are shown on Sheet 2.

15.14.6 Spherical Error Probability Calculation.xls

This algorithm computes the SEP. Sample results are shown in Tables 14.1 and 14.2, which are derived from Sheet 6, and in Fig. 13.2 in Chapter 13, which is derived from Chart 1.

15.14.7 Spherical Error Probability Compare.xls

This algorithm computes and compares the SEP by using the three-moments and the two-moments matching algorithms. For the case of zero offset, it compares the results with the exact values obtained by using the inverse error function. Sample results are shown in Tables 14.3 and 14.4, which are derived from Sheets 5 and 6.

15.15 Instructions for Using the Programs

The algorithms have been tested and are accurate to the precision indicated. Invariably, they have been chosen as perhaps the best available from the standpoint of computational speed and numerical stability over a wide range of parameters. More important, each Excel macro has been designed to be self-contained and easy to use. The user need only enter the clearly labeled input data and then press the RUN button on the first (primary) worksheet. The output results are clearly displayed on the same spreadsheet. If applicable, there may be graphical plots in addition to supporting secondary spreadsheets.

The software may be downloaded from the AIAA Web site for the reader's private use. (See the "Supporting Materials" section at the end of this book for instructions on downloading.) The equations and the variable names used in the code follow very closely the corresponding ones used in each chapter. This practice eliminates the need for mathematical specifications and documentation of the software.

If the worksheet is protected, then use the password "Aerospace." The tabulated results serve as benchmarks that the reader may wish to retain to check the algorithms.

Appendix A: A Novel Algorithm for Computing the Sun Vector

This appendix describes the computation of the sun vector using an approach different from the one presently employed in sources such as the *Astronomical Almanac*.[A.1] (See the "Explanatory Supplement to the Astronomical Almanac"[A.2] for construction of the Jet Propulsion Laboratory (JPL)/Solar, Lunar and Planetary (SLP) files.) Just as the planetary and lunar ephemerides in the JPL/SLP files are based on a least-squares fit to observational data and subsequent numerical integration of the dynamical equations of motion, this algorithm draws its input information from tables of the sun vector in the *Astronomical Almanac*. The following process describes how the computation is done.

The fundamental problem is to obtain the coefficients A', B', C', A'', B'', C'', A''', and C''' in Eq. (6.36) of Chapter 6. The user need not be aware of this procedure in all its detail (because those coefficients have already been obtained and are shown in Table A.1) but merely needs to use the rather simple equation (6.36) to compute the sun vector—hence the inclusion of the procedure in an appendix.

Table A.1. Yearly Values of Custom-Fitted Coefficients

Year	Time of Vernal Equinox	Obliquity (deg)	A'	B'	C'	A''	B''	C''	A'''	C'''
1989	79.644695	23.440722	1.8	0.0285	15	0.1137	−0.015	8	0.0215	148
1990	79.888401	23.440592	1.8	0.0285	15	0.113	0.036	10.1	0.0214	149
1991	80.126336	23.440462	1.8	0.0285	15	0.114	−0.01	9.35	0.0205	149
1992	80.366728	23.440332	1.8	0.0285	15	0.1149	−0.005	8.4	0.0195	150
1993	79.611581	23.440202	1.8	0.0285	15	0.1148	0.028	8.5	0.02	149
1994	79.852792	23.440072	1.8	0.0285	15	0.1153	−0.009	8.96	0.0205	148
1995	80.093386	23.439942	1.8	0.0285	15	0.1192	0.031	10.65	0.0206	148.5
1996	80.33552	23.439812	1.8	0.0285	15	0.1208	0.018	10.43	0.0215	149
1997	79.579661	23.439682	1.8	0.0285	15	0.1182	0.021	10.36	0.021	150
1998	79.829564	23.439552	1.8	0.0285	15	0.1158	0.042	13.05	0.02	150
1999	80.073533	23.439422	1.8	0.0285	15	0.1159	0.019	12.8	0.0195	149
2000	80.316221	23.439292	1.8	0.0285	15	0.1147	0.0035	11.85	0.02	149
2001	79.56311	23.439161	1.8	0.0285	15	0.1132	0.042	11.8	0.0215	149
2002	79.802953	23.439031	1.8	0.0285	15	0.1125	−0.008	11.81	0.0214	149
2003	80.041595	23.438901	1.8	0.0285	15	0.1144	0.013	12.8	0.0205	150
2004	80.283758	23.438771	1.8	0.0285	15	0.115	0.025	11.95	0.02	150
2005	79.523172	23.438641	1.8	0.0285	15	0.1141	−0.015	11.37	0.0203	149
2006	79.767705	23.438511	1.8	0.0285	15	0.1136	0.05	13.85	0.0208	148
2007	80.00507	23.438381	1.8	0.0285	15	0.1166	0.0315	14.2	0.021	148

(1) Write the true longitude θ of the sun in the form

$$\begin{aligned}\theta = \phi - A'\left[\left(1-B'\right)-\cos\left(\phi - C'\right)\right] \\ - A''\left[\left(1-B''\right)-\cos\left(\phi - C''\right)\right] \\ + A'''\cos 2\left(\phi - C'''\right)+\cdots\end{aligned} \tag{A.1}$$

where

$$\phi \equiv \varpi(t - t_{VE}) \tag{A.2}$$

t is the day plus fraction thereof from January $0^{d}.0$ in the year of interest, t_{VE} is the UT (universal time) of the vernal equinox in the year of interest, and ϖ is the rate of daily change of the geometric mean longitude of the sun (0.985647359 deg per 24 h).

(2) Obtain the right ascension α of the sun from the *Astronomical Almanac* at the end of every month in the mean of date coordinate system. We shall use year 2000 for illustration.

(3) For these times, compute θ_0 and α_0 according to the equations

$$\begin{aligned}\theta_0 &= \phi \\ \tan\alpha_0 &= \cos\varepsilon\,\tan\theta_0\end{aligned} \tag{A.3}$$

where ε is the obliquity of the ecliptic (the angle between Earth's equatorial plane and the plane of Earth's orbit around the sun). It is time-dependent, but a sufficiently accurate formula for its determination is

$$\varepsilon = 23^{\circ}.438251 - 0^{\circ}.000130(\text{Year} - 2008) \tag{A.4}$$

(4) Obtain and plot the residuals ($\alpha_0 - \alpha$) at these monthly intervals. These residuals typically do not exceed approximately 3.5 deg, as shown in Fig. A.1.

(5) Fit first harmonic trigonometric terms having approximately the same value and tangent near the vernal equinox and having approximately the same amplitude as the residual curve as shown in Fig. A.1. This procedure is used to determine A', B', and C' in Eq. (A.1), yielding

$$A' = 1.8, \qquad B' = 0.0285, \qquad C' = 15^{\circ} \tag{A.5}$$

These coefficients are retained to be the same for every year. That is, they are defined to be constants.

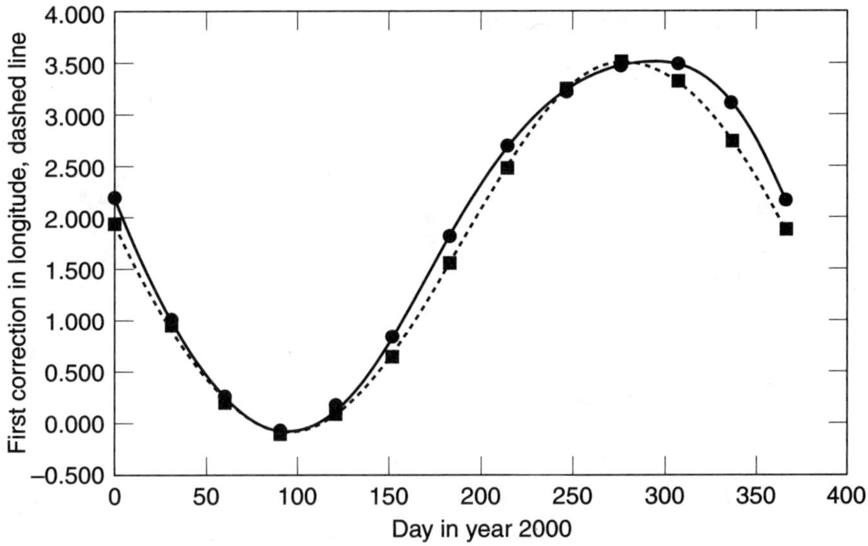

Figure A.1. Determination of first correction in longitude.

(6) Next, compute θ_1 and α_1 according to the equations

$$\theta_1 = \phi - A'\left[\left(1 - B'\right) - \cos\left(\phi - C'\right)\right] \tag{A.6}$$

$$\tan\alpha_1 = \cos\varepsilon \, \tan\theta_1$$

(7) Obtain and plot the residuals $(\alpha_1 - \alpha)$ at these monthly intervals. These residuals typically do not exceed approximately 0.25 deg, as shown in Fig. A.2. Note that these residuals are an order of magnitude smaller than the previous residuals $(\alpha_0 - \alpha)$.

(8) Fit first harmonic trigonometric terms by adjusting A'', B'', and C'' so that the resultant residual curve after this step (see Fig. A.3) has only second and higher harmonic terms. This procedure is used to determine A'', B'', and C'' in Eq. (A.1), yielding

$$A'' \approx 0.115, \qquad B'' \approx 0.0135, \qquad C'' \approx 11^\circ \tag{A.7}$$

Note that we have used the "very approximate" sign (≈) instead of the usual approximate sign (≅) in Eq. (A.7) to indicate that the variations are somewhat large. This relation is still better than the order of magnitude sign (~) often used in asymptotic analysis. These coefficients change from year to year. Throughout the nineteen-year period from 1989 to 2007, A'' varies somewhat sinusoidally between 0.113 and 0.1208, B'' varies somewhat sinusoidally between –0.021 and

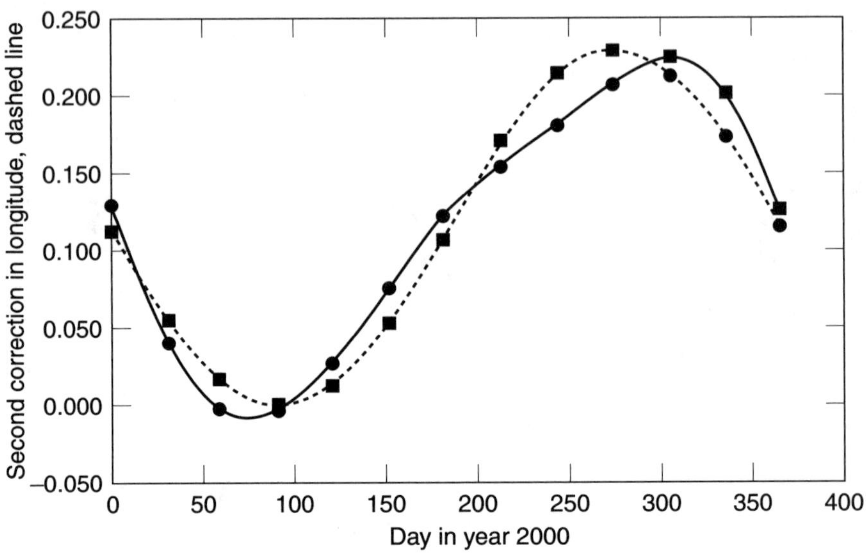

Figure A.2. Determination of second correction in longitude.

0.05, and C'' varies secularly plus somewhat sinusoidally between 8 and 14.2 deg. (The term "somewhat" here means roughly; that is, not close enough to sinusoidally to be represented by a sine function.)

(9) Next, compute θ_2 and α_2 according to the equations

$$\begin{aligned}\theta_2 &= \phi - A'\left[\left(1-B'\right)-\cos\left(\phi - C'\right)\right] \\ &\quad - A''\left[\left(1-B''\right)-\cos\left(\phi - C''\right)\right] \\ \tan\alpha_2 &= \cos\varepsilon\,\tan\theta_2\end{aligned} \tag{A.8}$$

(10) Obtain and plot the residuals ($\alpha_2 - \alpha$) at these monthly intervals. These residuals typically do not exceed approximately 0.025 deg, as shown in Fig. A.3. Note that these residuals are also an order of magnitude smaller than the previous residuals ($\alpha_1 - \alpha$).

(11) Fit second harmonic trigonometric terms to the residual curve as shown in Fig. A.3. This procedure is used to determine A''' and C''' in Eq. (A.1), yielding

$$A''' \approx 0.02, \qquad C''' \approx 149^\circ \tag{A.9}$$

These coefficients change very little from year to year. During the nineteen-year period from 1989 to 2007, A''' varies somewhat sinusoidally between 0.0195 and 0.0215, and C''' varies somewhat sinusoidally between 148 and 150 deg (the same meaning of "somewhat" as mentioned previously also applies here).

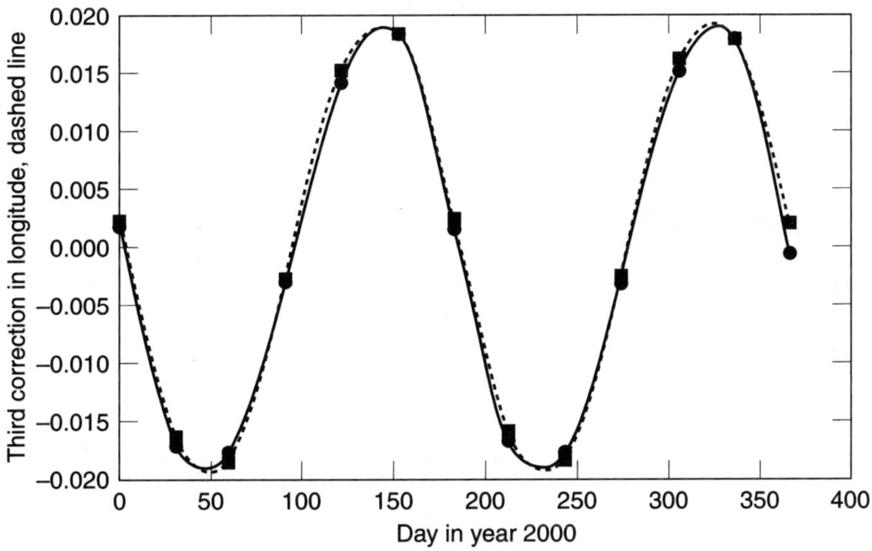

Figure A.3. Determination of third correction in longitude.

(12) Finally, compute θ_3 and α_3 according to the equations

$$\begin{aligned}\theta_3 = \phi - A'\left[\left(1-B'\right)-\cos\left(\phi-C'\right)\right]\\ - A''\left[\left(1-B''\right)-\cos\left(\phi-C''\right)\right]\\ + A'''\cos 2\left(\phi-C'''\right)\end{aligned} \quad \text{(A.10)}$$

$$\tan\alpha_3 = \cos\varepsilon\,\tan\theta_3$$

(13) Obtain and plot the residuals ($\alpha_3 - \alpha$) at these monthly intervals. These residuals typically do not exceed approximately 0.0025 deg, as shown in Fig. A.4. Note that these residuals are also an order of magnitude smaller than the previous residuals ($\alpha_2 - \alpha$).

(14) Perform these steps for every year from 1989 to 2007. The values of the coefficients A', B', C', A'', B'', C'', A''', and C''' are shown in Table A.1, which also includes the values of the time of vernal equinox and the obliquity of the ecliptic used to obtain them.

However, it is inconvenient to use these values on a yearly basis in Eq. (A.1). Moreover, this prevents us from using the equation outside this period. We recall that the coefficients A', B', and C' are set to be constant. Consequently, one simplification is to replace the coefficients A'', B'', A''', and C''' by their average values and replace C''' by the best linear fit as shown in Figs. A.5 through A.9.

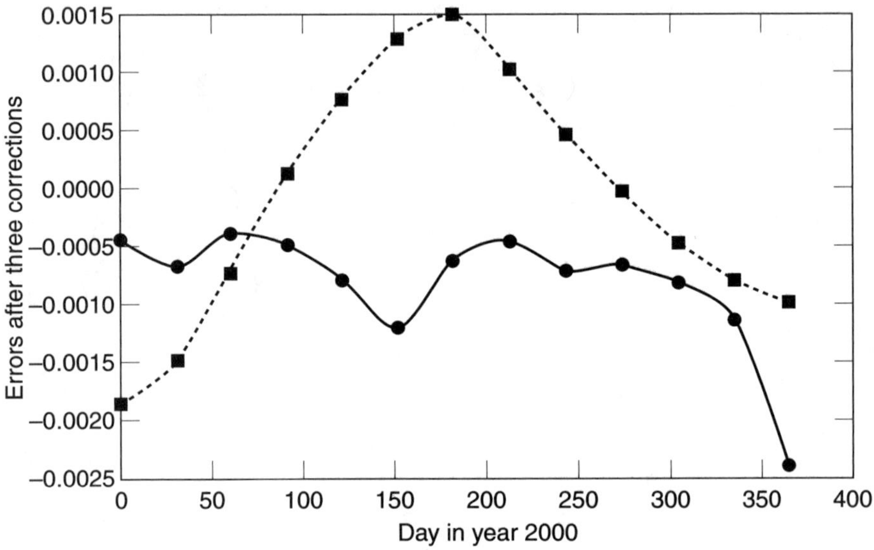

Figure A.4. Residual errors for year 2000 with custom-fitted coefficients.

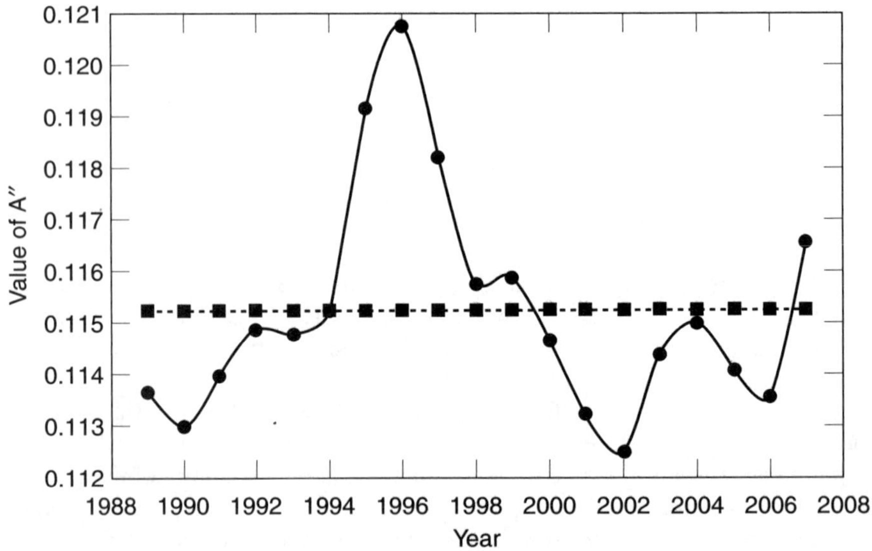

Figure A.5. Average fit to A''.

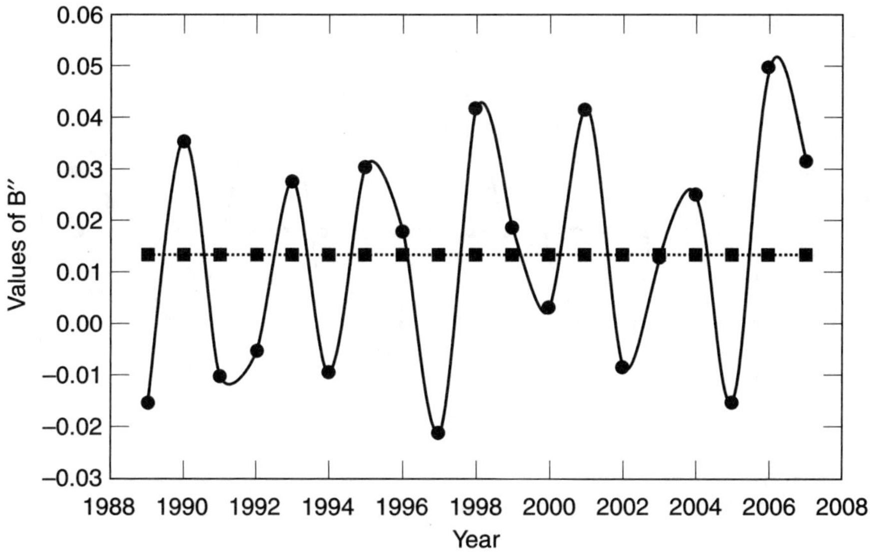

Figure A.6. Average fit to *B″*.

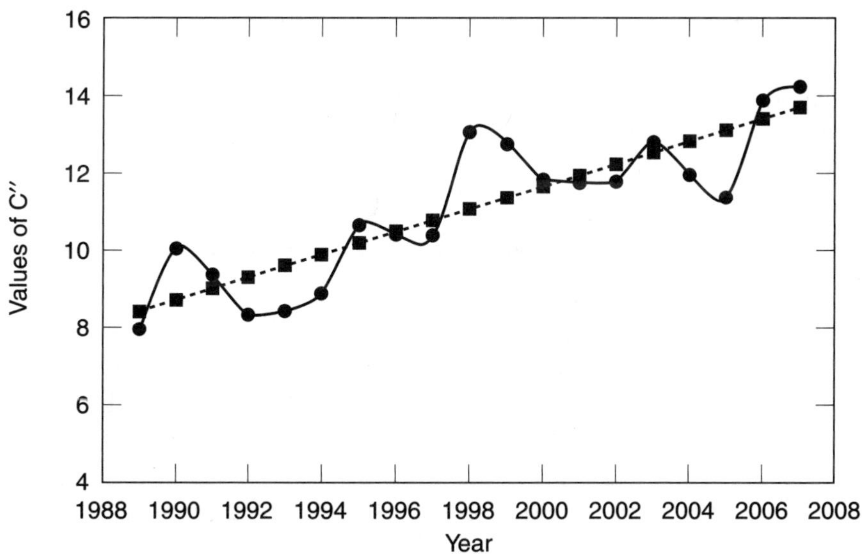

Figure A.7. Linear fit to *C″*.

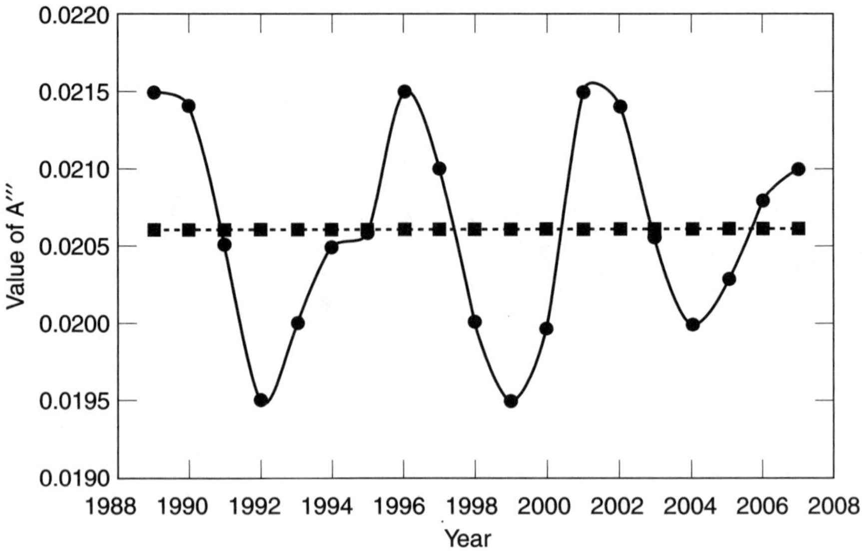

Figure A.8. Average fit to *A′′′*.

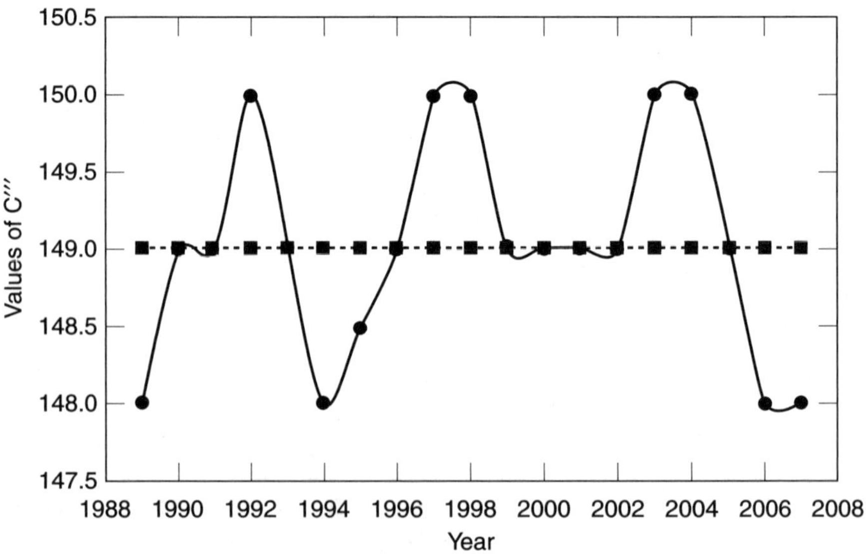

Figure A.9. Average fit to *C′′′*.

Thus, we have

$$A'' = 0.1152474, \quad B'' = 0.0134737, \quad A''' = 0.0206053, \quad C''' = 149^o$$
$$C'' = 8^o.207369 + 0^o.2857368(\text{Year} - 1988) \tag{A.11}$$

Hence, Eq. (A.1) becomes

$$\begin{aligned} \theta &= \phi - 1.7487 + 1.8\cos\left(\phi - 15^o\right) \\ &\quad - 0.113694591 + 0.1152474\cos\left(\phi - C''\right) \\ &\quad + 0.0206053\cos 2\left(\phi - 149^o\right) + \cdots \\ &= \phi - 1.862394591 + 1.8\cos\left(\phi - 15^o\right) \\ &\quad + 0.1152474\cos\left(\phi - C''\right) \\ &\quad + 0.0206053\cos 2\left(\phi - 149^o\right) + \cdots \\ C'' &= 8^o.207369 + 0^o.2857368(\text{Year} - 1988) \end{aligned} \tag{A.12}$$

Once the longitude θ is obtained from Eq. (A.12), the right ascension α and declination δ of the sun are computed by using the following equations:

$$\tan\alpha = \cos\varepsilon \tan\theta \tag{A.13}$$

$$\sin\delta = \sin\varepsilon \sin\theta \tag{A.14}$$

Equation (A.12) is strictly applicable for the nineteen-year period 1989 to 2007. However, we wish to use it outside this time interval. To do this, we need the time of the vernal equinox in other years. Table 6.1 of Chapter 6 gives this information for the 100 years from 1961 to 2060.

As a test of goodness of fit, the right ascension and declination of the sun in the year 2008 are computed using Eq. (A.12) and then compared to the corresponding values in the 2008 *Astronomical Almanac* (just published as of this writing). The residual errors are plotted in Fig. A.10. (In Figs. A.10 through A.15, solid lines show residual right ascension error; dashed lines, residual declination error.) We observe that the sun vector is accurate to approximately 5×10^{-3} deg. These residuals are approximately twice the errors (0.0025 deg) obtained by using the custom-fitted values of the coefficients A', B', C', A'', B'', C'', A''', and C''' shown in Table A.1 for the years 1989 to 2007.

Testing was also performed for some years prior to this period. We chose the years 1966, 1977, and 1988 because they are regularly spaced 11 years apart to avoid any synchronized idiosyncracies resulting from commensuration with the

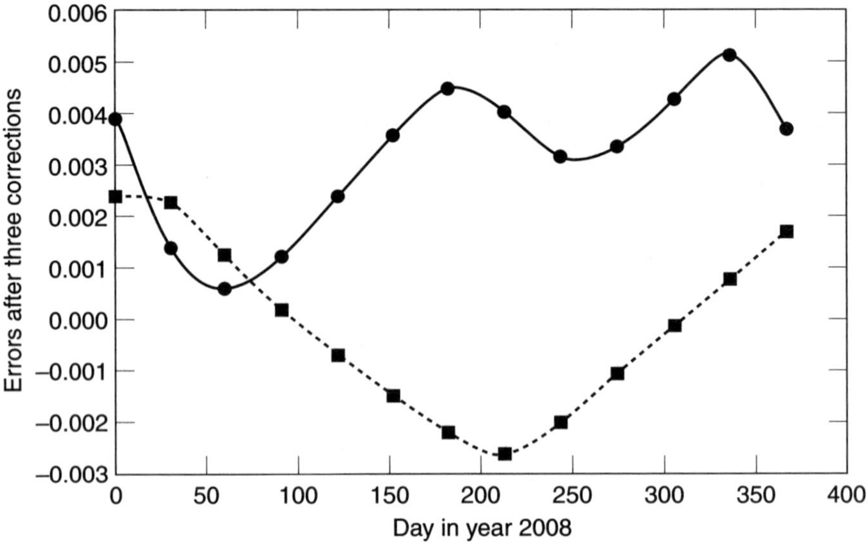

Figure A.10. Residual errors for the year 2008 with simplified average coefficients.

four-year cycle of the leap years. In addition, we have included the year 1999,which is within the time period 1989 to 2007. The residual errors are plotted in Figs. A.11 through A.14. Again, we observe that the sun vector is accurate to approximately 5×10^{-3} deg for all four years tested.

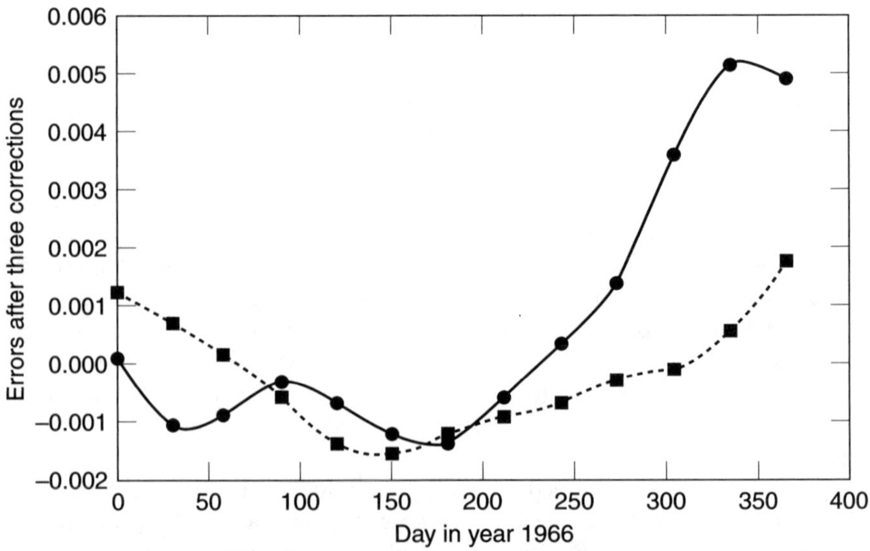

Figure A.11. Residual errors for the year 1966 with simplified average coefficients.

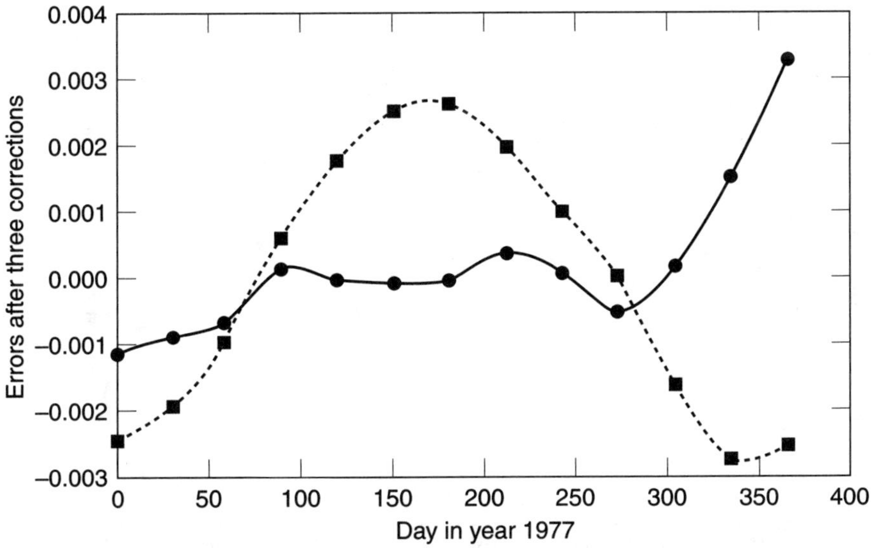

Figure A.12. Residual errors for the year 1977 with simplified average coefficients.

Specifically, for the year 1999, let us compare the errors obtained by using the simplified average values of the coefficients A', B', C', A'', B'', C'', A''', and C''' with those obtained using the custom-fitted values shown in Table A.1. The errors for the latter case are shown in Fig. A.15 and are seen to be half those of the former case shown in Fig. A.14.

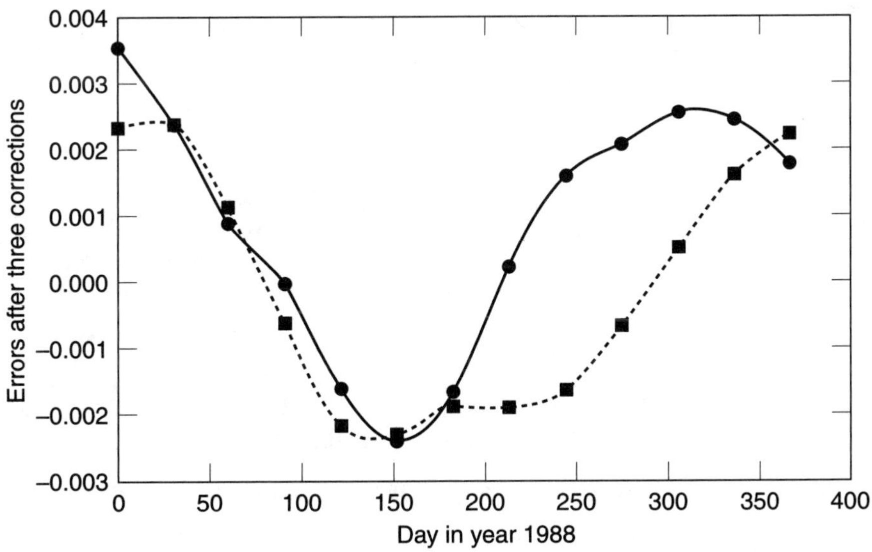

Figure A.13. Residual errors for the year 1988 with simplified average coefficients.

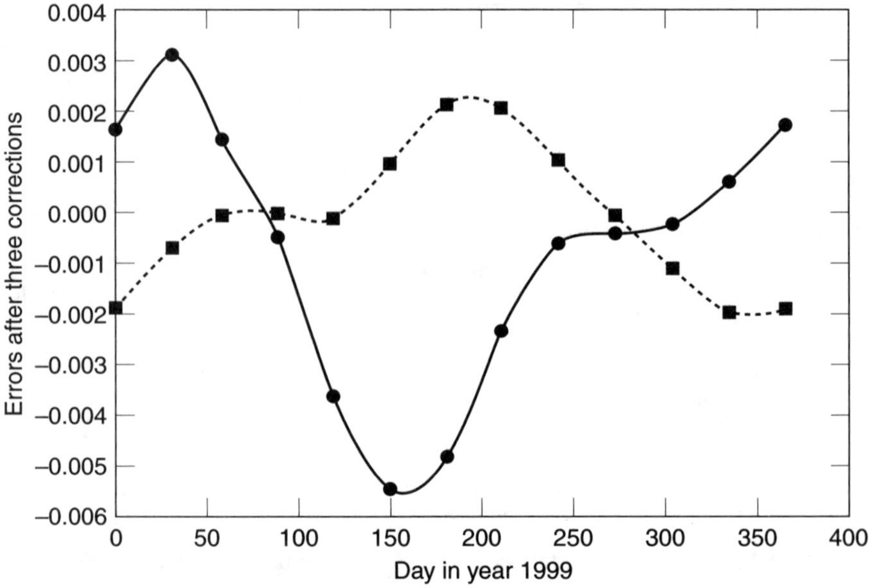

Figure A.14. Residual errors for the year 1999 with simplified average coefficients.

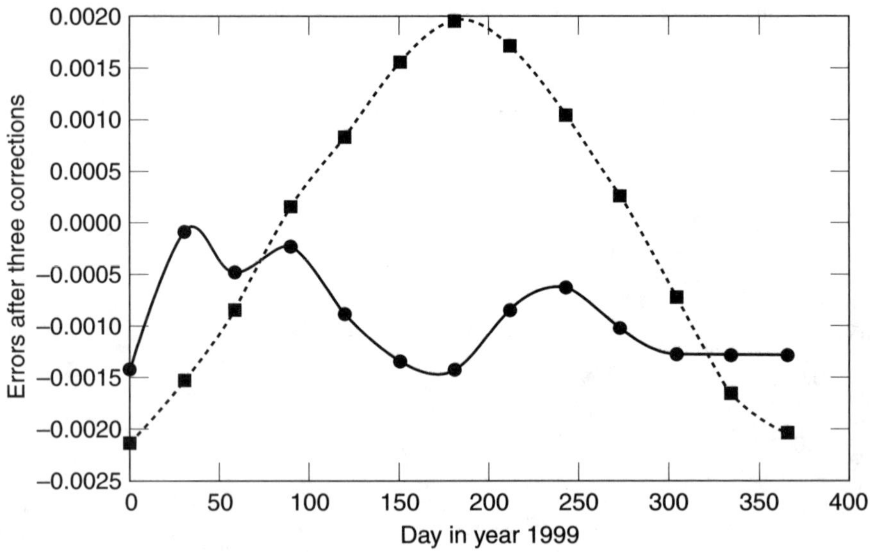

Figure A.15. Residual errors for the year 1999 with custom-fitted coefficients.

From the above testing, it is seen that Eq. (A.12) may be used with incurred errors not exceeding approximately 5×10^{-3} deg for at least 23 years prior to the period 1989 to 2007. Judging from this, it is expected that this equation may also be used likewise for at least 23 years beyond the year 2007 (i.e., the year 2030). It is probable that we can justifiably use this equation up to the year 2060 with accuracies of 5×10^{-2} deg. We know we can indefinitely use Eq. (A.12) with only the first three terms on the first line and not incur errors of more than approximately 2.5×10^{-1} deg.

A rigorous justification of the algorithm previously discussed is as follows: We begin with Eq. (A.13), which relates the longitude θ and obliquity ε to the right ascension α of the sun. Let us rewrite Eq. (A.1) in a slightly different form as

$$\begin{aligned}
&\theta = \theta_0 + (\Delta\theta)_1 + (\Delta\theta)_2 + (\Delta\theta)_3 + \cdots \\
&\theta_0 = \phi \equiv \varpi\left(t - t_{VE}\right) \\
&(\Delta\theta)_1 \equiv - A'\left[\left(1 - B'\right) - \cos\left(\phi - C'\right)\right] \\
&(\Delta\theta)_2 \equiv - A''\left[\left(1 - B''\right) - \cos\left(\phi - C''\right)\right] \\
&(\Delta\theta)_3 \equiv A''' \cos 2\left(\phi - C'''\right)
\end{aligned} \tag{A.15}$$

In Eq. (A.15), $(\Delta\theta)_1$, $(\Delta\theta)_2$, and $(\Delta\theta)_3$ are respectively referred to as the first, second, and third corrections in longitude.

Similarly, we shall also write the right ascension as

$$\alpha = \alpha_0 + (\Delta\alpha)_1 + (\Delta\alpha)_2 + (\Delta\alpha)_3 + \cdots \tag{A.16}$$

In Eq. (A.16), $(\Delta\alpha)_1$, $(\Delta\alpha)_2$, and $(\Delta\alpha)_3$ are respectively referred to as the first, second, and third corrections in right ascension corresponding to the first, second, and third corrections in longitude $(\Delta\theta)_1$, $(\Delta\theta)_2$, and $(\Delta\theta)_3$.

As in Eq. (A.3), let α_0 be the value of the right ascension corresponding to θ_0. That is,

$$\tan\alpha_0 = \cos\varepsilon \, \tan\theta_0 \tag{A.17}$$

Let $(\Delta\alpha)_{\text{no cor}}$ denote the error in the right ascension with no correction term in Eq. (A.15). Thus,

$$(\Delta\alpha)_{\text{no cor}} \equiv \alpha_0 - \alpha \tag{A.18}$$

Let θ_1, α_1, and $(\Delta\alpha)_1$ be sequentially defined by

$$\theta_1 \equiv \theta_0 + (\Delta\theta)_1 \tag{A.19}$$

$$\tan\alpha_1 \equiv \cos\varepsilon \tan\theta_1 \tag{A.20}$$

$$\alpha_1 \equiv \alpha_0 + (\Delta\alpha)_1 \tag{A.21}$$

Let $(\Delta\alpha)_{1\text{st cor}}$ denote the error in the right ascension with the first correction $(\Delta\theta)_1$ in Eq. (A.15). Thus,

$$(\Delta\alpha)_{1\text{st cor}} \equiv \alpha_1 - \alpha \tag{A.22}$$

We note that Eq. (A.21) may be written as

$$\alpha_1 - \alpha = \alpha_0 - \alpha + (\Delta\alpha)_1 \tag{A.23}$$

By using Eqs. (A.18) and (A.22), we obtain

$$\left(\Delta\alpha\right)_{1\text{st cor}} = \left(\Delta\alpha\right)_{\text{no cor}} + (\Delta\alpha)_1 \tag{A.24}$$

In Eq. (A.15), we wish to choose the coefficients A', B', and C' in $(\Delta\theta)_1$ so that $(\Delta\alpha)_{1\text{st cor}}$ is one order of magnitude smaller than $(\Delta\alpha)_{\text{no cor}}$. This may be accomplished by choosing

$$\left(\Delta\alpha\right)_{1\text{st cor}} = \lambda\left(\Delta\alpha\right)_{\text{no cor}} \tag{A.25}$$

where λ is some small number, say $\lambda \approx 0.1$. From Eqs. (A.24) and (A.25), it follows that

$$-\left(\Delta\alpha\right)_1 = \left(1-\lambda\right)\left(\Delta\alpha\right)_{\text{no cor}} \tag{A.26}$$

For convenience, let us write Eq. (A.26) as

$$-\left(\Delta\alpha\right)_1 = \mu\left(\Delta\alpha\right)_{\text{no cor}} \tag{A.27}$$

where μ is defined as

$$\mu \equiv 1 - \lambda \tag{A.28}$$

Because we choose $\lambda \approx 0.1$, therefore $\mu \approx 0.9$.

Next, by substituting Eqs. (A.19) and (A.21) into (A.20), we have

$$\tan\left[\alpha_0 + (\Delta\alpha)_1\right] \equiv \cos\varepsilon \tan\left[\theta_0 + (\Delta\theta)_1\right] \tag{A.29}$$

Suppose $|\tan B| << |\tan A|$ and also $|B| << 1$ in radians. Then, we have

$$\begin{aligned} \tan(A+B) &\equiv \frac{\tan A + \tan B}{1 - \tan A \tan B} = \frac{\tan A + B + O(B^2)}{1 - B\tan A + O(B^2)} \\ &= (\tan A + B)(1 + B\tan A) + O(B^2) = \tan A + B(1 + \tan^2 A) + O(B^2) \\ &= \tan A + B\sec^2 A + O(B^2) \approx \tan A + B\sec^2 A \end{aligned} \tag{A.30}$$

Note that we insert the "very approximate" sign before the last term in Eq. (A.30) when B is small but not very small (e.g., 3.5 deg = 0.06 rad).

By using the approximation (A.30) in Eq. (A.29), we obtain

$$\tan\alpha_0 + (\Delta\alpha)_1 \sec^2\alpha_0 \approx \cos\varepsilon \tan\theta_0 + (\Delta\theta)_1 \cos\varepsilon \sec^2\theta_0 \tag{A.31}$$

In view of Eq. (A.17), therefore we obtain the following relation between $(\Delta\alpha)_1$ and $(\Delta\theta)_1$:

$$(\Delta\alpha)_1 \approx (\Delta\theta)_1 \cos\varepsilon \frac{\sec^2\theta_0}{\sec^2\alpha_0} \tag{A.32}$$

$$(\Delta\theta)_1 \approx \frac{1}{\cos\varepsilon}\frac{\sec^2\alpha_0}{\sec^2\theta_0}(\Delta\alpha)_1 = \frac{1}{\cos\varepsilon}\frac{(1+\tan^2\alpha_0)}{\sec^2\theta_0}(\Delta\alpha)_1 \tag{A.33}$$

By substituting Eq. (A.16) into (A.31), we find it follows that

$$\begin{aligned} (\Delta\theta)_1 &\approx \frac{1}{\cos\varepsilon}\frac{(1+\cos^2\varepsilon\tan^2\theta_0)}{\sec^2\theta_0}(\Delta\alpha)_1 = \frac{1}{\cos\varepsilon}\frac{\left[\cos^2\varepsilon(1+\tan^2\theta_0)+\sin^2\varepsilon\right]}{\sec^2\theta_0}(\Delta\alpha)_1 \\ &= \frac{1}{\cos\varepsilon}\left(\cos^2\varepsilon + \frac{\sin^2\varepsilon}{\sec^2\theta_0}\right)(\Delta\alpha)_1 = \frac{1}{\cos\varepsilon}(\cos^2\varepsilon + \sin^2\varepsilon\cos^2\theta_0)(\Delta\alpha)_1 \\ &= (\cos\varepsilon + \sin\varepsilon\tan\varepsilon\cos^2\theta_0)(\Delta\alpha)_1 \end{aligned} \tag{A.34}$$

Equation (A.34) gives the relation between the first correction $(\Delta\theta)_1$ in longitude and the first correction $(\Delta\alpha)_1$ the right ascension throughout the year.

Because the average value of $\cos^2\theta_0 = 1/2$ in the interval $[0,2\pi]$, we can write Eq. (A.34) on the average as

$$
\begin{aligned}
(\Delta\theta)_1 &\approx \left(\cos\varepsilon + \frac{1}{2}\sin\varepsilon \tan\varepsilon \right)(\Delta\alpha)_1 \\
&\approx \left(\cos 23^o.44 + \frac{1}{2}\sin 23^o.44 \tan 23^o.44 \right)(\Delta\alpha)_1 \\
&\approx (0.9175 + 0.0863)(\Delta\alpha)_1 \approx 1.0038(\Delta\alpha)_1
\end{aligned}
\tag{A.35}
$$

Thus we have

$$
(\Delta\theta)_1 \approx (\Delta\alpha)_1 \tag{A.36}
$$

Note that, in deriving the relation (A.34), we did not assign any value to μ. That is, Eq. (A.34) holds for all values of μ, and it depends specifically on the value of the ecliptic $\varepsilon \approx 23.44$ deg. But it must not be used indiscriminately, because the applicability of Eq. (A.30) must be assured beforehand.

We recall that, to determine the first correction $(\Delta\theta)_1$ in longitude, we matched the curve to have approximately the same value and curvature near the vernal equinox and the same amplitude as the residual curve $(\Delta\alpha)_{\text{no cor}}$ as shown in Fig. A.1. This led to values of the coefficients A', B', and C'given by Eq. (A.5). It is easily verified that these values yield $\mu \approx 0.9$. That is, we chose the first correction $(\Delta\theta)_1$ in longitude θ to be approximately 90% of the residual error $(\Delta\alpha)_{\text{no cor}}$ in the right ascension with no correction term in Eq. (A.15). This is clearly borne out in Fig. A.1, whose residual error when multiplied by 0.9 yields Fig. A.16, which depicts the closeness $(\Delta\theta)_1 \approx (\Delta\alpha)_1$. This is why, as illustrated in Fig. A.2, the residual error $(\Delta\alpha)_{\text{1st cor}}$ in the right ascension with the first correction term $(\Delta\alpha)_1$ in Eq. (A.15) is equal to approximately 10% of $(\Delta\alpha)_{\text{no cor}}$. This result was obtained by design.

The second procedure was to obtain values of the coefficients A'', B'', and C'' so that the resultant residual curve after this step (see Fig. A.3) would have only second and higher harmonic terms. This was achieved by interlacing the residual error $(\Delta\alpha)_{\text{1st cor}}$ curve with the harmonic curve so that there resulted four intersecting points with approximately the same excursions in between. The third procedure was to obtain the coefficients A''' and C'''. This was achieved by equating the third correction $(\Delta\theta)_3$ in longitude to the residual error $(\Delta\alpha)_{\text{2nd cor}}$ in the right ascension with the first two correction terms $(\Delta\alpha)_1$ and $(\Delta\alpha)_2$ in Eq. (A.15). Again, these steps were done by design.

Finally, even though we do not show them, it is truly amazing that the plots corresponding to Figs. A.1, A.2, and A.3 for all other years in the period 1989 to 2007 are almost exactly the same in shape as those for the illustrative year 2000 shown in this appendix.

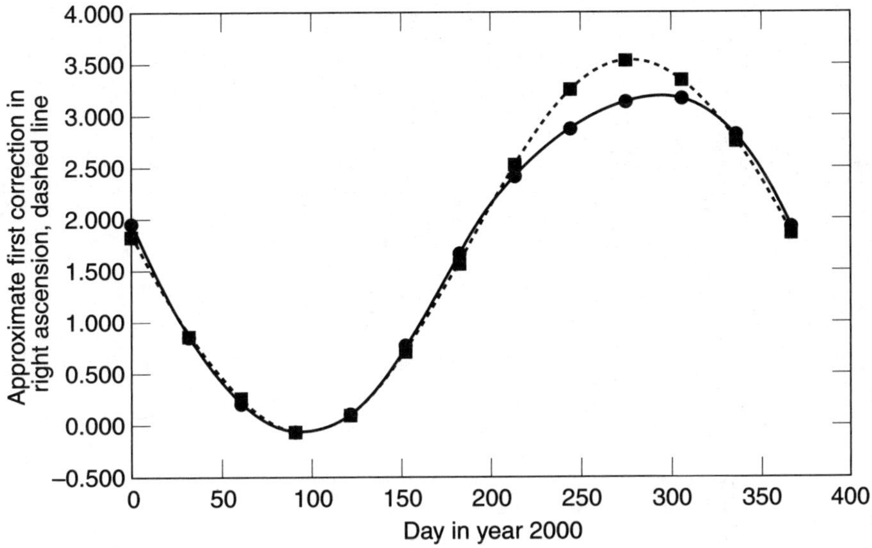

Figure A.16. Closeness of first correction in longitude to first correction in right ascension.

A.1 References

A.1. "The Astronomical Almanac for the Year 2007," prepared jointly by the Nautical Almanac Office, United States Naval Observatory and Her Majesty's Almanac Office, United Kingdom Hydrographic Office, Published jointly by the U.S. Government Printing Office.

A.2. "Explanatory Supplement to the Astronomical Almanac," prepared jointly by the Nautical Almanac Office, United States Naval Observatory and Her Majesty's Almanac Office, United Kingdom Hydrographic Office, edited by P. Kenneth Seidelmann (University Science Books, Mill Valley, CA, 1992).

Appendix B: Enhanced Method of Computing Collision Probability

In this approach, we divide the elliptical doughnut illustrated in Fig. 8.8 of Chapter 8 (reprinted here as Fig. B.1) into six subregions obtained by parallel planes intersecting its surface. If $|C| \le (3A/4)$, then we choose these planes perpendicular to the x-axis, and they are given by

$$x_1 = -(A+\rho),\ x_2 = -A,\ x_3 = -(A-\rho),$$
$$x_4 = (A-\rho),\ x_5 = A,\ x_6 = (A+\rho) \tag{B.1}$$

For any value of x between any two of these planes, the cross section of the doughnut is approximated by a circle using the method of equivalent cross-section areas (MECSA) described in Chapter 5. This approximation is justified because in most cases, the collision cross-sectional dimensions are small compared to the standard deviation. The accuracy of this method has already been demonstrated throughout a wide range of collision parameters. Then, for each subregion, we may use Eq. (9.17) with the appropriate values of u and v given by Eqs. (9.18) and (9.19).

B.1 Subregion Between Planes x_1 and x_2

For this subregion, it may be shown that

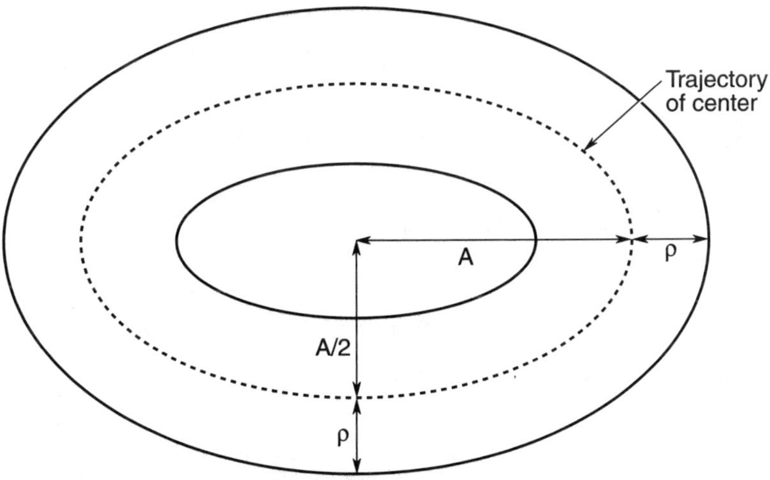

Figure B.1. Subregions of an elliptical doughnut obtained by the intersection of parallel planes with its surface.

$$u = \frac{z(y_L - y_S)}{2\sigma^2}, \; v = \frac{(y_L + y_S)^2}{4\sigma^2} = 0 \tag{B.2}$$

where

$$z = \sqrt{\left[\rho^2 - (x - x_2)^2\right]}, \; y_L = (A/2 + \rho)\sqrt{\left[1 - \frac{x^2}{(A+\rho)^2}\right]}, \; y_S = -y_L \tag{B.3}$$

The collision probability P_{12} is obtained according to the expression

$$P_{12} = \frac{1}{\sqrt{2\pi}\,\sigma} \sum e^{-v/2}(1 - e^{-u/2}) e^{-(x-C)^2/2\sigma^2} \Delta x \tag{B.4}$$

B.2 Subregion Between Planes x_2 and x_3

For this subregion, it may be shown that

$$u = \frac{\rho(y_L - y_S)}{2\sigma^2}, \; v = \frac{(y_L + y_S)^2}{4\sigma^2} \tag{B.5}$$

where

$$y_L = (A/2 + \rho)\sqrt{\left[1 - \frac{x^2}{(A+\rho)^2}\right]}, \; y_S = 0 \tag{B.6}$$

The collision probability P_{23} is obtained according to the expression

$$P_{23} = \frac{2}{\sqrt{2\pi}\,\sigma} \sum e^{-v/2}(1 - e^{-u/2}) e^{-(x-C)^2/2\sigma^2} \Delta x \tag{B.7}$$

B.3 Subregions Between Planes x_3 and x_4

For this subregion, it may be shown that

$$u = \frac{z(y_L - y_S)}{2\sigma^2}, \; v = \frac{(y_L + y_S)^2}{4\sigma^2} \tag{B.8}$$

where

$$y_L = (A/2+\rho)\sqrt{\left[1-\frac{x^2}{(A+\rho)^2}\right]},\ y_S = (A/2-\rho)\sqrt{\left[1-\frac{x^2}{(A-\rho)^2}\right]} \tag{B.9}$$

The collision probability P_{34} is obtained according to the expression

$$P_{34} = \frac{2}{\sqrt{2\pi}\,\sigma}\sum e^{-v/2}(1-e^{-u/2})e^{-(x-C)^2/2\sigma^2}\,\Delta x \tag{B.10}$$

B.4 Subregion Between Planes x_4 and x_5

For this subregion, it may be shown that

$$u = \frac{\rho(y_L - y_S)}{2\sigma^2},\ v = \frac{(y_L + y_S)^2}{4\sigma^2} \tag{B.11}$$

where

$$y_L = (A/2+\rho)\sqrt{\left[1-\frac{x^2}{(A+\rho)^2}\right]},\ y_S = 0 \tag{B.12}$$

The collision probability P_{45} is obtained according to the expression

$$P_{45} = \frac{2}{\sqrt{2\pi}\,\sigma}\sum e^{-v/2}(1-e^{-u/2})e^{-(x-C)^2/2\sigma^2}\,\Delta x \tag{B.13}$$

B.5 Subregion Between Planes x_5 and x_6

For this subregion, it may be shown that

$$u = \frac{z(y_L - y_S)}{2\sigma^2},\ v = \frac{(y_L + y_S)^2}{4\sigma^2} = 0 \tag{B.14}$$

where

$$z = \sqrt{\left[\rho^2 - (x-x_5)^2\right]},\ y_L = (A/2+\rho)\sqrt{\left[1-\frac{x^2}{(A+\rho)^2}\right]},\ y_S = -y_L \tag{B.15}$$

The collision probability P_{56} is obtained according to the expression

$$P_{56} = \frac{1}{\sqrt{2\pi}\,\sigma} \sum e^{-v/2}(1 - e^{-u/2}) e^{-(x-C)^2/2\sigma^2} \Delta x \tag{B.16}$$

However, if $|C| > (3A/4)$, then we choose the dividing planes perpendicular to the y-axis, and they are given by

$$\begin{aligned} &y_1 = -(A/2 + \rho),\ y_2 = -A,\ y_3 = -(A/2 - \rho), \\ &y_4 = (A/2 - \rho),\ y_5 = A/2,\ y_6 = (A/2 + \rho) \end{aligned} \tag{B.17}$$

B.6 Subregion Between Planes y_1 and y_2

For this subregion, it may be shown that

$$u = \frac{z(x_L - x_S)}{2\sigma^2},\ v = \frac{(x_L + x_S + 2C)^2}{4\sigma^2} = 0 \tag{B.18}$$

where

$$z = \sqrt{\left[\rho^2 - (y - y_2)^2\right]},\ x_L = (A + \rho)\sqrt{\left[1 - \frac{y^2}{(A/2 + \rho)^2}\right]},\ x_S = -x_L \tag{B.19}$$

The collision probability P_{12} is obtained according to the expression

$$P_{12} = \frac{1}{\sqrt{2\pi}\,\sigma} \sum e^{-v/2}(1 - e^{-u/2}) e^{-y^2/2\sigma^2} \Delta y \tag{B.20}$$

B.7 Subregion Between Planes y_2 and y_3

For this subregion, it may be shown that

$$u = \frac{\rho(x_L - x_S)}{2\sigma^2},\ v_L = \frac{(x_L + x_S + 2C)^2}{4\sigma^2},\ v_S = \frac{(x_L + x_S - 2C)^2}{4\sigma^2} \tag{B.21}$$

where

$$x_L = (A+\rho)\sqrt{\left[1-\frac{y^2}{(A/2+\rho)^2}\right]},\ x_S = 0 \tag{B.22}$$

The collision probability P_{23} is obtained according to the expression

$$P_{23} = \frac{1}{\sqrt{2\pi}\,\sigma}\sum(e^{-v_L/2}+e^{-v_S/2})(1-e^{-u/2})e^{-y^2/2\sigma^2}\,\Delta y \tag{B.23}$$

B.8 Subregions Between Planes y_3 and y_4

For this subregion, it may be shown that

$$u = \frac{\rho(x_L - x_S)}{2\sigma^2},\ v_L = \frac{(x_L + x_S + 2C)^2}{4\sigma^2},\ v_S = \frac{(x_L + x_S - 2C)^2}{4\sigma^2} \tag{B.24}$$

where

$$x_L = (A+\rho)\sqrt{\left[1-\frac{y^2}{(A/2+\rho)^2}\right]},\ y_S = (A-\rho)\sqrt{\left[1-\frac{y^2}{(A/2-\rho)^2}\right]} \tag{B.25}$$

Note that, because of the second equation in (B.25), we cannot allow ρ to take on the value of $A/2$.

The collision probability P_{34} is obtained according to the expression

$$P_{34} = \frac{1}{\sqrt{2\pi}\,\sigma}\sum(e^{-v_L/2}+e^{-v_S/2})(1-e^{-u/2})e^{-y^2/2\sigma^2}\,\Delta y \tag{B.26}$$

B.9 Subregion Between Planes y_4 and y_5

For this subregion, it may be shown that

$$u = \frac{\rho(x_L - x_S)}{2\sigma^2},\ v_L = \frac{(x_L + x_S + 2C)^2}{4\sigma^2},\ v_S = \frac{(x_L + x_S - 2C)^2}{4\sigma^2} \tag{B.27}$$

where

$$x_L = (A+\rho)\sqrt{\left[1 - \frac{y^2}{(A/2+\rho)^2}\right]}, \; x_S = 0 \tag{B.28}$$

The collision probability P_{45} is obtained according to the expression

$$P_{45} = \frac{1}{\sqrt{2\pi}\,\sigma} \sum (e^{-v_L/2} + e^{-v_S/2})(1 - e^{-u/2}) e^{-y^2/2\sigma^2} \Delta y \tag{B.29}$$

B.10 Subregion Between Planes y_5 and y_6

For this subregion, it may be shown that

$$u = \frac{z(x_L - x_S)}{2\sigma^2}, \; v = \frac{(x_L + x_S - 2C)^2}{4\sigma^2} = 0 \tag{B.30}$$

where

$$z = \sqrt{\left[\rho^2 - (y - y_5)^2\right]}, \; x_L = (A+\rho)\sqrt{\left[1 - \frac{y^2}{(A/2+\rho)^2}\right]}, \; x_S = -x_L \tag{B.31}$$

The collision probability P_{56} is obtained according to the expression

$$P_{56} = \frac{1}{\sqrt{2\pi}\,\sigma} \sum e^{-v/2}(1 - e^{-u/2}) e^{-y^2/2\sigma^2} \Delta y \tag{B.32}$$

By summing P_{12}, P_{23}, P_{34}, P_{45}, and P_{56}, we obtain the probability of collision for the elliptical doughnut volume of interest. The results are accurate to one or two significant digits.

Appendix C: Derivation of Density Relations

Approximately one-third of the results in this appendix (equations marked by "*") were obtained by Dennis in his paper[C.1] on statistical distribution of satellites. However, it would be disruptive to quote his results, and then also derive additional relations, which are needed for the main text. Thus, for the sake of continuity and completeness, all of the relevant relations will be presented here.

Consider n_{total} satellites, each with a circular orbit of radius R and inclination i_s. Suppose the ascending node is statistically uniform in the equatorial plane. Moreover, in a given orbital plane, suppose the phase is also statistically uniform. For a given satellite, we have the relation

$$\sin\theta = \sin i_s \sin\phi_s \tag{C.1*}$$

where θ is the satellite latitude and ϕ_2 is the argument of latitude. Let $f_{\phi s}(\phi_s)d\phi_s$ denote the probability of finding a satellite having argument of latitude between ϕ_s and $(\phi_s + d\phi_s)$. Then, the assumption of uniform phase yields

$$f_{\phi_s}(\phi_s) = \frac{1}{2\pi} \tag{C.2*}$$

Let $f_\theta(\theta)d\theta$ denote the probability of finding a satellite between θ and $(\theta + d\theta)$. Therefore,

$$f_\theta(\theta) = 2 f_{\phi_s}(\phi_s)\frac{d\phi_s}{d\theta} \tag{C.3*}$$

in which the factor of 2 is included to account for both ascending and descending satellites at a given latitude. Differentiation of Eq. (C.1) yields

$$\frac{d\phi_s}{d\theta} = \frac{\cos\theta}{\sin i_s \cos\phi_s} \tag{C.4*}$$

Hence, we obtain

$$f_\theta(\theta) = \frac{\cos\theta}{\pi \sin i_s \cos\phi_s} \tag{C.5*}$$

Let dn denote the number of satellites between latitudes θ and $(\theta + d\theta)$. Therefore, we have

$$dn = n_{\text{total}} f_{\theta}(\theta) d\theta = \frac{n_{\text{total}} \cos\theta}{\pi \sin i_s \cos\phi_s} d\theta \tag{C.6}$$

Suppose the satellites at radius R are distributed over a thin layer of thickness h. Then, the volume dv of the toroidal ring between latitudes θ and $(\theta + d\theta)$ is

$$dv = 2\pi R^2 h \cos\theta d\theta \tag{C.7}$$

Hence the total density $\rho_{\text{total}}(\theta)$ of both ascending and descending satellites at latitude θ is given by

$$\rho_{\text{total}}(\theta) = \frac{dn}{dv} = \frac{n_{\text{total}}}{2\pi^2 R^2 h \sin i_s \cos\phi_s} \tag{C.8}$$

Let L denote the circumference of the orbit (i.e., $L = 2\pi R$). Therefore, Eq. (C.8) becomes

$$\rho_{\text{total}}(\theta) = \frac{2n_{\text{total}}}{L^2 h \sin i_s \cos\phi_s} \tag{C.9}$$

If we set $\phi_s = 0$, we obtain the total density at the equator $\rho_{\text{eq,total}}$:

$$\rho_{\text{eq,total}} = \frac{2n_{\text{total}}}{L^2 h \sin i_s} \tag{C.10}$$

Equation (C.9) may also be written as

$$\rho_{\text{total}}(\theta) = \frac{\rho_{\text{eq,total}}}{\cos\phi_s} \tag{C.11}$$

Let $\rho(\theta)$ and ρ_{eq} respectively denote the density of ascending (or descending) satellites at latitude θ at the equator. It follows from Eq. (C.11) that

$$\rho(\theta) = \frac{\rho_{\text{eq}}}{\cos\phi_s} \tag{C.12}$$

Next, by using the identity $\sin^2\phi_s = 1 - \cos^2\phi_s$, we note that Eq. (C.1) yields

$$\sin i_s \cos\phi_s = \sqrt{\left(\sin^2 i_s - \sin^2\theta\right)} \tag{C.13}$$

Hence Eq. (C.5) becomes

$$f_\theta(\theta)\frac{\cos\theta}{\pi\sqrt{\left(\sin^2 i_s - \sin^2\theta\right)}} \tag{C.14*}$$

Let θ'' be defined by

$$\left.\begin{aligned} \theta'' &= i_s \quad \text{for} \quad i_s < \pi/2 \\ \theta'' &= (\pi - i_s) \quad \text{for} \quad i_s < \pi/2 \end{aligned}\right\} \tag{C.15}$$

Let θ' be any latitude such that $0 \le \theta' < \theta''$. Therefore, the probability of finding a satellite between latitude θ' and θ'' is

$$\begin{aligned} P(\theta',\theta'') &= \int_{\theta'}^{\theta''} f_\theta(\theta)\,d\theta = \frac{1}{\pi}\int_{\theta'}^{\theta''} \frac{\cos\theta}{\sqrt{\left(\sin^2 i_s - \sin^2\theta\right)}}\,d\theta \\ &= \frac{1}{\pi}\cos^{-1}\left(\frac{\sin\theta'}{\sin i_s}\right) \end{aligned} \tag{C.16}$$

Hence, the number of satellites between latitudes θ' and θ'' is

$$n(\theta',\theta'') = n_{\text{total}}P(\theta',\theta'') = \frac{n_{\text{total}}}{\pi}\cos^{-1}\left(\frac{\sin\theta'}{\sin i_s}\right) \tag{C.17}$$

Let $v(\theta', \theta'')$ denote the volume of the toroidal ring of thickness h between latitudes θ' and θ''. Therefore, we have

$$v(\theta',\theta'') = \frac{2\pi}{3}\left[(R+h)^3 - R^3\right]\left(\sin\theta'' - \sin\theta'\right) \tag{C.18}$$

Hence, the average density in the toroidal ring is

$$\bar{\rho}_{\text{total}}(\theta',\theta'') = \frac{n(\theta',\theta'')}{v(\theta',\theta'')} = \frac{3n_{\text{total}}\cos^{-1}\left(\dfrac{\sin\theta'}{\sin i_s}\right)}{2\pi^2\left[(R+h)^3 - R^3\right](\sin\theta'' - \sin\theta')} \tag{C.19}$$

Equations (C.17) through (C.19) are valid for any finite toroidal ring.

C.1 Reference

[C.1] N. G. Dennis, "Probabilistic Theory and Statistical Distribution of Earth Satellites," *J. Br. Interplanet. Soc.* **25**, 333–376 (1972).

Appendix D: Instantaneous Probability of Collision, Continued

In Chapter 13, we dismissed the option of transforming the ellipsoid V'' into a sphere V''' of equal volume. If we had done this, we would have obtained an analytical solution instead of Eq. (13.30), which is semianalytical. This appendix takes up the analysis that was omitted.

In the (x, y, z) coordinate system, let the combined covariance C describing the relative position uncertainties be defined by

$$C = \begin{bmatrix} \sigma_x^2 & \rho_{xy}\sigma_x\sigma_y & \rho_{xz}\sigma_x\sigma_z \\ \rho_{xy}\sigma_x\sigma_y & \sigma_y^2 & \rho_{yz}\sigma_y\sigma_z \\ \rho_{xz}\sigma_x\sigma_z & \rho_{yz}\sigma_y\sigma_z & \sigma_z^2 \end{bmatrix} \tag{D.1}$$

As in Chapter 5, we shall take the origin to be at the secondary object. Hence, the instantaneous probability of collision at time t is given by

$$P = \iiint_V \frac{1}{\sqrt{(2\pi)^3 |C|}} e^{-\frac{1}{2}\mathbf{r}^T C^{-1}\mathbf{r}} dx\, dy\, dz \tag{D.2}$$

where V is a sphere of radius R centered at the primary object whose coordinates are (x_p, y_p, z_p). If we rotate to principal axes (x', y', z'), then we have

$$C' = \begin{bmatrix} \sigma_{x'}^2 & 0 & 0 \\ 0 & \sigma_{y'}^2 & 0 \\ 0 & 0 & \sigma_{z'}^2 \end{bmatrix} \tag{D.3}$$

Then, the collision probability (D.2) becomes

$$P = \iiint_{V'} \frac{1}{(2\pi)^{3/2}\sigma_{x'}\sigma_{y'}\sigma_{z'}} e^{-\frac{1}{2}\mathbf{r}'^T (C')^{-1}\mathbf{r}'} dx'\, dy'\, dz' \tag{D.4}$$

where V' is also a sphere of radius R centered at the primary object. Let (x_p', y_p', z_p') denote the coordinates of the center of mass of the primary in this system.

We next wish to map the ellipsoids of constant pdf

$$\frac{x'^2}{\sigma_{x'}^2}+\frac{y'^2}{\sigma_{y'}^2}+\frac{z'^2}{\sigma_{z'}^2}=k^2 \tag{D.5}$$

into spheres of constant pdf having the equation

$$\frac{x''^2}{\sigma_{z'}^{\ 2}}+\frac{y''^2}{\sigma_{z'}^{\ 2}}+\frac{z''^2}{\sigma_{z'}^{\ 2}}=k^2 \tag{D.6}$$

The constant k is a label for the corresponding ellipsoid or sphere in the two sets. This mapping is accomplished by the following transformation:

$$x''=\frac{\sigma_{z'}}{\sigma_{x'}}x', \qquad y''=\frac{\sigma_{z'}}{\sigma_{y'}}y', \qquad z''=z' \tag{D.7}$$

In the (x'', y'', z'') system, the pdf becomes isotropic and the collision probability given in Eq. (C.4) is

$$P=\frac{1}{(2\pi)^{3/2}\ \sigma_{z'}^{\ 3}}\iiint_{V''} e^{-\left(x''^2+y''^2+z''^2\right)/2\sigma_{z'}^{\ 2}}\,dx''\,dy''\,dz'' \tag{D.8}$$

where V'' is an ellipsoid with semiaxes a, b, and c centered at the primary respectively defined to be along the z'', y'', and x'' axes. Let (x_p'', y_p'', z_p'') denote the coordinates of the center of mass of the primary in the $(x'', y''\ z'')$ system. Therefore, by Eq. (D.7), we have

$$V''=\frac{\sigma_{z'}^{\ 2}}{\sigma_{x'}\sigma_{y'}}V', \quad c=\frac{\sigma_{z'}}{\sigma_{x'}}R, \quad b=\frac{\sigma_{z'}}{\sigma_{y'}}R, \quad a=R, \quad x_p''=\frac{\sigma_{z'}}{\sigma_{x'}}x_p', \quad y_p''=\frac{\sigma_{z'}}{\sigma_{y'}}y_p', \quad z_p''=z_p' \tag{D.9}$$

If we had labeled the principal axes (x', y', z') so that $\sigma_{x'}\geq\sigma_{y'}\geq\sigma_{z'}$, then Eq. (13.25) would yield $c \leq b \leq a$.

Up to this step, we have not made any approximations. Suppose we now approximate the ellipsoid V'' with a sphere V''' of the same volume with radius ρ. Then, we have

$$V'''=V'', \qquad \rho=\sqrt[3]{abc}=\sqrt[3]{\frac{\sigma_{z'}^{\ 2}}{\sigma_{x'}\sigma_{y'}}}R, \qquad x_p'''=x_p'', \qquad y_p'''=y_p'', \qquad z_p'''=z_p'' \tag{D.10}$$

Thus, the collision probability in Eq. (D.8) is approximated by

$$P = \frac{1}{(2\pi)^{3/2}\,\sigma_{z'}^{\;3}} \iiint_{V'''} e^{-\left(x''^2 + y''^2 + z''^2\right)/2\sigma_{z'}^{\;2}}\, dx''\, dy''\, dz'' \tag{D.11}$$

Equation (D.11) is the integral of a three-dimensional isotropic Gaussian pdf over a sphere of radius ρ. This integral may be explicitly written as

$$P = \frac{1}{\sqrt{2\pi}\sigma_{z'}} \int_{y_p''-\rho}^{y_p''+\rho} e^{-y''^2/2\sigma_{z'}^{\;2}} \left[\frac{1}{2\pi\sigma_{z'}^{\;2}} \iint_{A'''} e^{-(x''^2+z''^2)/2\sigma_{z'}^{\;2}}\, dx''\, dz'' \right] dy'' \tag{D.12}$$

where A''' denotes the circular cross section of the sphere obtained by the intersection with a plane where y'' is a constant between $y'' = (y_p'' - \rho)$ and $y'' = (y_p'' + \rho)$. We note that the double integral I defined by

$$I \equiv \frac{1}{2\pi\sigma_{z'}^{\;2}} \iint_{A'''} e^{-(x''^2+z''^2)/2\sigma_{z'}^{\;2}}\, dx''\, dz'' \tag{D.13}$$

represents the integral of a two-dimensional isotropic Gaussian pdf over a circle with center at the point (x_p'', z_p'') in the (x'', z'')-plane. Let us denote the radius of this circle by ξ. Thus, this integral is precisely the Rician integral that we have already obtained in the form of the convergent infinite series in Eq. (5.21) in Chapter 5. If we retain only the first term in the series, Eq. (5.26) yields

$$I \simeq e^{-v/2}\left(1 - e^{-u/2}\right) \tag{D.14}$$

where, by Eqs. (5.22) and (5.23),

$$u \equiv \left(\frac{\xi}{\sigma_{z'}}\right)^2 > 0 \tag{D.15}$$

$$v \equiv \left(\frac{x_p''^2 + z_p''^2}{\sigma_{z'}^{\;2}}\right) > 0 \tag{D.16}$$

Let us introduce a new variable ζ defined by

$$\zeta = y'' - y''_p \tag{D.17}$$

From the definitions of ρ and ξ, it follows from the Pythagorean theorem that

$$\rho^2 = \xi^2 + \zeta^2 \tag{D.18}$$

Therefore, in view of Eqs. (D.15) and (D.16), the collision probability (D.12) may be written as

$$P = \frac{\alpha}{\sqrt{2\pi}\sigma_{z'}} \int_{y''_p-\rho}^{y''_p+\rho} e^{-y''^2/2\sigma_{z'}^2} \left[1 - e^{-(\rho^2-\zeta^2)/2\sigma_{z'}^2}\right] dy'' \tag{D.19}$$

$$\alpha \equiv e^{-(x''^2_p + z''^2_p)/2\sigma_{z'}^2} \tag{D.20}$$

By invoking Eq. (D.17), we may simplify Eq. (D.19) as

$$\begin{aligned}
P &= \frac{\alpha}{\sqrt{2\pi}\sigma_{z'}} \int_{y''_p-\rho}^{y''_p+\rho} e^{-y''^2/2\sigma_{z'}^2} dy'' - \frac{\alpha}{\sqrt{2\pi}\sigma_{z'}} \int_{y''_p-\rho}^{y''_p+\rho} e^{-y''^2/2\sigma_{z'}^2} e^{-(\rho^2-\zeta^2)/2\sigma_{z'}^2} dy'' \\
&= \frac{\alpha}{\sqrt{2\pi}\sigma_{z'}} \left[\int_0^{y''_p+\rho} e^{-y''^2/2\sigma_{z'}^2} dy'' - \int_0^{y''_p-\rho} e^{-y''^2/2\sigma_{z'}^2} dy''\right] - \frac{\beta}{\sqrt{2\pi}\sigma_{z'}} \int_{-\rho}^{+\rho} e^{-(y''_p\zeta)/\sigma_{z'}^2} d\zeta \\
&= \frac{\alpha}{2}\left[erf\left((y''_p+\rho)/(\sqrt{2}\sigma_{z'})\right) - erf\left((y''_p-\rho)/(\sqrt{2}\sigma_{z'})\right)\right] + \frac{\beta\sigma_{z'}}{\sqrt{2\pi}\,y''_p}\left[e^{-(y''_p\rho)/\sigma_{z'}^2} - e^{(y''_p\rho)/\sigma_{z'}^2}\right] \quad for \quad y''_p \neq 0 \\
&= \alpha erf\left(\rho/(\sqrt{2}\sigma_{z'})\right) - \sqrt{\frac{2}{\pi}}\frac{\beta\rho}{\sigma_{z'}} \quad for \quad y''_p = 0
\end{aligned} \tag{D.21}$$

$$\beta \equiv e^{-(x''^2_p + y''^2_p + z''^2_p + \rho^2)/2\sigma_{z'}^2} \tag{D.22}$$

Thus, Eq. (D.22) is an analytical solution for the instantaneous collision probability, obtained if we invoke the transformation of the ellipsoid V'' to a sphere V''' of equal volume. If we use this equation to compute the probabilities for the same cases shown in Table 13.3 for the case of the sphere offset from an isotropic Gaussian pdf, we obtain the results shown in Table D.1.

Comparison with Table 13.3 shows clearly the superiority of the semianalytical solution in Eq. (13.30). We need not even show additional evidence such as the analog of Table 13.5 to substantiate this conclusion.

Table D.1. Comparison with Numerical Solution of Nonzero Offset Isotropic Gaussian pdf

$\sigma_x, \sigma_y, \sigma_z$	Displacement x_0, y_0, z_0 of Sphere	Radius of Sphere	Probability (Numerical Integration)	Probability (Equivalent Volume)	Percent Error for Equivalent Volume
1,1,1	0.5,0,0	0.5	2.74×10^{-02}	2.72×10^{-02}	–0.73
1,1,1	1,0,0	0.5	1.92×10^{-02}	1.87×10^{-02}	–2.54
1,1,1	0.5,0,0	1	1.80×10^{-01}	1.75×10^{-01}	–2.42
1,1,1	1,0,0	1	1.32×10^{-01}	1.21×10^{-01}	–8.97
1,1,1	1,0,0	2	6.03×10^{-01}	4.48×10^{-01}	–25.67
1,1,1	2,0,0	1	3.86×10^{-02}	2.69×10^{-02}	–30.25
1,1,1	2,0,0	2	3.01×10^{-01}	9.99×10^{-02}	–66.75
1,1,1	5,0,0	1	4.91×10^{-06}	7.41×10^{-07}	–84.90
1,1,1	10,0,0	1	1.01×10^{-20}	3.83×10^{-23}	–99.62

Index

L

M

N

P

Supporting Materials

To download the programs described in this book as well as any software updates, please see this page on AIAA's Web site:

http://www.aiaa.org/publications/supportmaterials

Follow the instructions provided and enter the following password: **collision**